Understanding Dental Caries

Michel Goldberg
Editor

Understanding Dental Caries

From Pathogenesis to Prevention and Therapy

Springer

Editor
Michel Goldberg
UMR-S 1124
INSERM
Paris
France

ISBN 978-3-319-30550-9 ISBN 978-3-319-30552-3 (eBook)
DOI 10.1007/978-3-319-30552-3

Library of Congress Control Number: 2016941182

Printed on acid-free paper

This Springer imprint is published by Springer Nature
The registered company is Springer International Publishing AG Switzerland

Preface

Dental and periodontal diseases are two major public health pathologies. Teeth injuries include enamel and dentin carious lesions and periodontal disorders. Carious lesions are the most widespread dental pathologies. They may be limited to simple occlusal fissures or located solely in the proximal aspect, or they expand to complex class II and/or cervical lesions.

In the United States, over 50 % of 5–9-year-old children have at least one cavity and/or one restoration of decayed teeth [(D) and/or filled (F)]. That proportion increases to 78 % among 17-year-old children. The World Health Organization (WHO) estimation of global DMFT [decayed, missing, filled teeth] for 12-year-old children has reported that in the 188 countries included in their database, on a global basis, about 240 millions of teeth are injured in this age group [*Bagramian RA, Garcia-Godoy F, Volpe AR. The global increase in dental caries. A pending public health crisis. Am J Dent 2009*; *22*: *3–8*]. These evaluations underline the significance of dental caries and its correlation with dental practice. In contrast, severe periodontitis was limited to only 5–20 % of the adult population.

Younger and older patients are the targets of dental carious decay, well recognized as a major health problem in most industrialized countries, affecting 60–90 % of school-aged children and the vast majority of adults (*Petersen et al., The global burden of oral diseases and risks to oral health. Bulletin of the WHO 2005*; *83*: *661–669*). Patients with three DMFT constitute 51 % of the patients at the age of 12, while the other patients displayed higher values. Therefore, most dental practitioners are implicated in their everyday practice by the treatment of dental caries.

Clearly, this implies also that carious lesion is more than likely the most prominent pathology of the mouth, and the importance of carious lesions is fundamental both for patients and for dental practitioners. This underlines also the significance of understanding dental caries, their pathogenesis, prevention, and subsequent therapies.

The present book focuses most exclusively on the carious lesion, going from the initial pathogenesis of the lesion, mild enamel alteration, to deep dentin lesions, which appear as a major pathology with pulpal irreversible incidences. The therapies and prevention of the enamel decay are analyzed in the first part of this book.

After a brief description concentrating on the structure and epidemiology of the diverse forms of enamel alterations, carious lesions are reported. We describe successively enamel softening and analyze the etching pattern of acidic effects on enamel. Doing so, we moved from the superficial etching to the initial enamel carious lesion. Bacterial films and acidic biofilms of the dental plaque lead to the formation of active and/or inactive lesions. The methods used for an accurate diagnosis of the carious lesion were improved during the past few years, and a specific chapter concludes the first part of the book, by reporting new diagnostic methods.

Another group of chapters is devoted to the carious dentin and to active or inactive lesions, superficial or deep, reaching the dental pulp and/or located exclusively in the cervical region. How the patient brush and eliminate the dental plaque is another topic. Which toothpastes are used, the evolution, and/or the stabilization of the lesion are factors involved in the carious progression. Eventually, non-carious cervical lesions may regenerate, and it is well documented that some cervical pathology remineralize spontaneously. In addition, we note that 8–13 % among adult patients are affected by the increasing problem of dental erosions.

Finally, new trends in resin infiltrations of the initial lesion, minimal invasive therapies aiming to stabilize the carious lesion, and strategies devised to prevent the expansion of the lesion are control and preventive measures restraining the broad field of cariology.

Fluoride is considered to be the main tool of carious prevention. At some high doses, it induces pathologic fluorosis, but if added in minimal quantity in controlled assays, different forms of fluoride prevents the evolution of carious lesions, contributing to remineralization of the initial lesion or to their stabilization. Other preventive therapies have been elaborate, and we focused on the differences that appear between prevention and minimal restorative dentistry.

The different chapters of this book were written as requested by different researchers and clinicians recognized to be the best in their specific domain. We wish sincerely to acknowledge their outstanding contributions, and I wish to thank them warmly for what they did for the dental community.

Paris, France
January 2016

Michel Goldberg

Contents

Part I

The Carious Enamel

Understanding Dental Caries – from Pathogenesis to Prevention and Therapy

1

Nigel Pitts

Abstract

This chapter provides an overview demonstrating the pivotal importance of understanding the caries process in enamel (and then, for a subset of lesions which ever progress, beyond that, into the dentine) if we are to best prevent and control dental caries over the life course in both patients and populations. There is a need also to understand the complexities and opportunities in the detection, assessment and diagnostic steps in order to inform decision-making and effective, personalised care planning. Modern caries care, provided at the right times on the basis of caries risk, should ensure that the disease is controlled and that tooth structure is preserved whenever possible.

1.1 The Carious Enamel

1–1 *Dental caries: structure, diagnosis, which treatment is appropriate.*

1.2 Introduction

This chapter provides an overview demonstrating the pivotal importance of understanding the caries process in enamel (and then, for a subset of lesions which ever progress, beyond that, into the dentine) if we are to best prevent and control dental caries over the life course in both patients and populations. It sets the scene for the detail that follows in subsequent chapters. Aside from appreciating the science around enamel structure which underpins caries prevention and control, there is also a need also to understand the complexities and opportunities in the detection, assessment and diagnostic steps employed by clinicians examining their patients. Rather than just finding "holes to fill", dentists of today need to carefully assess tooth sites and assess both lesion severity and activity. This is in order to inform their decision-making in selecting from an ever-widening choice of preventive and minimally invasive care options. The goal is to achieve effective, personalised and risk-based care planning with a long-term perspective. Modern caries care, provided at the right times on the basis of caries risk, should ensure caries is controlled and

N. Pitts
Dental Innovation and Translation Centre,
Kings College London Dental Institute, London, UK
e-mail: nigel.pitts@kcl.ac.uk

M. Goldberg (ed.), *Understanding Dental Caries*, DOI 10.1007/978-3-319-30552-3_1

that tooth structure is preserved whenever possible. The era of "automatic" decisions to restore all lesions detected should now be past, but change can be frustratingly slow in many countries and systems.

1.3 Structure

One important element of understanding the healthy structure of enamel as well as carious enamel is to appreciate the long-term clinical value of the sound tissue. In terms of coping with a lifetime of thermal, chemical and physical challenges in a hostile wet environment, tooth enamel is still superior in its physical properties to any of the currently available artificial alternatives. This reality underpins the guiding philosophy to protect and preserve as much natural tooth structure and specifically enamel as possible. Even though we have at our disposal the clinical technology to cut enamel very rapidly and efficiently, this should only be done as a last resort (Pitts 2004a, b; Ismail et al 2013).

The following series of chapters describe and illustrate the unique, highly organised structure of the enamel, the hardest mineralised tissue in the human body. This varies from the important superficial aprismatic surface enamel, which matures for a period following eruption into the oral environment, to the deeper bulk of the prismatic enamel – which is comprised of prismatic enamel (carbonated hydroxyapatite) and interprismatic enamel.

Knowledge of the sound structure is important in understanding the differing initial mechanisms of the caries process (producing net sub-surface demineralisation after long alternating periods of de- and remineralisation) as opposed to the direct surface loss of tissue which is associated with erosive tooth wear. In caries, there is a critical interplay between the superficial structure of the enamel and the covering complex biofilm which, when cariogenic, can shift ecologically to produce and retain a low pH at the tooth surface (see Chapter I-4- by Phil Marsh). It is this interplay and the periods of repeated de- and remineralisation that give rise to the macroscopically intact "surface zone" of the initial caries lesion. Preserving this zone has tremendous clinical value in maintaining the potential to arrest and reverse lesions.

1.4 Diagnosis

The evidence-based consensus statements from the ICW-CCT, a major international consensus workshop on caries clinical trials (Pitts and Stamm 2004), clearly differentiated three important and different elements and terms related to caries diagnosis. These were caries: *detection, assessment and diagnosis*.

Detection is concerned with the clinical decision as to whether a tissue is classified as sound or carious (and may record degrees of caries severity, which can be staged), *assessment* characterises the behaviour of a lesion (i.e. is this lesion *active* now or is it *arrested*), and finally *diagnosis* represents the human summation by the clinician of all information available (from clinical visual and radiographic assessments as well as from any other special tests which may be employed) to decide the disease status of a particular tooth surface (Pitts and Stamm 2004; Longbottom et al 2009).

The wide variation in the way in which the terminology around caries diagnosis was used in the literature, and specifically the ambiguity associated with many of the different criteria used and reporting for caries clinical trials and research, gave rise after this meeting to the creation in 2002 of a harmonised system built, on integrating the best evidence. This is the "ICDAS", an *I*nternational *C*aries *D*etection and *A*ssessment *S*ystem (www.icdas.org/). This system was developed to facilitate caries epidemiology, research and appropriate clinical management (Pitts 2004a, b; Ismail et al 2007) and has been developed over the years into a number of approved options. The system has also been incorporated into a number of international conventions and recommendations from bodies such as the FDI World Dental Federation (Fisher and Glick 2012) and the American Dental Association (ADA 2015).

The ICDAS criteria were built around the evidence relating the clinical visual appearance of the enamel (and dentine) to the histological extent of the lesion within the tooth tissue. Critically, the very first clinical visual changes in the enamel can only be seen when the tooth is clean and has been dried with compressed air, ideally for 5 s. White spot lesions visible only when dry extend less far into the enamel than those visible when the enamel is wet with saliva, due to changes in the refractive index masking the initial lesion. In the latter case, the lesion may extend across the full thickness of the enamel, and defence reaction changes may be visible in the underlying dentine. It is therefore important to examine teeth which are clean and dry and to use sharp eyes, rather than sharp probes (which have been found many years ago to cause iatrogenic damage whilst not contributing significantly more diagnostic information than visual-alone examination).

Whilst clinical examination is the foundation for assessing caries, for teeth in anatomical contact, there remain fundamental limitations in assessing approximal caries and also in understanding the depth of penetration of some occlusal lesions. For these reasons dental radiography, and particularly the bitewing projection, has become ubiquitous in many countries as part of a routine examination. The use of radiography in addition to clinical visual examination provides the most comprehensive clinical picture of caries status (Pitts and Kidd 1992a; b).

Although there have been some debates and concerns about using ionising radiation too frequently in low caries populations (particularly in Scandinavia), the evidence supporting the use and clinical utility of properly timed radiographs for planning both preventive and operative care remains. The International Caries Detection and Assessment System (ICDAS), which classifies carious lesions, has been developed into a comprehensive International Caries Classification and Management System (ICCMS™). This includes methods for staging of the caries process which combines the findings from both radiographic and visual examinations (Pitts and Ekstrand 2013). This helps dentists manage caries most effectively in their patients when assessed for caries risk. It should be further appreciated that there are a range of other method and technologies which have been developed to act diagnostic aids to clinicians. These are considered in a forthcoming chapter (Chapter I-5- by Neuhaus and Lussi, 2016).

In terms of assessing enamel caries, the *depth of penetration* through the enamel is an important consideration. This information helps determine what kind of treatments and care strategies may be required and are appropriate for each lesion. It also helps in the monitoring of lesion development and, conversely, in establishing the degree of success obtained when seeking to stop further progression of a lesion. The so-called diagnostic threshold (or cut point) at which caries is recognised as disease has dramatic affects at both the individual patient level and at the population health level (Selwitz et al. 2007). There is a need for more clarity and consistency on this issue, both internationally and across dental "silos".

Caries *activity* information is prized highly by both clinicians and researchers, but despite this there are evidence gaps and surprisingly few systems currently available to help dentists with this type of caries assessment task (ICDAS website; Pitts 2011). New systems, such as using bioluminescence in order to identify increases in free calcium associated with actively demineralising lesions, show promise for future clinical practice.

1.5 Which Treatment Is Appropriate (When)

The importance (and for many years the neglect of) considering the decision-making process in treatment planning has come to the fore over the last decade. Rather than simple no-drill vs. drill (binary decisions), clinicians today have to consider a wide range of factors at the population, patient, tooth and service levels.

The context for making treatment decisions in caries care is also changing. Factors which are operating in the background include international agreements to phase down the use of dental amalgam on environmental grounds and to phase up prevention (United Nations Environment Programme 2013), as well as the widespread desire for preventive interventions to link oral and systemic health improvements with the so-called NCDs. A current example is a systematic re-examination of evidence around the role of sugar in caries and the desire to link caries improvements to those in diabetes, obesity and heart disease (Moynihan and Skelly 2014). This has led to new WHO Guidelines on Sugar Intake for Adults and Children (World Health Organisation 2015).

A further influence on decision-making is an increasing awareness of the need to try to reduce health inequalities in caries (Pitts et al. 2011a, b) and, therefore, to consider caries risk by population subgroups. These various threads have led to a renewed interest in international public health advocacy for caries prevention and control, through groupings such as the Alliance for a Cavity-Free Future (www.allianceforacavity-freefuture.org/), and also a parallel push for social movements in caries prevention which links with public/private collaborations (Bonecker et al. 2012).

There has been a focus in recent years on achieving consensus on exactly what a graduating dentist should know about caries. The elements across pathogenesis, prevention and therapy are key parts of this knowledge and skill set. Europe has led the way with a core cariology curriculum which was built by research and education organisations working together to build consensus (Schulte et al. 2011). This process also generated specific guidance on caries risk assessment, diagnosis and the synthesis of all information into a care plan (Pitts et al. 2011a, b) which established that nonoperative and surgical treatments should be deemed to have equal "value", but the surgical treatment should only be used as a last resort. This European resource material has been debated, fine-tuned and localised in a range of territories including Colombia (Martignon et al. 2014), Malaysia and most recently the USA (Fontana et al. 2016).

Since 2010 the ICDAS Foundation (a registered charity) has been working internationally to build the International Caries Classification and Management System, *ICCMS™*. This is a health outcomes focused system that aims to maintain health and preserve tooth structure, by using a simple form of the ICDAS caries severity and activity *classification* model in order to derive an appropriate, personalised, preventively based, risk-adjusted and tooth-preserving *management* plan for each patient (Pitts NB et al. on behalf of the participating authors of the International Caries Classification and Management System (ICCMS™) Implementation Workshop, 2013). An international consensus workshop held at Kings College London in 2013 laid the groundwork for the incremental development of this guide for practitioners and educators. The guide is available in a number of formats and languages, including a short quick reference guide, from the ICDAS website ((www.icdas.org/). The relationships between ICDAS, ICCMS and the more recent Global Collaboratory for Caries Management – GCCM are shown in Fig. 1.1.

The best evidence for deciding which treatment is appropriate and when has been assembled by a group of 75 international academics and practitioners in a cyclical format with four main elements which together lead to beneficial patient outcomes (see Fig. 1.2). These elements are:

1. HISTORY – which provides a patient-level caries risk assessment
2. CLASSIFICATION – caries staging and activity assessment
3. DECISION-MAKING – both synthesis and diagnoses
4. MANAGEMENT – personalised caries prevention, control and tooth-preserving operative care

Leading to OUTCOMES assessed in the domains of health maintenance, disease control, patient-centred quality metrics and wider impacts on systems and society.

Important features of the ICCMS™ are that it is risk based. For some years there have been groups advocating the CAMBRA philosophy (Caries Management by Risk Assessment), and

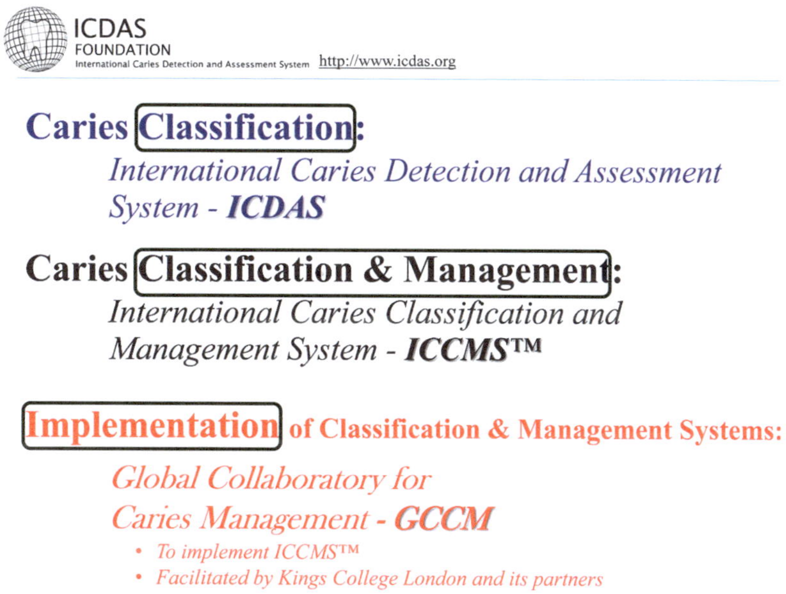

Fig. 1.1 Interrelationships and definitions of *ICDAS* and *ICCMS* and *GCCM*

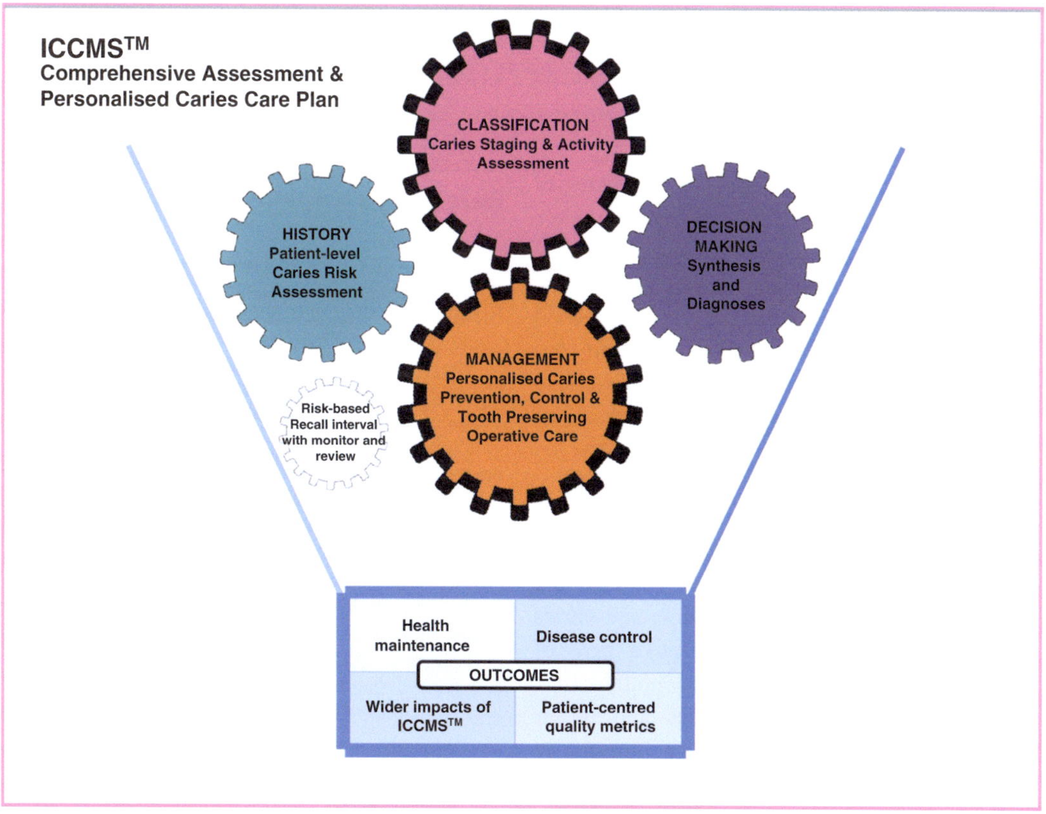

Fig. 1.2 ICCMS™: Overview of the comprehensive assessment and personalised caries care plan

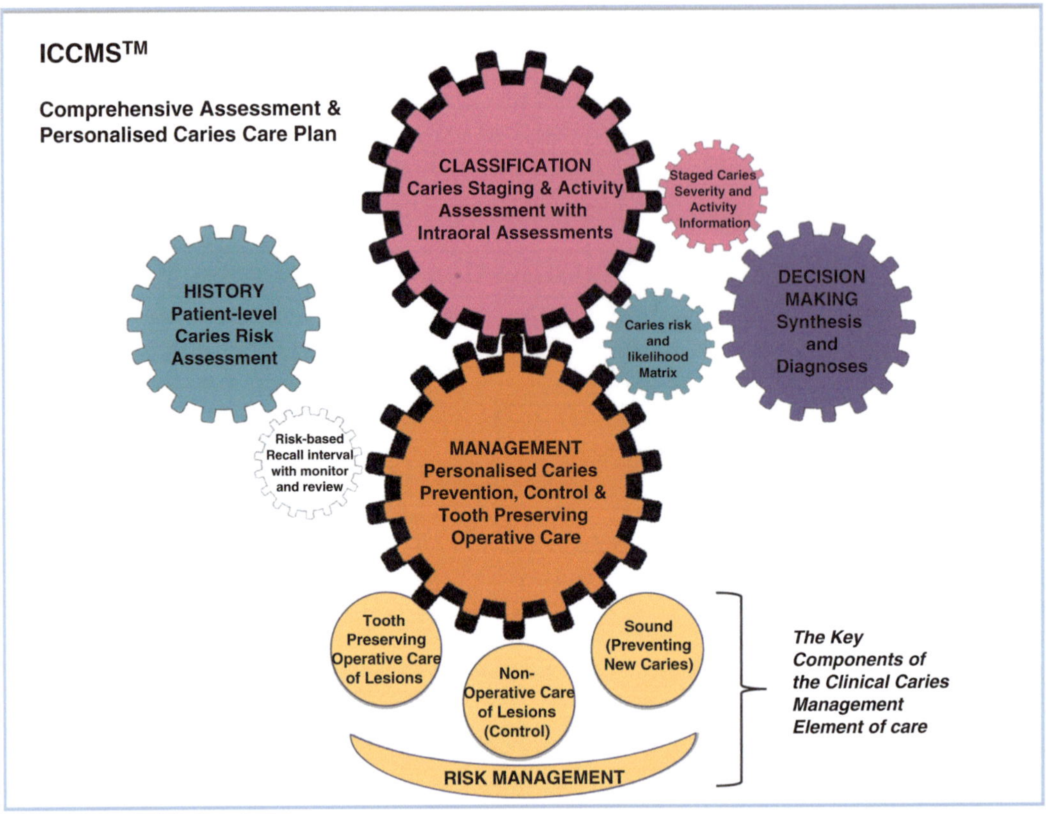

Fig. 1.3 ICCMS™ – Detail showing the key components of the clinical caries management element of care

in terms of planning appropriate recall strategies for patients, the UK National Health Service's National Institute for Clinical Excellence (NICE) convened a guideline development group to look at the evidence in this area. They recommended that for dental recall, the interval between routine dental examinations should be personalised and risk based (NICE 2004). For caries management this means monitoring and review is required.

Figure 1.3 shows the key components of the clinical caries management element of care. These are all underpinned by risk management strategies and comprise (a) preventing new caries for sound surfaces; (b) nonoperative care of lesions, that is, caries control using remineralisation strategies including fluorides and newer methods; and (c) as a last resort – tooth-preserving operative care of lesions that cannot be arrested or reversed or are to extensive when a patient is first seen.

References

Alliance for a Cavity Free Future – ACFF. http://www.allianceforacavityfreefuture.org/.

Bonecker M, Pucca GA, Bella Costa P, Pitts NB. A social movement to reduce caries prevalence in the world. Braz Oral Res. 2012;26(6):491–2 (São Paulo).

Fisher J, Glick M. A new model for caries classification and management: the FDI World Dental Federation Caries Matrix. JADA. 2012;143:546–51.

Fontana M, et al. Development of a core curriculum in cariology for US Dental Schools. J Am Dental Educ Assoc. 2016 (in press).

Ismail AI, Sohn W, Tellez M, Amaya A, Sen A, Hasson H, Pitts NB. The International Caries Detection and Assessment System (ICDAS): an integrated system for measuring dental caries. Community Dent Oral Epidemiol. 2007;35:170–8.

Ismail AI, Tellez M, Pitts NB, Ekstrand KR, Ricketts D, Longbottom C, Eggertsson H, Deery C, Fisher J, Young DA, Featherstone JDB, Evans RW, Zeller GG, Zero D, Martignon S, Fontana M, Zandona A. Caries management pathways preserve dental tissues and promote oral health. Community Dent Oral Epidemiol. 2013;41:e12–40.

Longbottom C L, Huysmans MC, Pitts NB, Fontana M. Glossary of key terms. Monogr Oral Sci. 2009;21:209–16.

Martignon S, Marin LM, Pitts N, Jácome S. Consensus on domains, formation objectives and contents in cariology for undergraduate dental students in Colombia. Eur J Dent Educ. 2014;18(4):222–33.

Minamata Convention on Mercury. United Nations Environment Programme, adopted October 10th 2013. http://www.mercuryconvention.org/Convention/tabid/3426/Default.aspx. Accessed 27 Oct 2014.

Moynihan PJ, Skelly SA. Effect on caries of restricting sugar intake: systematic review to inform WHO guidelines. J Dent Res. 2014;93:8–18.

NICE Clinical Guideline 19. Dental recall: recall interval between routine dental examinations National Institute for Clinical Excellence (NICE), Department of Health, London October 2004. www.nice.org.uk/CG019NICEguideline, ISBN: 1-84257-801-4.

Pitts NB. Modern perspectives on caries activity and control. J Am Dent Assoc. 2011;142(7):790–2.

Pitts NB (Editorial). "ICDAS" – an international system for caries detection and assessment being developed to facilitate caries epidemiology, research and appropriate clinical management. Community Dent Health. 2004b;21:193–8.

Pitts NB. Are we ready to move from operative to non-operative/preventive treatment of dental caries in clinical practice? Caries Res. 2004a;38:294–304.

Pitts NB, Ekstrand KR. International Caries Detection and Assessment System (ICDAS) and its International Caries Classification and Management System (ICCMS™) – methods for staging of the caries process and enabling dentists to manage caries. Community Dent Oral Epidemiol. 2013;41:e41–52.

Pitts NB, Kidd EAM. The prescription and timing of bitewing radiography in the management of dental caries: contemporary recommendations. Br Dent J. 1992a;172:225–7.

Pitts NB, Kidd EAM. Some of the factors to be considered in the prescription and timing of bitewing radiography in the diagnosis and management of dental caries. J Dent. 1992b;20:74–84.

Pitts NB, Stamm J. ICW-CCT statements. J DentRes. 2004;83(Special Issue C):125–8.

Pitts N, Amaechi B, Niederman R, Acevedo A-M, Vianna R, Ganss C, Ismail A, Honkala E. Global oral heath inequalities dental caries task group – research agenda. Adv Dent Res. 2011a;23:211–20.

Pitts N, Melo P, Martignon S, Ekstrand K, Ismail A. Caries risk assessment, diagnosis and synthesis in the context of a European Core Curriculum in Cariology. Eur J Dent Educ. 2011b;15 Suppl 1:23–31.

Pitts NB, Ismail AI, Martignon S, Ekstrand K, Douglas G, Longbottom C and Contributing co-authors on behalf of the Participating Authors of the International Caries Classification and Management System (ICCMS™) Implementation Workshop, held June 2013. ICCMS™ Guide for Practitioners and Educators, December 2014. https://www.icdas.org/uploads/ICCMS.Guide_Full_Guide_With_Appendices_UK.pdf. Accessed 31 Oct 2015.

Schulte AG, Pitts NB, Huysmans M-C, Splieth C, Buchalla W. European cariology core curriculum. Caries Res. 2011;45:336–45.

Selwitz RH, Ismail AI, Pitts NB. Dental caries. Lancet. 2007;369:51–9.

The International Caries Detection and Assessment System (ICDAS): https://www.icdas.org/.

World Health Organization. Guideline: sugars intake for adults and children. Geneva: World Health Organization; 2015. http://apps.who.int/iris/bitstream/10665/149782/1/9789241549028_eng.pdf. Accessed 4 Nov 2015.

Young DA, Nový BB, Zeller GG, Hale R, Hart TC, Truelove EL. American Dental Association Council on Scientific Affairs. The American Dental Association Caries Classification System for Clinical Practice. JADA. 2015;146(2):79–86.

2 Enamel Softening (Dental Erosion)

Michel Goldberg

Abstract

For many years, most of the published reports of enamel softening dealt with consequences of acid or chelator etching. It occurs without bacterial involvement. The 2–5 nm thick outer enamel surface layer is mainly concerned. Limited crystallite dissolution is due to abrasion, attrition, abfraction, or erosion. More than likely, enamel dissolution is due to acidic demineralization. At early stages, it is a reversible process. Preventive strategies include dietary counseling, stimulation of salivary flow, optimization of fluoride regimens, modification of erosive beverages, and adequate oral hygiene measures.

2.1 Introductory Remarks

For many years, most of the published reports were dealing with three well-identified enamel-induced pathologies, which have been specifically studied and compared. They included three groups of major studies studying *enamel softening* getting worse and becoming a more severe *acid or chelator etching* and ultimately being converted into *carious lesions*. The etio-pathologic complexity of the early enamel lesions was increased, whereas a parallel decreased of carious lesions was noted.

M. Goldberg
University Paris Descartes, Sorbonne, Paris Cité
and INSERM UMR-S1124, 45 rue des Saints Pères,
Cedex 06, 75270 Paris, France
e-mail: mgoldod@gmail.com

Dental enamel is the most highly mineralized structure of the skeleton. The percentage of inorganic components of enamel is greater than in bone and dentin. It is the actual target of specifically defined aggressions directed toward the enamel structure. Due to the presence of an outer aprismatic layer, dental erosions, attritions, abfractions, and abrasion became the most prominent lesions during the past decades. Such phenomena are obviously in continuity with enamel softening. After an acid attack, or following the action of chelators, the presence of a prismatic enamel layer is determinant for an etching pattern, beneath the dental plaque, which is responsible for the progression of carious lesions within enamel. The cascade of enamel decays leads from one type of superficial alteration to more severe deterioration.

The comparison between the three enamel alterations provides a better understanding of the carious process, the specific topic of this book.

M. Goldberg (ed.), *Understanding Dental Caries*, DOI 10.1007/978-3-319-30552-3_2

Hence, analysis of enamel softening opens gates on enamel etching and shed lights on the early stages of the enamel carious lesion.

2.2 Dental Erosion

Tooth wear or dental erosive lesion involves multifactorial causes. There is an interplay between chemical, biological, and behavioral factors. Erosion as a pathology entity results from the *chemical loss of dental hard tissue by an acid, without bacterial involvement*. Attrition (physical wear through tooth-tooth contact) and abrasion (physical wear produced by the interaction between a tooth surface and another material) are two other well-recognized factors. Dental erosion is exclusively a surface phenomenon, whereas in contrast, the initial carious lesion implicates both surface and subsurface modifications.

Erosion is due to structural feature of the tooth, physiological properties of saliva, and intrinsic and extrinsic acidic sources (Lussi et al. 2011). The critical pH below which enamel dissolves is about 5.5. Erosion starts by initial softening of the enamel surface, followed by a loss of volume with a softened layer persisting at the surface of the remaining tissue. Exposure to acids combined with insufficient salivary flow results in enhanced dissolution. Enamel tends to dissolve more slowly than dentin.

During the initial stage of dental erosion, the loss of tooth hard tissue affects up to 80 % of the adults and ~ 50 % of the children (more recent evaluations indicate a prevalence of erosion as high as 68 %). Enamel dissolution is due to acidic demineralization. At these early stages, it is a reversible process. Soft drink consumption of acidic food and drinks is correlated with the decrease of milk consumption, and in addition, this points at calcium deficiency.

2.3 Crystallite Dissolution

Hydrogen ions or chelating agents begin their deleterious effects by dissolving enamel crystal, either in the center of crystallites (central dissolution affecting a screw-like structure, due to the presence of defective Burger vectors) or at the lateral border and eventually at the edge of the crystallite. This outer screw dislocation occurs at the edge of the crystallite. The prism sheath (organic extracellular matrix) and the prism core are dissolved, leaving apparent a honeycomb structure mostly identifiable after acid etching. Differences in the behavioral, biological, and chemical factors may contribute to explain why some individuals display more erosion than others.

If the acidic impact persists (e.g., longer periods of interaction and/or increased concentrations), further dissolution of the enamel occurs. The dissolution becomes irreversible and leads to a severe alteration associated with a reduction of enamel thickness.

The erosion may be also dietary or result from chronic regurgitation. Soft drinks have an erosive potential. The effects of soft drinks on enamel can be evaluated by measuring the amount of calcium or phosphate ions released by enamel. There was no significant correlation between the % SMHC (percentage of superficial microhardness changes) and the other variables tested for a number of drinks leading to enamel surface softening. The pH seems to have more influence on the erosive potential of these drinks. Increased protective and defensive factors can restore or prevent loss of calcium and phosphate from enamel.

Tooth brushing, citric acid, or orange juice may remove the superficial part of the softened enamel (Figs. 2.1a, 2.2, and 2.4a). The thickness of the softened layer varied between 254 and 323 nm, depending on the acid used and its concentration. In any case, it is obvious that soft drink consumption increases the potential for enamel erosion.

Remineralization agents induced reduced caries and appropriately promote subsurface deposits. Acid neutralization may be obtained by buffering components of the diet. In addition to an early diagnosis of dental erosion, the detection of isolated factors like sports drinks may be implicated in multifactorial erosions. The significance of the mechanisms involved constitutes prerequisites, which are mandatory to initiate preventive and therapeutic measures.

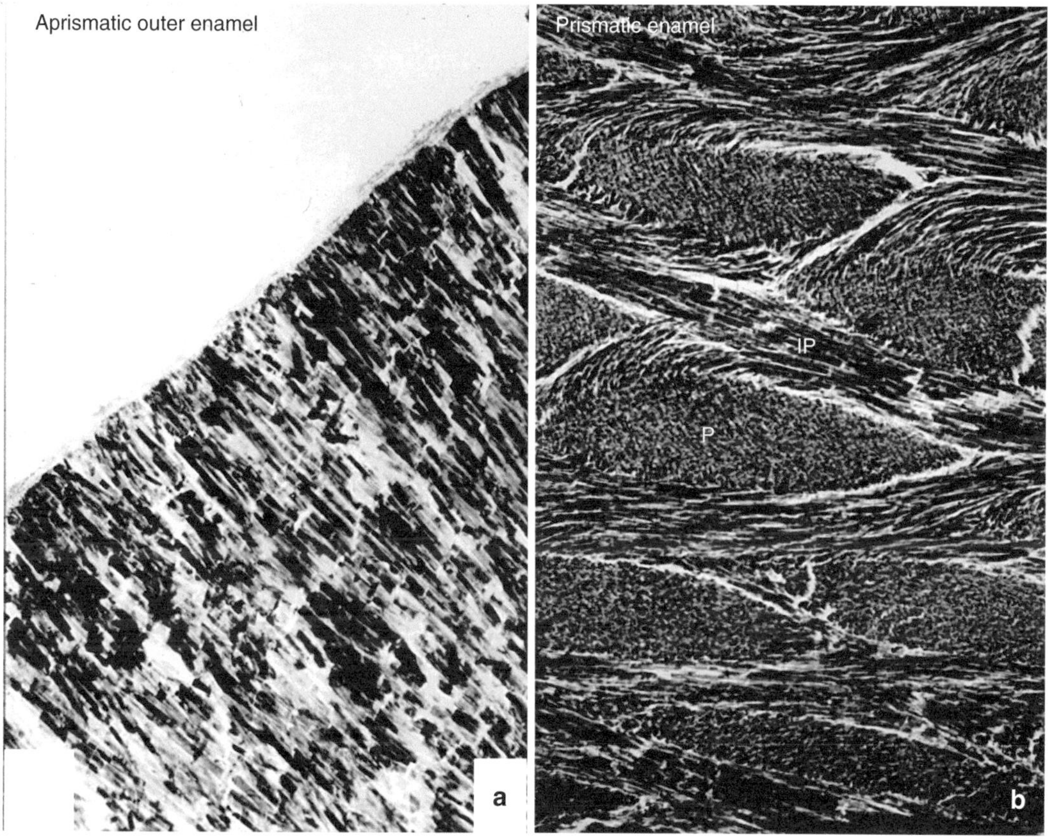

Fig. 2.1 Rat's molar enamel. (**a**) Normal aprismatic outer enamel/hydroxyapatite crystals are parallel, forming a continuous palisade-like structure. (**b**) Beneath the surface, enamel displays a prismatic structure, where prisms (*P*) (or rods) alternate with interprismatic enamel (*IP*) (interrod enamel)

2.3.1 Four Types of Physical and Chemical Dental Erosions Have Been Reported

Imfeld (1996a, b) has defined different types of tissue losses. According to Ganss (2006), each type of alteration bears its own specificity.

1. *Abrasion* is located on the incisal or occlusal surfaces and depends on the abrasiveness of the individual diet. The most abrasive agents are toothpaste, as shown by clinical data and *in vitro* studies. Both patient factors and material factors influence the prevalence of abrasion.
2. *Attrition* results from the action of the antagonistic teeth. It has also been named *demastication*. It is a mixture of abrasion and attrition.
3. *Abfraction* is located mainly in the cemento-enamel region where microfractures occur (also defined as fatigue wear). Wedge-shaped defects are related to abfractions or wedge-shaped non-carious cervical lesions. Analyses that demonstrate theoretical stress concentration at the cervical areas of the teeth have not yet been actually proven. However, there are some strong arguments favoring this possibility. The non-carious stress-induced cervical lesion or abfractions are observed in the buccal surface at the cemento-enamel junction of the teeth, with prevalence ranging in humans from 27 to 85 % (Sarode and Sarode 2013)
4. *Erosion* results from the action of acids or chelators acting on plaque-free tooth surfaces. The loss of tooth structure is due to acid dissolution without involvement of bacteria.

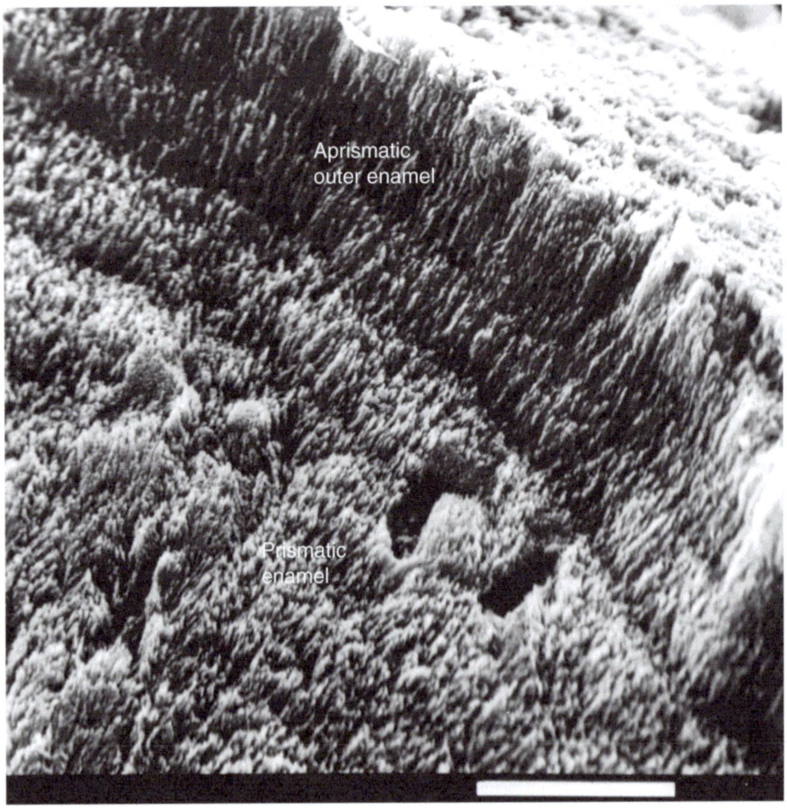

Fig. 2.2 Human enamel. The surface outer enamel layer looks laminated. This is not the case for the prismatic enamel located underneath

Regurgitated gastric acids or extrinsic components (soft drinks, acidic fruits) may act as extrinsic agents. Erosion is related to enamel surface softening. Repeated direct removal of a softened enamel layer favors more rapid demineralization and tissue loss (Figs. 2.3b and 2.4b).

2.3.2 Structure and Chemistry of Dental Erosion

Table 2.1

Structurally, the outer layer of enamel (aprismatic zone) consists of parallel crystals forming a palisade-like structure (Figs. 2.1a and 2.3b). The free ending of the crystals, located beneath a glycoprotein structure, which is controlled by the dental plaque, melts in response to the acidic extracellular gel or displays corroded extremities with enlarged inter-crystallite spaces. With effects that are time dependent and concentration dependent, the 5–15 μm thick aprismatic layer disappears gradually; and consequently the overall enamel thickness is reduced. The 3–5 μm prismatic enamel, which is now exposed by the erosion, displays a scalloped profile with numerous indentations and a drastic calcium and phosphate loss that is important near the new surface. The loss is gradually reduced until it reaches the original enamel level. The inner prismatic enamel is not altered, and both the enamel shape and thickness are undamaged.

The thickness of the softened outermost enamel and dentin layers is estimated to be 2–5 μm. Citric acid erosion caused a mean substance loss of 16.0 μm (SD ± 2.5 μm). Remineralization of re-hardened enamel is apparently similar to the original structure (Feagin et al. 1969).

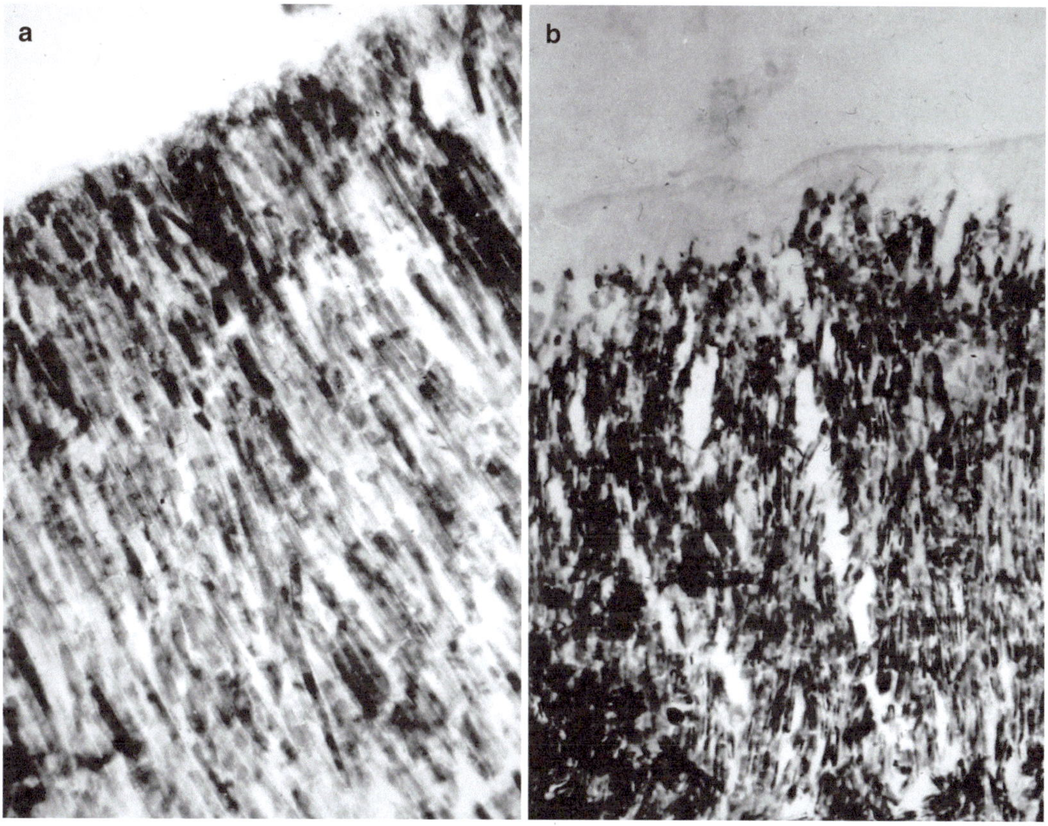

Fig. 2.3 (**a**) The outer enamel layer displays some interruptions or defects after softening. (**b**) The surface of corroded enamel displays structural alterations at the tip of crystallites and, at some locations, between crystallites

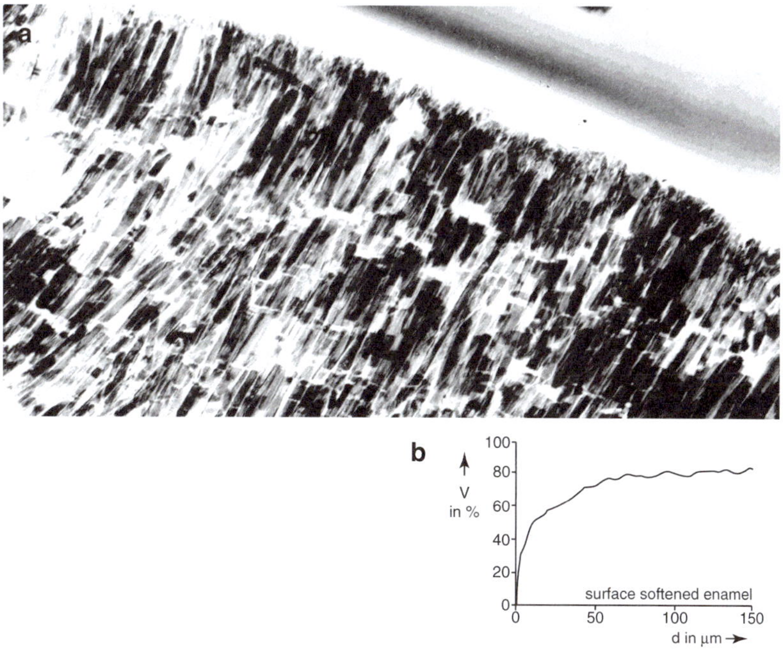

Fig. 2.4 (**a**) At the surface, crystallite endings look irregular with a scalloped profile. (**b**) There is a gradual mineral increase after the mineral loss due to the softening agent in the outer enamel surface. The percentage of mineral reaches a "normal" value at 50 µm under the enamel surface

Table 2.1 Composition percentage in enamel and dentine

Component	Enamel percent by volume	Dentine percent by volume
Carbonated hydroxyapatite	85	47
Water	12	20
Protein and lipid	3	33

See references by: Curzon and Featherstone (1983); De Carvalho Sales-Peres et al. (2007); Featherstone and Lussi (2006); and Lussi and Jaeggi (2008)

The mineral part of teeth is a calcium-deficient carbonated hydroxyapatite. Substitutions in the crystal lattice render the mineral phase more acid soluble. The direct attack by hydrogen ion combines with the carbonate and phosphate release of the crystal surface, leading to direct surface etching. The citrate ion can also form complex with the calcium removed from the crystal surface. The substitutions in the mineral crystal lattice disturb the structure. The carbonate content of "sound" enamel is approximately 3 %, while in dentine it is 5–6 %. Therefore the mineral is even more acid soluble in dentine. Crystals in dentine are smaller than in enamel; consequently the dissolution process needs shorter periods of time in dentine compared with enamel.

Chemical factors explain erosive attack. Addition of calcium and phosphate salts to erosive drinks show protection of surface softening. Biological factors such as saliva, acquired dental pellicle, and tooth structure and positioning are related to dental erosion development. Behavioral factors also play role in erosion. Frequent tooth brushing and good oral hygiene are important in the etiology of dental erosion. Sport and increased gastroesophageal reflux enhance the risk of developing dental erosion.

2.3.3 Intrinsic Causes of Erosion

Gastric juice entering the mouth causes dental erosion. This disease affects reflux (suppress disease), eating disorders, and concern about 65 % of the western population. In such case, the erosion is mostly palatal, due to reflux disease, regurgitation, anorexia, bulimia, and rumination (Eisenburger 2009).

Micro- and nanoindentations, indentation length, and surface hardness measurements, according to Knoop or Vickers, have identified rhomboid indentation of about 30–40 μm length. They have been recorded immediately and are not time dependent. Surface profilometry allows determining by scanning electron microscopy the tendency of the stylus to penetrate the fragile outer layer. Altogether, other methods such as SEM and ESEM, surface hardness measurements, surface profilometry, iodide permeability test, atomic force microscopy, nanoindentations, and ultrasonic measurement of enamel thickness may provide insights on the effects of acid solutions on enamel softening and the subsequent erosion (Fig. 2.4b).

Preventive strategies of patients suffering from erosion include dietary counseling, stimulation of salivary flow, optimization of fluoride regimens, modification of erosive beverages, and adequate oral hygiene measures (Magalhaes et al. 2009).

References

Curzon MEJ, Featherstone JDB. Chemical composition of enamel. In: Lazzari EP, editor. Handbook of experimental aspects of oral biochemistry. CRC Press; Inc. Boca Raton, Florida. 1983. p. 123–35.

De Carvalho Sales-Peres SH, Magalhaes AC, De Andrade Moreira Machado MA, Buzalaf MAR. Evaluation of the erosive potential of soft drinks. Eur J Dent. 2007;1:10–3.

Eisenburger M. Degree of mineral loss in softened human enamel after acid erosion measured by chemical analysis. J Dent. 2009;37:491–4.

Feagin F, Koulourides T, Pigman W. The characterization of enamel surface demineralization, remineralization, and associated hardness changes in human and bovine material. Arch Oral Biol. 1969;14:1407–17.

Featherstone JDB, Lussi A. Understanding the chemistry of dental erosion. In: Lussi A, editor. Dental erosion. Monogr Of Oral Sci, vol 20. Basel: Karger; 2006. p. 66–76.

Ganss C. Definition of erosion and links to tooth wear. In: Lussi A, editor. Dental erosion Monogr Oral Sci, vol 20. Basel: Karger; 2006. p 9–16.
Imfeld T. Prevention of progression of dental erosion by professional and individual prophylactic measures. Eur J Oral Sci. 1996a;104:215–20.
Imfeld T. Dental erosion. Definition, classification and links. Eur J Oral Sci. 1996b;104:151–5.
Lussi A, Jaeggi T. Erosion- diagnosis and risk factors. Clin Oral Investig. 2008;12 Suppl 1:S5–13.
Lussi A, Schlueter N, Rakhmatullina E, Ganss C. Dental erosion- an overview with emphasis on chemical and histopathological aspects. Caries Res. 2011;45 Suppl 1:2–12.
Magalhaes A-C, Wiegand A, Rios D, Honorio HM, Buzalaf MAR. Insights into preventive measures for dental erosion. J Appl Oral Sci. 2009;17:75–86.
Sarode GS, Sarode SC. Abfraction: a review. J Oral Maxillofacial Pathol. 2013;17:222–7.

Enamel Etching

3

Michel Goldberg

Abstract

After the deterioration due to an acid or chelating solution, enamel crystal dissolution starts either as screw dislocations in the central part of the crystallite (dissolution of the hollow-core type), or the initial dissolution begins at defects located in the edge of the crystallite (edge dislocation). A thin layer is dissolved by the acid and eliminated near the enamel surface. In the inner prismatic zone, the rods disappeared, leaving a continuous network of interprismatic enamel (type 1 etching pattern), or the interprismatic enamel is dissolved and rods persist (type 2 etching pattern). An amorphous flat surface may be observed where rods and interrods are both dissolved (type 3 etching pattern). Using chelators, rods protrude on 20–50 μm in length, whereas interrods are dissolved. Enamel etching is due to acid corrosion, a phenomenon occurring in the absence of bacteria. Used at the chair side, this method increases resin adhesion on dental enamel and has clinical implications.

3.1 The Acid-Etched Enamel: Clinical Usefulness

In 1955, Buonocore published that enamel treatment with phosphoric acid alters chemically the surface and creates a suitable relief. The change induced on a smooth flat surface is modified into indented crenels and provides an increased adhesion of acrylic filling materials to dental enamel. Enamel etching is a method of reducing the manual preparation of a tooth, namely, undercuts and bevels. It increases the adhesive properties of resin composites on the prepared enamel surface. It allows both the bonding of orthodontic brackets, adhering to the enamel surface for a short period of time, and the attachment of restorative material, aiming to produce a more stable bond. After this pioneer publication, the acid-etched enamel method became widely accepted. Different types of dissolution were induced, depending on enamel structure and maturation. To summarize the findings, the formation of microporosities allows the resin penetration

M. Goldberg
University Paris Descartes, Sorbonne, Paris Cité and INSERM UMR-S1124, 45 rue des Saints Pères, Cedex 06, 75270 Paris, France
e-mail: mgoldod@gmail.com

M. Goldberg (ed.), *Understanding Dental Caries*, DOI 10.1007/978-3-319-30552-3_3

between enamel crystallites and tags inside rods or interrods. In dentin, a hybrid layer is formed including collagen fibrils, with protruding resin tags that penetrate inside the dentinal tubules, enlarged after acidic peritubular dissolution. Altogether the etching effects on dentin provide micromechanical retentions. These structures contribute to increase the adhesive properties of resins applied on etched enamel but also to dentin.

3.2 Effects of Acid or Chelating Solutions on Dental Enamel

The anatomical distribution of the different enamel layers contributes specifically to the etching pattern after the attack by an acid or chelating solution. Differences in size and orientation of crystallites appear between (1) the outer aprismatic layer (superficial surface layer); (2) the bulk of the prismatic layer, including rods and interrods; and (3) the thin inner aprismatic enamel located at the dentinoenamel junction. The resulting pattern implies massive differences in the etching properties after acid dissolution of sound enamel.

A thin layer of the superficial aprismatic enamel is totally dissolved and disappears (4–15 μm). Then gradually, the demineralization pattern that is found is gradually restored, and finally in the bulk of enamel, mineralization is identical to what was found in "normal" enamel.

Monocrystals (hydroxyapatite crystals) are composed by cuboidal structures, with a = b = 9.4 Å and a shorter c-axis about 6.9 Å. Monocrystals are closely connected, forming lattices associated as regular structures, also called Burger's circuit or vector. Slight disturbances in the regular assembly of monocrystals constitute the initial points of acidic attack. The crystal dissolution starts either as screw dislocations in the central part of crystallite section (dissolution of the hollow-core type), or the initial dissolution begins at defects located in the edge of the crystallite (edge dislocation) (Arends and Jongebloed. 1979 and Figs. 3.1, 3.2, 3.3, and 3.4).

Measurements of the overall size of the crystallite on transverse sections have been reported to be 700 nm × 300 nm (mean value: L+l : 2=500 nm) (263 Å±22 x 683 Å±34- Daculsi et al. 1984). They appear as long ribbons with a length over a few millimeters, starting at the dentinoenamel junction and probably reaching at the surface the whole enamel thickness.

In the outer aprismatic layer, crystallites are parallel to each other and form a palisade-like structure. Acidic solutions or gels spread at the surface and dissolve the center of the crystal or enlarge the narrow intercrystalline structures. After a short period of time, the row of crystallites is reduced in height. The aprismatic layer disappears and the new surface created reaches the prismatic layer.

During enamel formation, ameloblast Tomes' processes fill structures that will become rod (or prisms) and mineralize (Figs. 3.3, 3.4, 3.5, 3.6, 3.7, and 3.8). At the rod periphery, the interrod material forms a continuous network. The width of the rods is about 3 μm and includes more than 1000 crystallites/rod unit, whereas the thinner interrod displays a mean thickness of 0.5 μm and contains about 100–300 tightly packed crystallites. In rods, the crystals are bending from the head to the tail. A thin layer of enamel matrix proteins, the so-called enamel sheath, separates rods and interrods. Depending on the location of the etched area at the enamel surface, rods and interrod crystallites form a 60°angle.

This structural organization implies that acid gel or solution dissolves primarily the mineralized crystallites when the crystals are exposed along their c-axis. It takes a little longer time when the crystals are angulated at 60° in the enamel structures. These differences are at the origin of the 3 different types described by Silverstone et al. (1975).

In 1975, Silverstone et al. described the effects of exposure of dental enamel to acid solutions (Figs. 3.7, 3.8, and 3.9):

1. The *type I etching pattern* displays dissolution of the prism core, whereas the prism periphery was relatively well preserved.

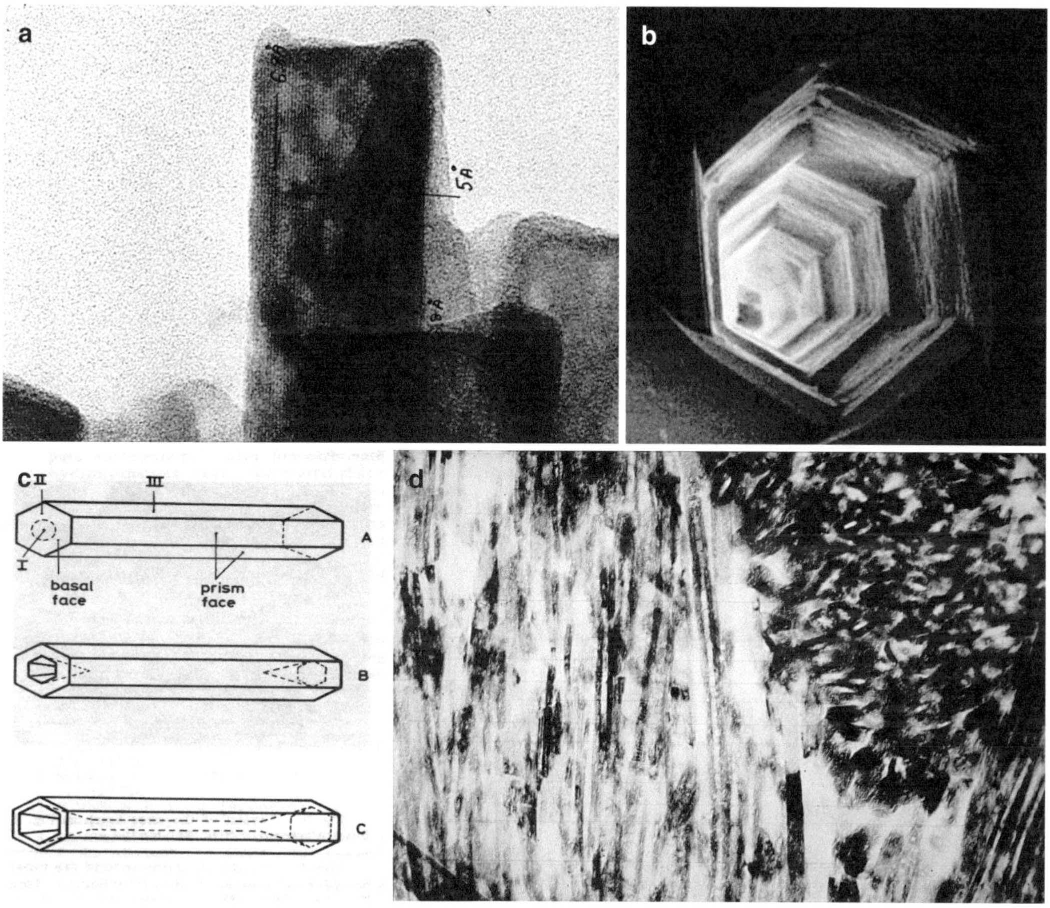

Fig. 3.1 (**a**) Crystallite of a mouse incisor. Alignments of hydroxyapatite monocrystals form a lattice, with – 5 Å–6.8 Å spacing. (**b**) Axial dissolution of a crystallite. (**c**) The acidic dissolution starts on the basal face (*A*), then increases in depth (*B*), and dissolves the central part of the crystals along the c-axis (*C*). (**d**) View on the longitudinal and central dissolution of enamel crystallites

2. A reverse pattern was observed in the *type 2 etching pattern*: the peripheral interrod enamel was dissolved, whereas the rods were less corroded.
3. A random pattern was seen with *type 3*, with an amorphous surface where the etching pattern was not clearly related to prism morphology.

The differences are not related to variations in chemical composition, but rather to the crystallite orientation. Variations of structure occur from place to place at the enamel surface and between sites on a single tooth surface (Silverstone et al. 1975).

Enamel etching with chelating solution dissolves essentially interrod enamel. The crystallites resulting from sucked residual rods are longer than after an acid attack. Their length varies between 20 μm and 50 μm (Fig. 3.10).

Enamel is a more complex structure, and in addition of aprismatic outer layer and rods and interrods of the prismatic zone, Hunter-Schreger's bands occupy the inner third of enamel, near the dentinoenamel junction. Rod twisting contributes to the thickening of rods. Longitudinal sections of rods cause the formation of parazones, whereas diazones contribute to the arrangement of packed rods in transverse sections. Parazones and diazones

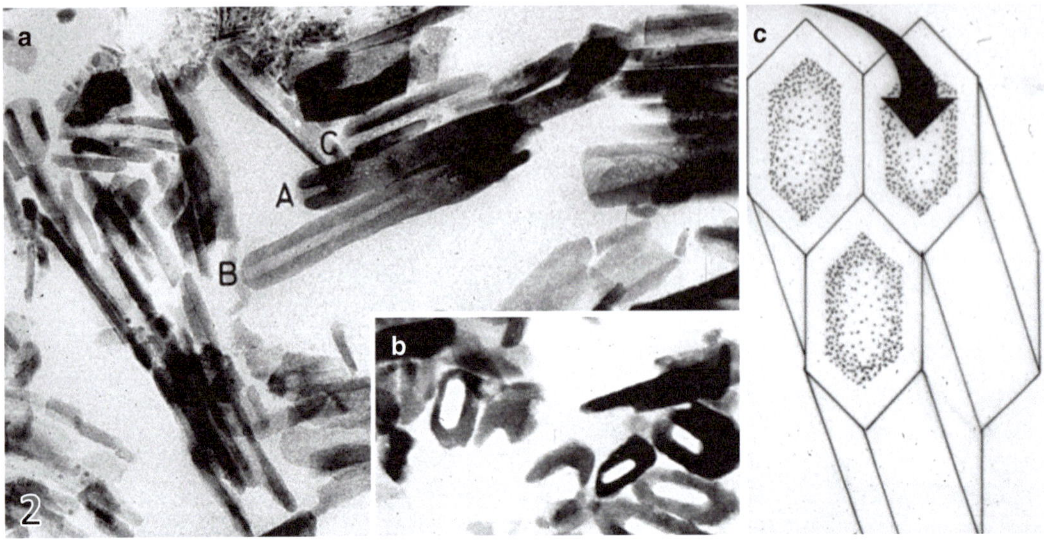

Fig. 3.2 Shows the successive steps of crystallite dissolution: (**a**) longitudinal dissolution; (**b**) dissolution in the central c-axis; (**c**) schematic drawing of the crystallite dissolution

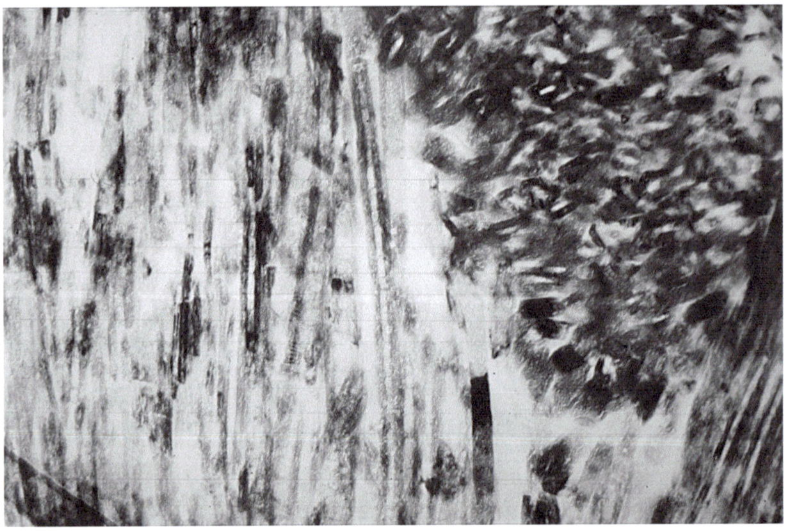

Fig. 3.3 Longitudinal (*left part of the figure*) and axial (*right part of the figure*) dissolution of enamel crystallites

display differences in crystallites orientation and consequently influence the etching pattern.

The Retzius lines are located at more or less regular distances within the mature enamel point at the bending of rods and potential differences in the crystal dissolution as well. The complex three-dimensional enamel organization is directly concerned by the pattern evidenced by etching procedures.

3.3 The Thickness of Enamel Layers After Etching

Acids or chelators contribute to destroy largely or totally the acid-etched enamel aprismatic surface. Consequently a 4 µm–15 µm outer layer is removed. The new outer surface is formed by softened enamel, with corroded crystallites. Depending on the rod/interrod orientation, either the center of rods is destroyed,

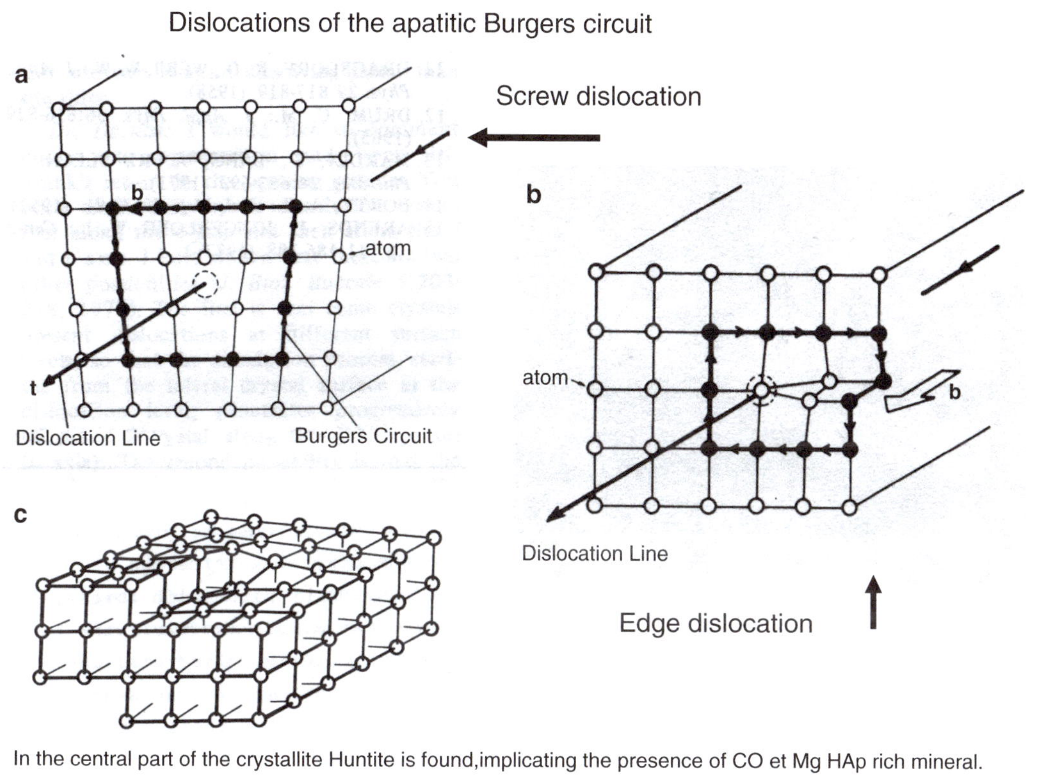

Fig. 3.4 Screw dislocation (**a**) and edge dislocation (**b**) of the apatitic Burgers circuit. In (**c**), huntite is found in the central part of crystallites. The huntite-rich central part implicates an elevated content of carbonate and magnesium

or it is the reverse, the interrod border being stable (type I or II). The depth of the new scalloped surface is about 10 μm. The thickness of the softened enamel is about 10–20 μm. Structural alterations occur in acid-etched enamel, forming band with an indented profile, with 10–15 μm softened enamel below the etched surface. This contributes to the adhesion of resins on the etched enamel. In deeper parts of prismatic enamel, changes may be detected after exposure up to 100 μm or more below the surface. The penetration of resin between corroded crystallites enhances the adhesive properties of the restorative material (Ryf et al. 2012, and Fig. 3.6).

Resin tags in enamel pretreated with various acid concentrations decrease significantly from 22 μm for 35 % H3PO4 to 12 μm for 20 % and 9 μm for 5, 10, and 65 % H3PO4. In contrast, tags of 5 μm were found when a 3 % concentration of H3PO4 was used. The length of the tags does not contribute to the bond strength of the specimens. The major role is related to the resin ability to penetrate between enamel crystallites and rods (Shinchi et al. 2000)

After etching, the enamel loss, enamel breakout, and adhesive remnants were detectable following bracket removal. The mean volume loss was 0.02 mm^3 (±O.03 mm^3) and a depth of 44.9 μm^3 (±48.3 μm). Composite remnants after debonding had a mean volume of 2.48 mm^3 (±0.92 mm^3) (Ryf et al. 2012).

As a consequence of acid and chelator effects on enamel, softening and different etching patterns reveal the intrinsic enamel architecture and its structural variations.

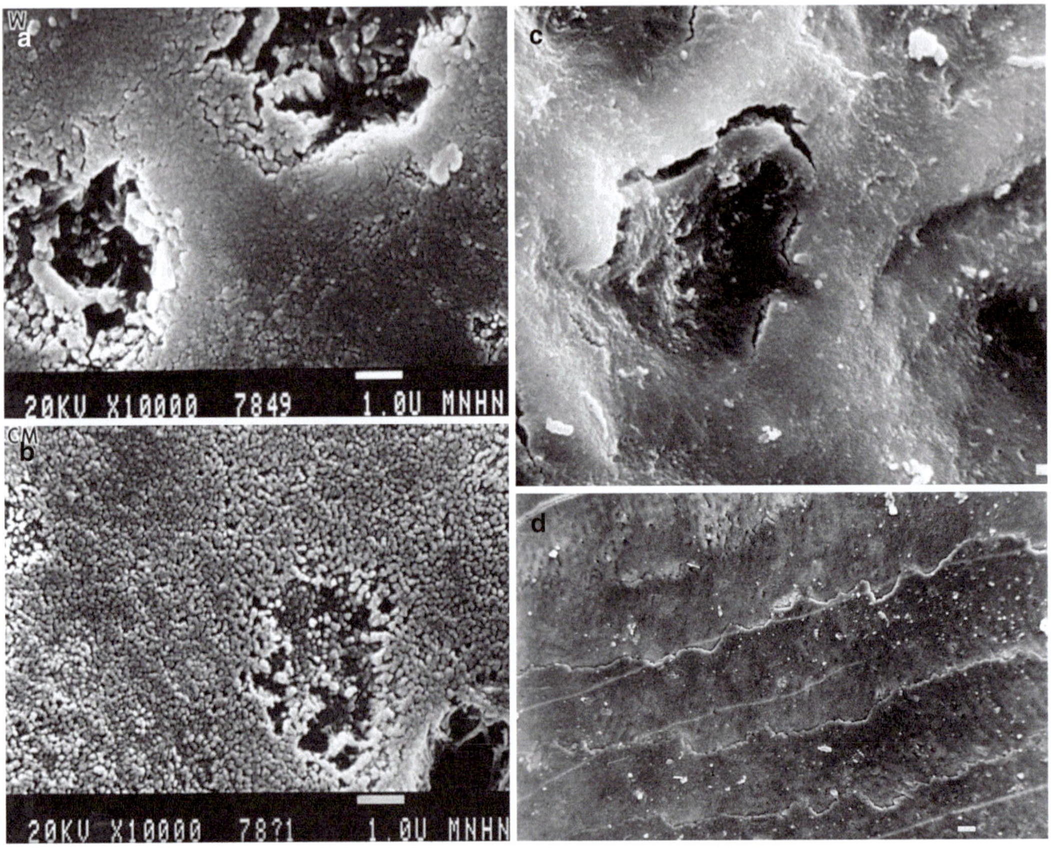

Fig. 3.5 (**a**) Human enamel surface cleaned with tape running water. Empty rods are open at the surface. (**b**) Human enamel surface cleaned with a chloroform/methanol, which dissolves extracellular matrix lipids. The organic material inside rods is eliminated and intercrystalline spaces are empty. (**c**) Untreated enamel surface. Rods (*r*) and interrods (*ir*) constitute irregularities at the surface. (**d**) Perikymata and prints of ameloblasts are visible on the enamel surface

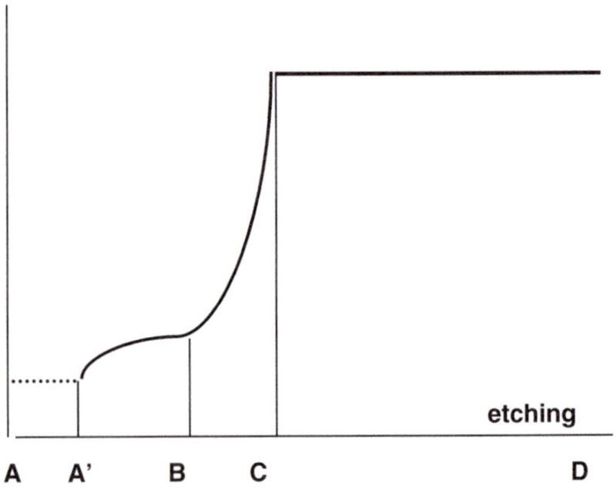

Fig. 3.6 The surface enamel located between A and A' has been totally dissolved and disappeared. The mineral percentage between A' and B is slowly increasing, and a more accentuate rise in mineral content occurs between B and C. Between C and D mineralization is unchanged despite the effect of acid etching

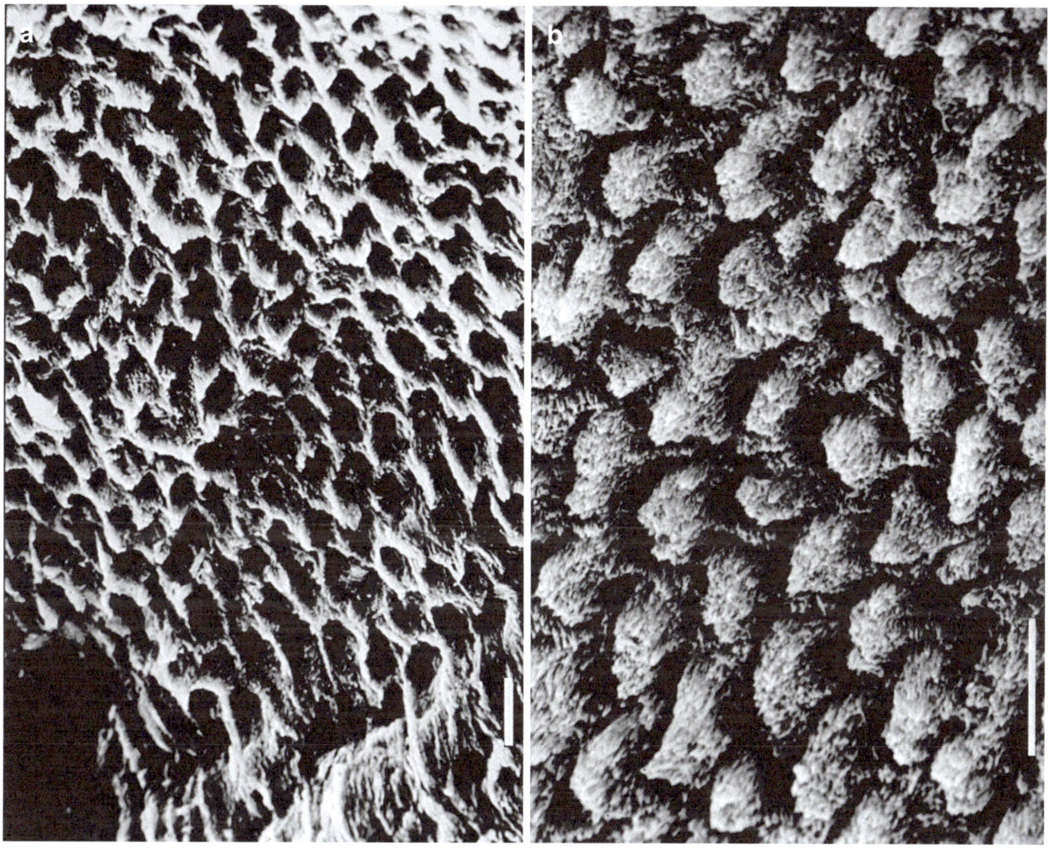

Fig. 3.7 Human enamel after acid etching observed with a scanning electron microscope (SEM). (**a**) Type 1 etching pattern. Rod enamel is dissolved, whereas interrod enamel forms a honeycomb. (**b**) Type 2 etching pattern. Interrod enamel is largely dissolved, whereas rods are less affected

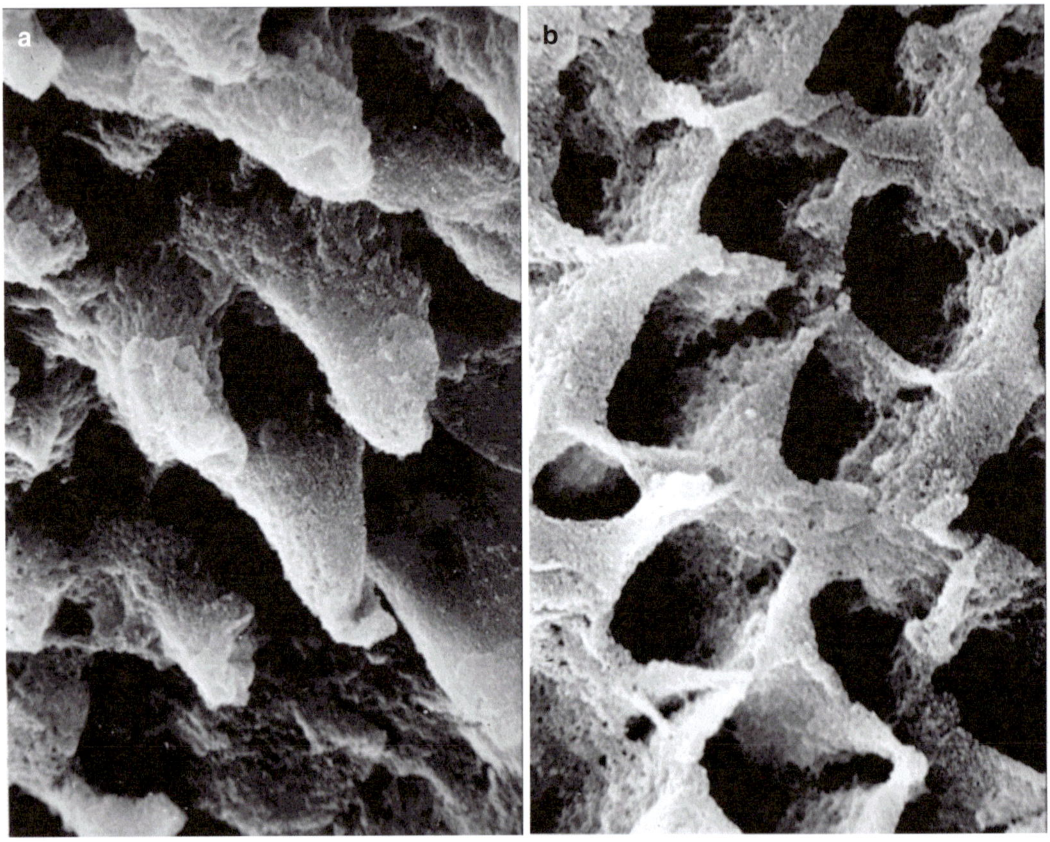

Fig. 3.8 Replica of resin restorations. In (**a**), the dissolution of rods allows the formation of tags within the rods (type 1). In (**b**), a reverse pattern is observed (type 2). Dissolution of interrod enamel allows the penetration of resin in the dissolved interrod network

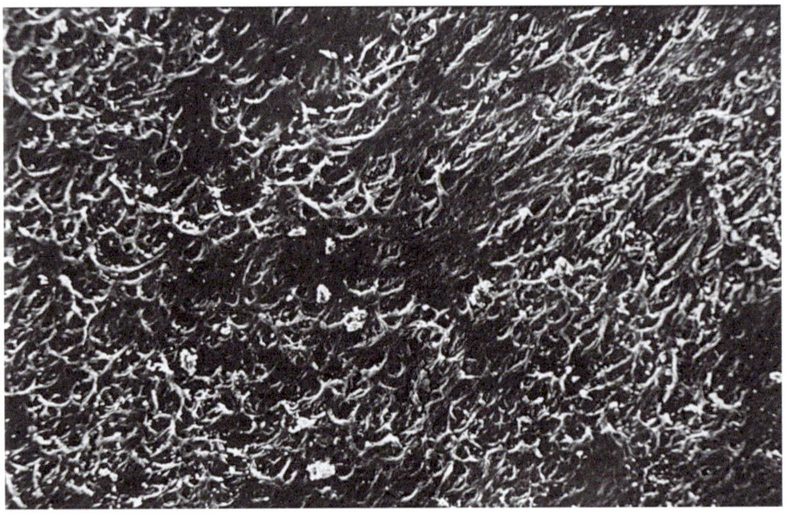

Fig. 3.9 Pattern 3 observed with the SEM after acid etching. The enamel surface is flat. No protruding structure contributes to the resin adhesion. This pattern may be due either to the fluoride level in enamel preventing dissolution or to the presence of an aprismatic structure

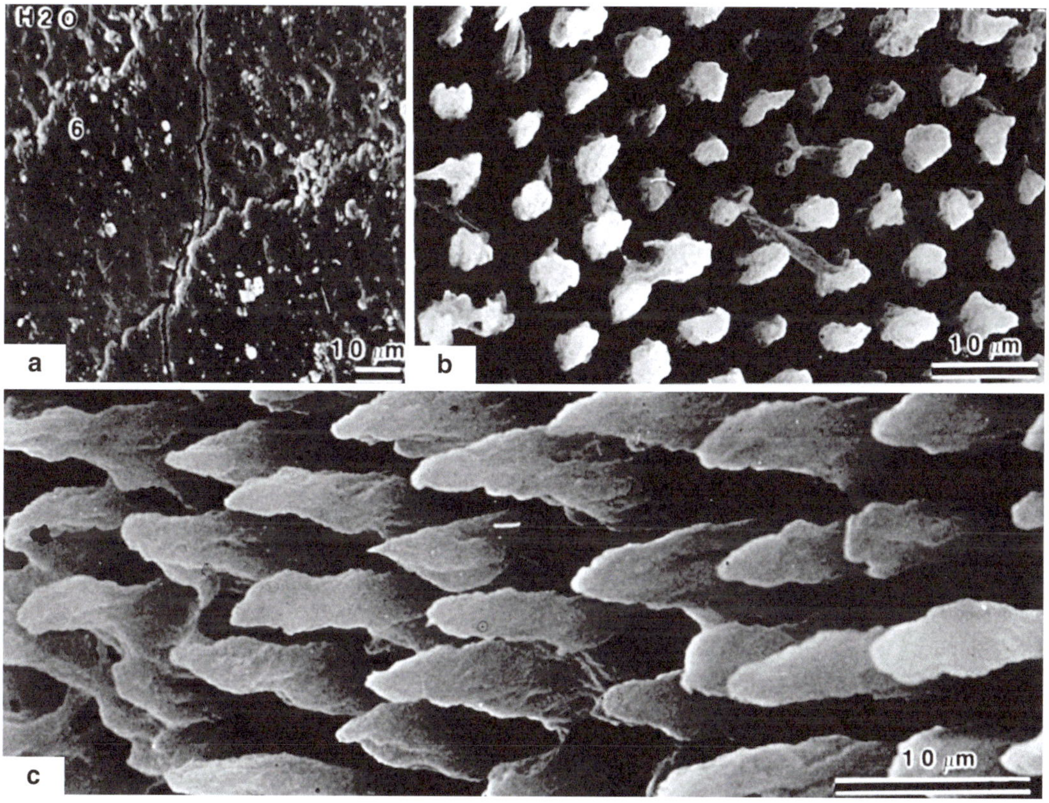

Fig. 3.10 (**a**) Enamel surface after tape water rinsing. (**b**) Action of a chelating solution on the enamel surface. Interrod enamel is dissolved but rods persist. (**c**) Long tags of corroded rods penetrate into the chelated enamel allowing good adhesion of the resin restoration

References

Arends J, Jongebloed WL. Ultrastuctural studies of synthetic apatite crystals. J Dent Res. 1979;58(B):837–42.

Buonocore MG. A simple method of increasing the adhesion of acrylic filling materials. J Dent Res. 1955;34:849–53.

Daculsi G, Menanteau J, Kerebel LM, Mitre D. Length and shape of enamel crystals. Calcif Tissue Int. 1984;36:550–5.

Ryf S, Flury S, Palaniappan S, Lussi A, Van Meerbeek B, Zimmerli B. Enamel loss and adhesive remnants following bracket removal and various clean-up procedures in vitro. Eur J Orthodontics. 2012;34:25–32.

Shinchi MJ, Soma K, Nakabayashi N. The effect of phosphoric acid concentration on resin tag length and bond strength of a photo-cured resin to acid-etched enamel. Dent Mater. 2000;16:324–9.

Silverstone LM, Saxton CA, Dogon IL, Fejerskov O. Variation in the pattern of acid etching of human dental enamel examined by scanning electron microscopy. Caries Res. 1975;9:373–87.

4 The Early Enamel Carious Lesion

Michel Goldberg

Abstract

The dental enamel comprises an outer aprismatic layer, a thick prismatic zone, and inner aprismatic enamel. Under the dental plaque, the initial carious lesion displays a surface zone, characteristic of the lesion, a subsurface (or body of the lesion), a dark zone, and a translucent zone. The major phenomenon of the initial enamel caries is the formation of a surface zone, resulting from the demineralization/remineralization processes. Anatomical entities such as rod endings at the enamel surface and Retzius striae play major roles in the initiation and development of the lesion. Enamel caries start by a central demineralization of rods, enlargement of enamel sheaths, and the formation of tunnels crossing the surface zone. The cone-shaped structure reaches the dentinoenamel junction, and the lesion spreads into dentin. The destruction occurs along the dentinoenamel junction and decreased the thickness of the mantle dentin.

4.1 Enamel Structure and Composition

The dental enamel is formed by an outer aprismatic layer (5–15 μm), covering the bulk of enamel, which is prismatic. The prismatic enamel includes rods (or prisms) and interrod enamel (interprismatic enamel). At the junction between rods and interrods, a thin layer of organic matrix constitutes specifically the enamel sheath (arch shaped), which is a non-mineralized interface between prism substructures. In the inner enamel, a thin scalloped aprismatic enamel layer intermingles with the mantle dentin at the dentinoenamel junction.

Enamel is the most highly mineralized structure (96 %), but contains also some organic matrix (0.6 %) and two forms of water (bound or free) (total 3.4 % and including 1 % free water). This allows some ions and molecules diffusion throughout the enamel structure and also additional limited resilience.

M. Goldberg
University Paris Descartes, Sorbonne, Paris Cité
and INSERM UMR-S1124, 45 rue des Saints Pères,
Cedex 06, 75270 Paris, France
e-mail: mgoldod@gmail.com

M. Goldberg (ed.), *Understanding Dental Caries*, DOI 10.1007/978-3-319-30552-3_4

4.2 The Early Carious Enamel Lesion

Dental biofilm is a site of bacterial proliferation and growth. It is also a location for acid production and a reservoir for calcium exchange between the tooth and saliva. Saliva reduces the cariogenic effects of acidogenic bacteria and influences tooth demineralization. The saliva and dental plaque contribute to remineralization. Such equilibrium is crucial for limiting the development of carious lesions. In some cases, enamel cavitation at some specific points leads to the initial development of carious lesions.

The buccal and lingual pits and occlusal fossae contain debris and particles of food. The proximal caries and smooth surface lesions are well identified. In the gingival sulcus, different types of plaques are detected: remnants of the enamel organ and pycnotic epithelial cells and heavy organic cuticles. Therefore, the early phase of enamel caries involves the presence of microorganisms in the plaque and the invasion of the organic cuticle. The formation of open cavities comes later.

The early enamel carious lesion (or white spot) is characterized by 4 successive zones, which have been identified in the approximate smooth enamel surfaces (Figs. 4.1, 4.2, and 4.3):

1. The most superficial "unaltered" *surface zone* (*the surface enamel layer*) (#20 µm–50 µm). The lesion remains covered by a surface layer, which seems relatively unaffected by the carious attack. Dissolution/precipitation mechanisms and protection by adsorbed agents provide some explanations clarifying the basis of porosity or solubility gradients. The formation of enamel caries does not imply initially a subsurface formation. The thickness of the surface layer develops during the progress of the carious lesion. However, the thickness of the surface layer seems to be fairly constant. The mineral-rich layer develops later. Inhibitors such as F or proteins play important role in the surface layer formation. After the initially surface-softened enamel where dissolution takes place (inhibitor action), a subsurface region is created where dissolution occurs. The point of entry of the "cariogenic agent" through the surface layer was found to be related to several Retzius striae. The surface zone has a pore volume of less that 5 %.

   In the surface zone of artificial carious lesions, tiny microchannels about 0.5–1.5 µm in diameter and roughly 100 µm in length have been observed (Goldberg et al. 1981). This suggests that these channels are involved in the lesion development, playing role in the diffusion processes. The microchannels originate in prisms in the perikymata of the surface enamel. They extend in the direction of Hunter-Schreger bands, mainly in connection with diazones. In conclusion, the initial

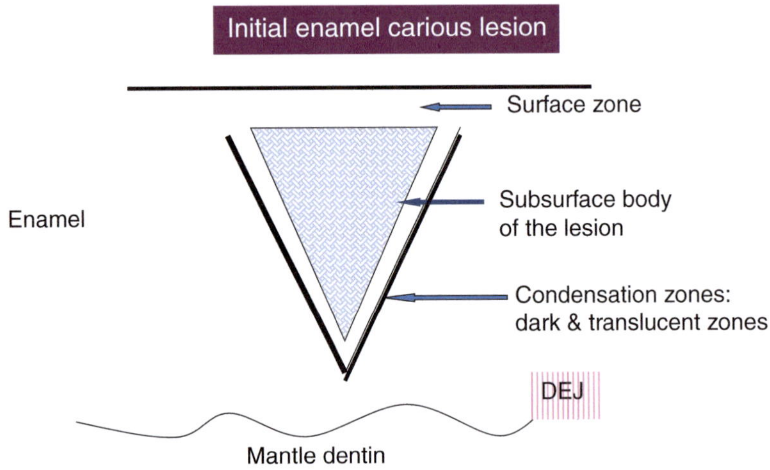

Fig. 4.1 Schematic drawing of the initial carious lesion including a surface zone, the subsurface lesion (or body of the lesion), the condensation zones (dark zone and translucent zone), and the normal enamel above the mantle dentin

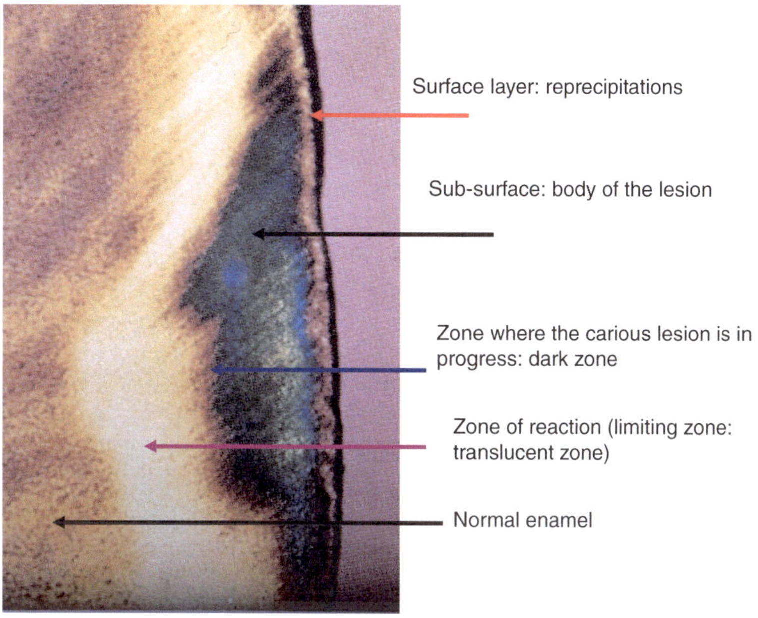

Fig. 4.2 Ground section of an initial carious enamel lesion. The surface layer is due to mineral re-precipitations. In the subsurface, the body of the lesion is triangular in shape, with a summit oriented toward the dentinoenamel junction. The lesion displays two borders: one dark zone that is in progress and a reaction zone (limiting or translucent zone)

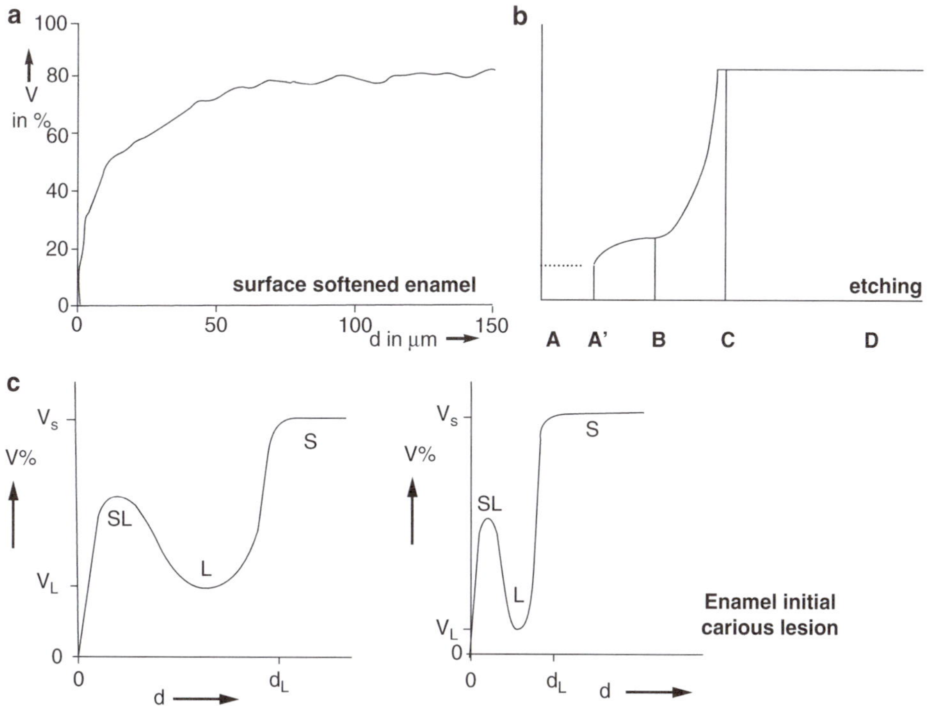

Fig. 4.3 Schematic percentage of mineral in volume: (**a**) in the softened enamel, (**b**) after acid etching, (**c**) in the initial carious lesion. *SL* surface layer, *L* body of the lesion, *S* normal enamel surface

artificial lesion formation is related to the organization and ultrastructure of enamel (Goldberg et al. 1981).

In a 40–50 mm-thick surface layer, an average of 9.9 % reduction in mineral content was found. In this zone, only the magnesium content was unchanged compared with adjacent surface zones.

2. The *subsurface* layer (or *body of the lesion*) (30 μm), which may appear either parallel to the surface or adopt a triangular shape, with a top oriented toward the dentinoenamel junction. The pore volume in the body of the lesion was approximately 10 %–25 % in the central part of the lesion and shows enhanced incremental lines. The Retzius striae are well marked. They demonstrate a pattern of cross-striations. Alternate radiolucent lines (slightly demineralized) and radio-opaque (more mineralized Retzius striae) were spaced 6–8 μm. For some authors, the demineralization process unmasked the Retzius striae. The lowest mineralization content was 29 % by volume. The lesion showed well-mineralized bands passing through the body of the lesion, giving a laminated appearance. Microchemical studies indicate a reduction of 24 % in mineral per unit volume compared with sound enamel. Magnesium was reduced by 20.1 %.
3. Two parallel inner zones: a *dark* zone seems to be hypomineralized. This is the second zone of alteration from normal enamel. Occurring in 85–90 % of the lesions, positive birefringence contrasts with the negative birefringence of the sound enamel. The pigmentation may be due to the arrest of microorganisms, which are present within the dissolved enamel parts. The dark zone contains a pore volume of 2–4 % of spaces and behaves as a molecular sieve. The mineral is reduced by 6 % per unit volume, with a loss of 12 % in magnesium.
4. The last identifiable zone is the *translucent* zone, with hyper (remineralized) mineralized layers and an increased crystalline volume. The translucent zone is not always present along the whole advancing front of the lesion. The width of the translucent zone was found to vary from 5–100 μm, with an average of 40 μm. It contains approximately 1 % of spaces, whereas the sound enamel contains about 0.1 % of spaces. These enlarged spaces are probably located at the periphery of prisms, where the orientation of crystallites changes abruptly. Microchemical studies reported that the fluoride content of the translucent zone is increased. There is an associated loss of magnesium, together with a lower carbonate content. The cone-shaped structure (triangular shaping into enamel) displays an apical part oriented toward the dentin.

See references (Silverstone and Poole 1969; Moreno and Zahradnik 1974; Goldberg et al. 1981; Thylstrup and Fejerskov 1986; Arends and Christoffersen 1986; Kidd and Fejerskov 2004).

This configuration is also detectable in artificial carious lesion, established on abraded labial surfaces of calf teeth, either on windows subjected to mild acid treatments or exposed to acid vapors. However, morphological, chemical composition, and physical property differences must be took into account in the interpretation of the results obtained with bovine teeth substrate when compared with human (Yassen et al. 2011).

The earliest visible change is a loss of transparency, enamel becoming opaque and chalky. Enamel caries may progress slowly (white spots) or become arrested (inactive lesions). In such case the carious lesion becomes brown or yellow. This is related to the presence of wide dark zones in arrested or inactive carious lesion, where it appears as a brown spot. This phenomenon may be controlled by spontaneous remineralization due to saliva and/or toothpastes.

4.3 Occlusal and Proximal Caries

Initial enamel caries may also develop in fissures or in deep occlusal invaginations. In occlusal fissures, a morphological classification has been reported (Newbrun 1983).

1. V type, wide at the top and gradually narrowing toward the bottom of the fissure. In occlusal fissures, 34 % of such lesions are concerned.
2. U type displays a constant width in the top and bottom of the fissure (14 %).
3. I type appears as a narrow space between cusps (19 %).
4. IK type, with a narrow space associated with a larger space in the bottom (26 %).
5. Other types (7 %).

Food debris and dental plaque accumulate in fissures and produce acid fermentable carbohydrates, which give rise to initial hard tissue dissolution and consequently to carious lesions. The carious lesion starts often at both sides of the fissure wall rather than at the base. The cone-shaped lesion penetrates nearly perpendicularly toward the dentinoenamel junction. These lesions precede cavitation and occur without apparent break in the enamel surface.

4.4 Microscopic Changes of Enamel (Figs. 4.4, 4.5, 4.6, and 4.7)

Enamel is destroyed by acid, probably lactic acid formed by *B. acidophilus*, and by the proteolytic action of bacteria (streptococci) upon a portion of the protein content. The proteolytic bacteria destroy the content of enamel rods more quickly than the enclosing enamel-rod sheath. Hence, the two structures may have different chemical contents.

After an initial loss of mineral, seen only at the surface layer, active enamel lesions involve surface erosion and subsurface porosity. Arrested or inactive enamel lesions are related to the surface zone, which acts as a diffusion barrier. A predominant calcium loss was seen in the subsurface along the Retzius striae. Lactic acid buffers plus diphosphonate may induce artificial caries-like lesions, which contribute to clarify the carious physiopathological process.

Enamel destruction consists (1) in enlarged prism junctions, (2) diffuse mineral destruction in the prism cores, and (3) destruction of the interprismatic substance (Frank 1990).

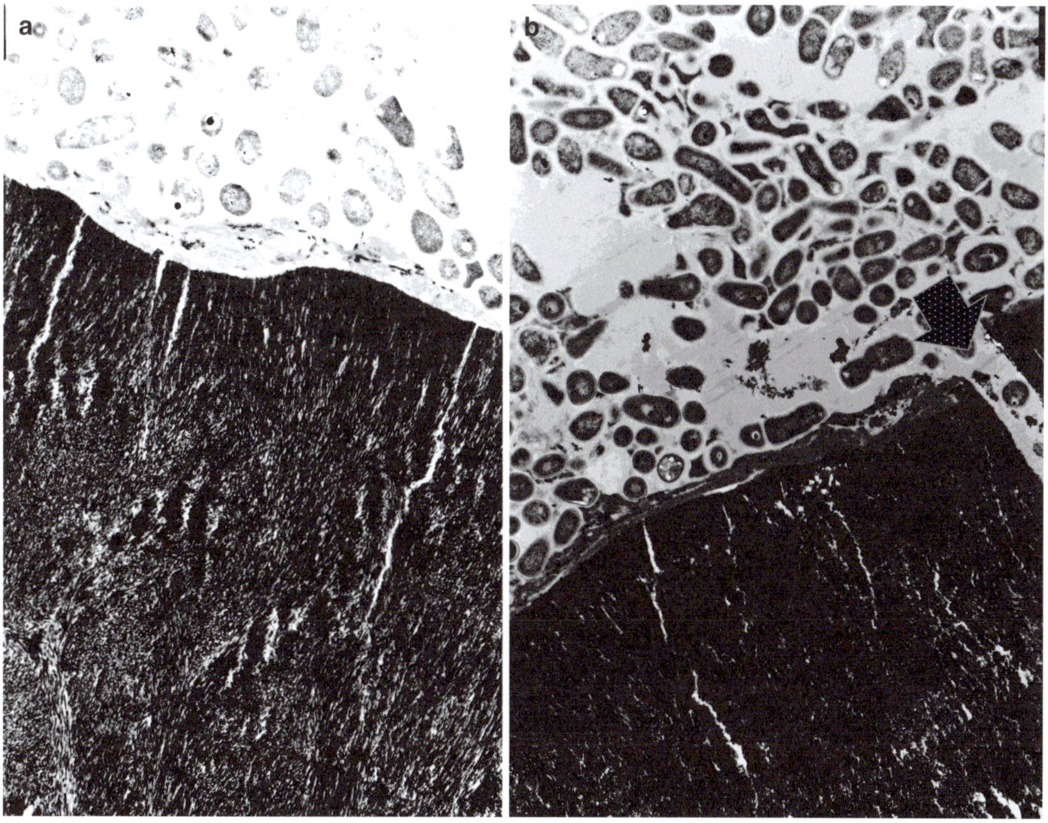

Fig. 4.4 (**a**) Bacteria and dental plaque above the surface of human enamel. (**b**) Dental plaque and on the right (*arrow*) a tubular structure connecting the surface and subsurface

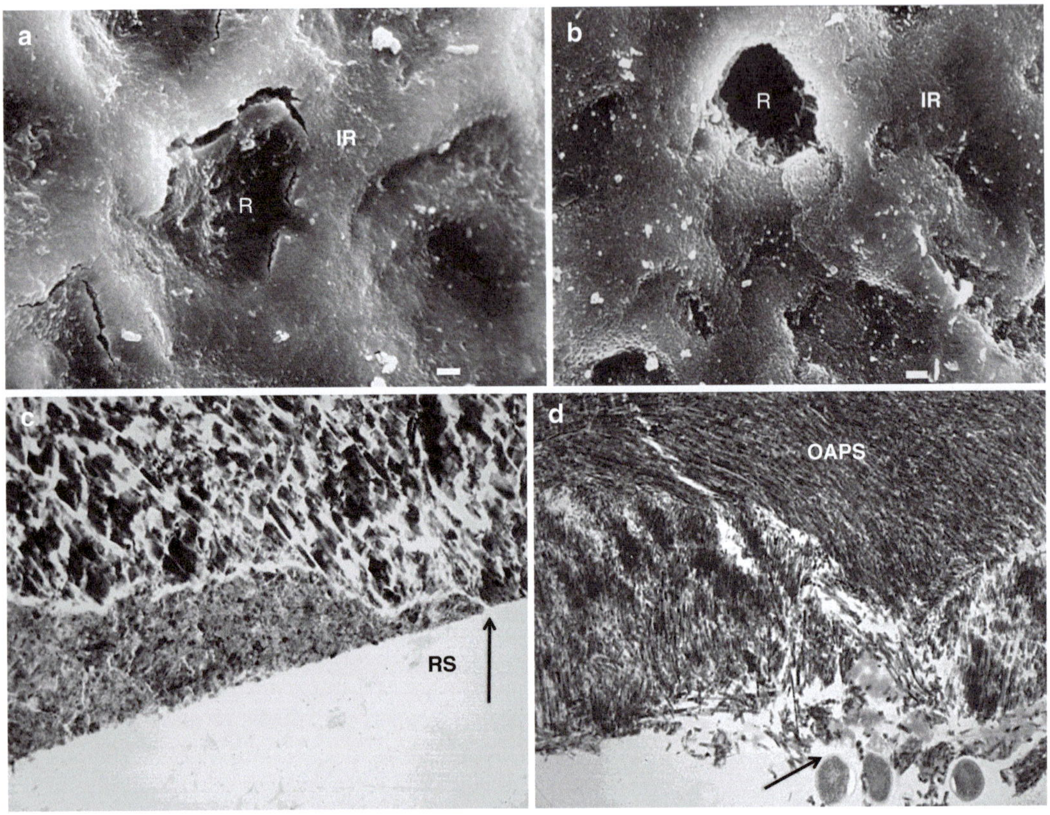

Fig. 4.5 (**a**) Enamel surface without specific treatment. *R* rod, *IR* interrod enamel. (**b**) The extracellular matrix associated to the apical end of ameloblast was removed by chemical treatment (chloroform/methanol or acid-induced cariogenic attack). *R* rod, *IR* interrod. (**c**) *RS* Retzius striae, indicated by the connection between two segments of the surface enamel (*arrow*). (**d**) At the junction, the Retzius striae located between two segments of the outer aprismatic enamel surface (OAPS) display the early formation of a carious invagination beneath the dental plaque and bacteria (*arrow*)

Diffusion of organic and phosphoric acids is higher in the surface zone than in the inner enamel. Enamel demineralization is under the control of acid conditions produced by the metabolism of cariogenic microorganisms. In the translucent zone, mineral is characterized by a 1.2 % loss. The dark zone shows positive birefringence. Spaces or pores display a 6 % average reduction per unit volume. In the body of the lesion, positive birefringence is seen, with enhanced Retzius striae. The prism structure shows a pattern of cross-striations (each 4 μm). There is a reduction of 24 % in mineral per unit volume.

The presence of a relatively sound surface layer (20 to 100 μm thick) is overlying the demineralized zone. Focal holes are seen with the SEM and reveal partial demineralization (about 8 % loss by volume). They may be at the origin of bacteria penetration within enamel. Accumulation of cell membrane debris taking origin from the residual Tomes' processes, water, and lipids altogether may constitute good substrates for the bacteria trapped into the dental plaque.

The kinetic of carious events is the following: following the Retzius striae, the prism sheaths, and the cross-striations of the rods, demineralization occurs before the prism core attack (Table 4.1).

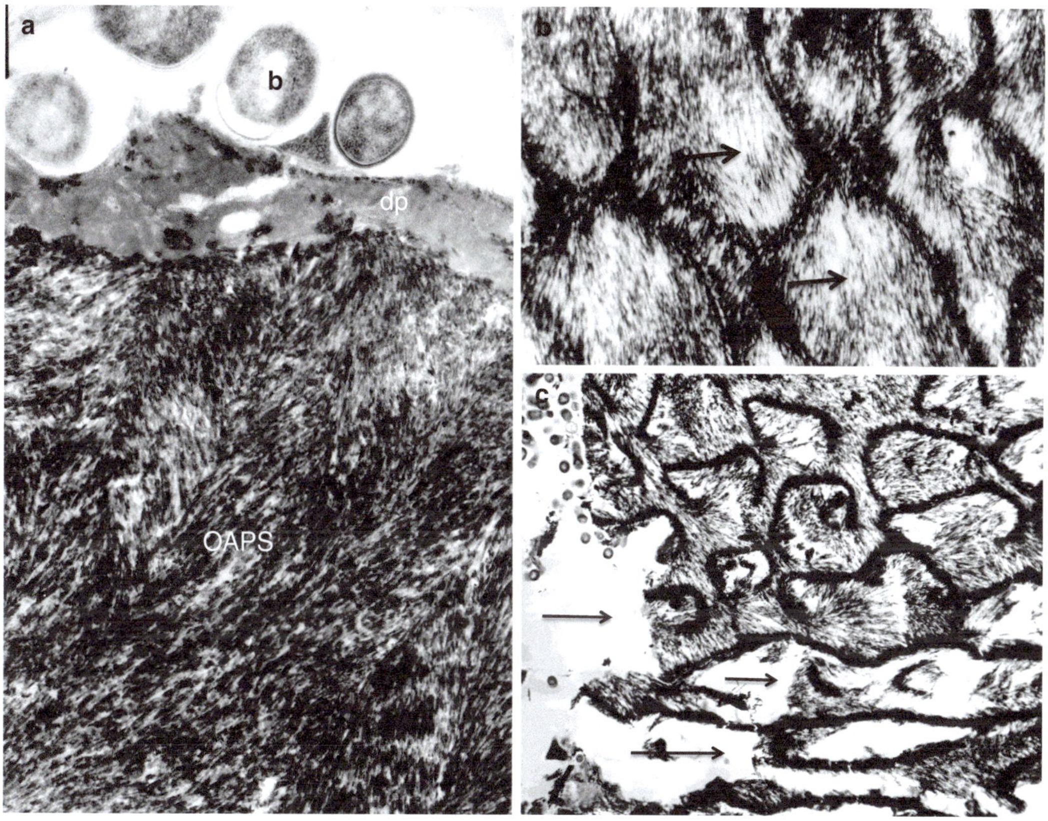

Fig. 4.6 (**a**) Outer aprismatic surface (*OAPS*) of human enamel beneath the dental plaque (*dp*) and bacteria (*b*) present in the oral cavity. (**b**) During the early stage of the carious decay, demineralization occurs inside rods (*arrows*). (**c**) Degradation of the prismatic enamel is concomitant with the formation of tubules where rods are demineralized and empty (*arrows*)

4.5 Ultrastructural Changes in Enamel

After the broadening of intercrystalline spaces, the area is filled with amorphous material, positively stained for carbohydrates.

According to Moreno and Zahradnik (1979), the first mineral lost in enamel demineralization is present in interprismatic regions. Individual crystals are subjected to partial dissolution, leading to enlargement of intercrystalline spaces. The progression of the lesion occurs through the cross-striations into enamel prisms and continues along enamel cores. By high-resolution electron microscopy (HREM), the dissolution phenomenon was identified as an initial disappearance of the lattice fringes and the formation of a central perforation in crystallites. Also the disappearance of lattice fringes in the lateral portion of the crystallites was seen to occur mostly in the subsurface prismatic region. Hence, the susceptibility of enamel to caries is spatially and temporally different during the progression of the carious lesion. Intracrystalline diffusion of acids contributes to induce rapid crystallite dissolution (Hayashi 1995). Eanes (1979) has reported that enamel apatite is imperfect, low in calcium and hydroxide ions, but rich in substitutional impurities. Ions such as F-, Cl-, Si-, and Zn2+ are found in high concentration near the surface, whereas CO $^{2-}{}_{3}$, Na+, and Mg2+ increase in the deeper parts of enamel.

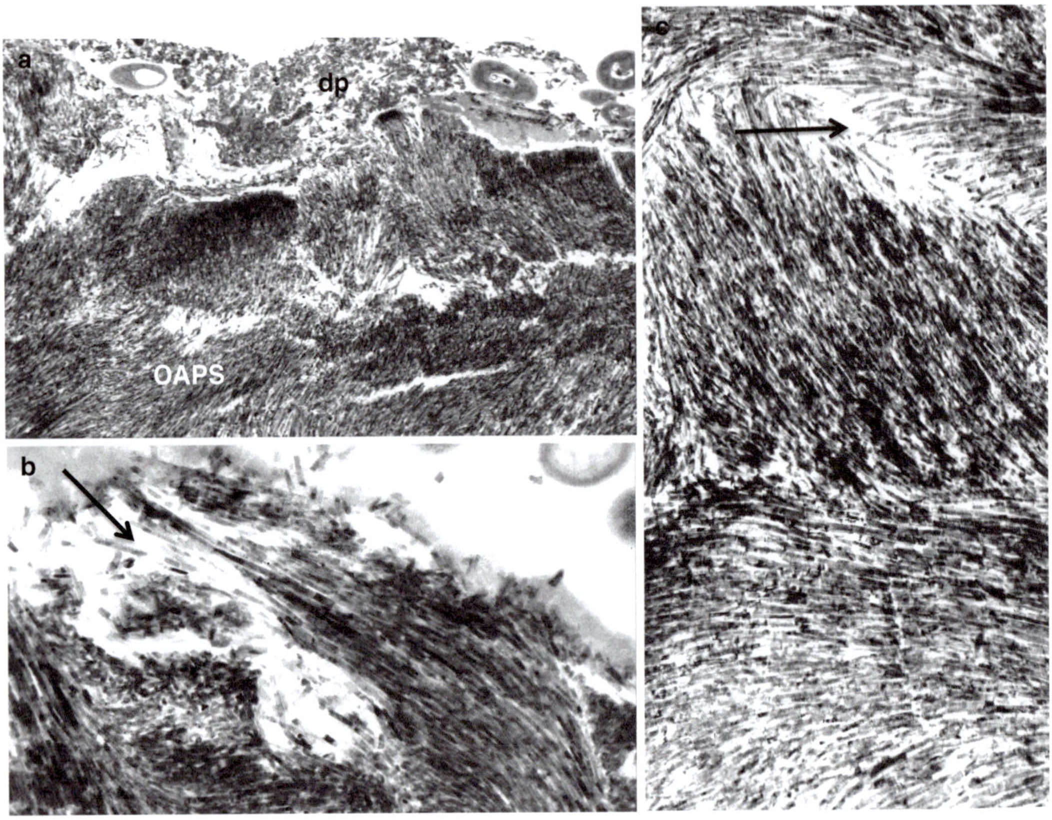

Fig. 4.7 (**a**) The dental plaque (*dp*) and bacteria cover the outer aprismatic surface (*OAPS*) enamel layer. The enamel profile is irregular and corroded, and the carious enamel lesion is initiated. (**b**) A tubule-like (*arrow*) cavity indicates the early stage of development of the carious lesion. (**c**) In addition, defective mineralization areas are seen inside rods (*arrow*)

Table 4.1 Summary of the mineral loss during the carious attack of an enamel surface (Newbrun 1983)

Zone	Birefringence	X-ray	Mineral loss
			In %
Translucent	–	Opaque	1.2
Dark	+	Opaque	6
Body of the lesion	+	Lucent	24
Surface layer	–	Opaque	10

Others such as K are evenly distributed. Thin perikymata exhibit dissolution, and empty Tomes' process pits and focal holes are enlarged. They may be at the origin of tubules crossing the surface zone and reaching the subsurface body of the lesion. The zones of reaction (dark and translucent zones) limit the diffusion of mineral in and out the initial lesion.

When the tubules reach the dentinoenamel junction (DEJ), the dental plaque spreads laterally along the DEJ. This is a carbohydrate-rich border, containing a higher percentage of proteoglycans and glycosaminoglycans (Goldberg et al. 2002) (Figs. 4.8, 4.9, 4.10, and 4.11).

Remineralization potential of saliva seems to be the property of saliva which counteracts demineralization produced by natural caries-like lesions or enamel pretreated with acid solution to produce "softened" enamel.

Alternatively, either the prism sheaths or the interprismatic substance is destroyed before the prisms themselves. Or there is also a possibility that the prisms are more susceptible to dissolution.

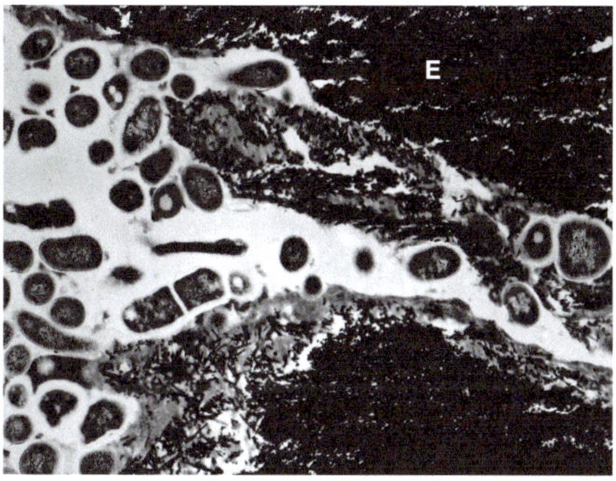

Fig. 4.8 Tubule-like structures cross the surface zone. Bacteria and plaque-like adhesive material are deposited along the tubule walls and contribute to the diffusion of the carious decay through enamel (*E*)

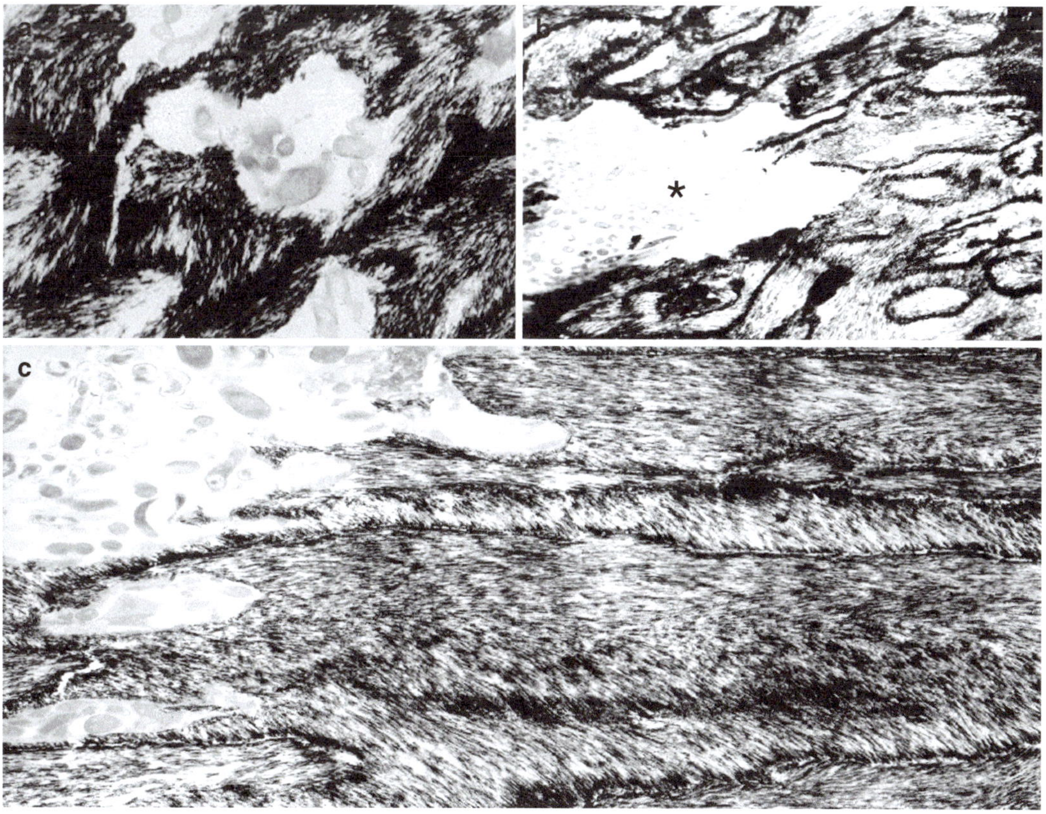

Fig. 4.9 Early enamel lesion formation. In (**a**), rods are partially demineralized and destroyed. In (**b**), rods and inter-rods melt and contribute to the initial cavity (*asterisk*). (**c**) Profile of the early formation of a carious cavity

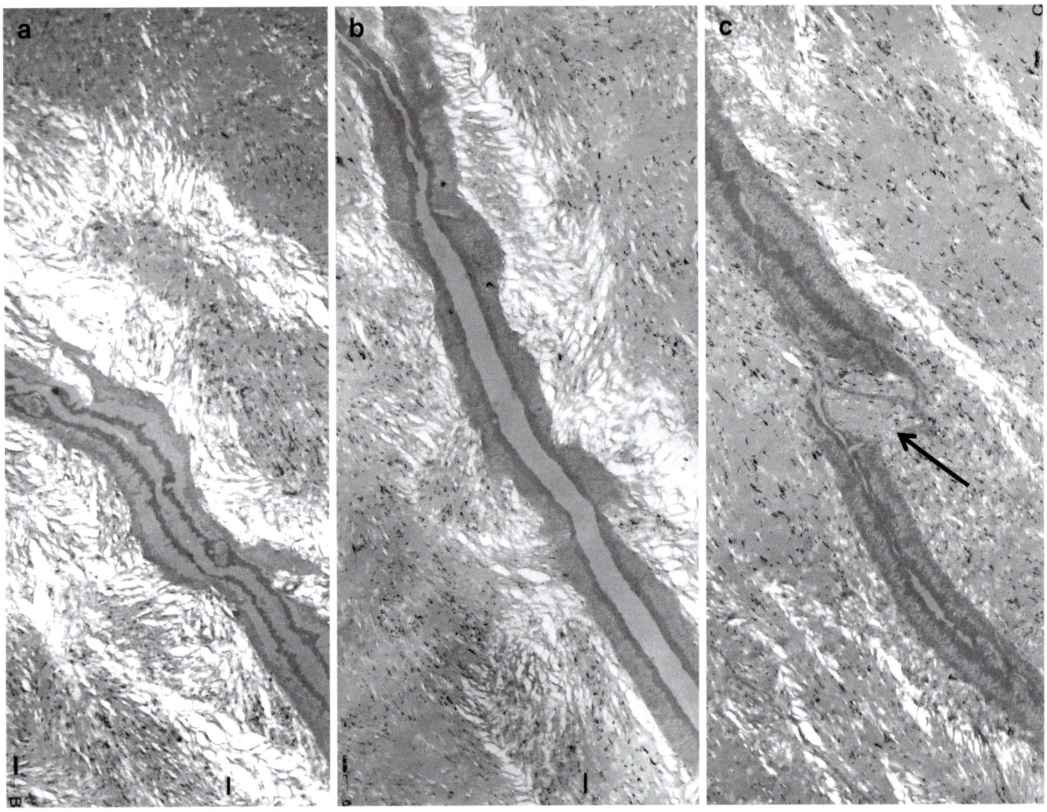

Fig. 4.10 (**a**–**c**) Tubule-like structure crossing the surface zone and contributing to mineral exchanges between the oral cavity and the subsurface body of the carious lesion. In (**c**), the tubule crosses Retzius striae (*arrow*)

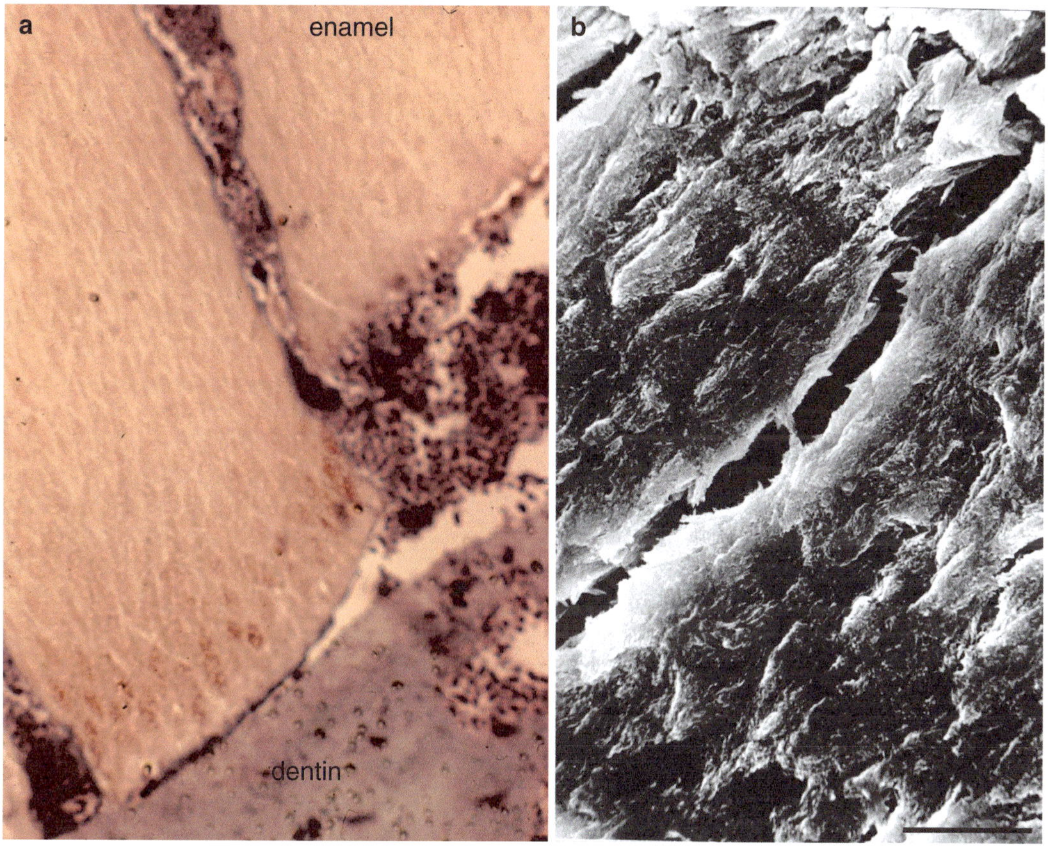

Fig. 4.11 (**a**) The tubule filled with bacteria crosses the whole thickness of enamel. The amelodentinal junction is enlarged and contributes to the diffusion of the carious decay toward the dentin surface. (**b**) Scanning electron microscopy of the enamel carious tubule shown in Fig. 4.10

References

Arends J, Christoffersen J. The nature of early caries lesions in enamel. J Dent Res. 1986;65:2–11.

Eanes ED. Enamel apatite: chemistry, structure and properties. J Dent Res. 1979;58:829–34.

Frank RM. Structural events in the caries process in enamel, cementum, and dentin. J Dent Res. 1990;69 (Spec Iss):559–66.

Goldberg M, Arends J, Septier D, Jongebloed WL. Microchannels in the surface zone of artificially produced caries-like enamel lesions. J Biol Buccale. 1981;9:297–314.

Goldberg M, Septier D, Bourd K, Hall R, Jeanny J-C, Jonet L, Colin S, Tager F, Chaussain-Miller C, Garabédian M, George A, Goldberg H, Menashi S. The dentino-enamel revisited. Connect Tissue Res. 2002;43:482–9.

Hayashi Y. High resolution electron microscopy of enamel crystallites demineralized by initial dental caries. Scanning Microsc. 1995;9:199–205.

Kidd EA, Fejerskov O. What constitutes dental caries? Histopathology of carious enamel and dentin related to the action of cariogenic biofilms. J Dent Res. 2004;83 Spec N°C:C35–8.

Moreno EC, Zahradnik RT. Chemistry of enamel subsurface demineralization in vitro. J Dent Res. 1974;53:226–35.

Moreno EC, Zahradnik RT. Demineralization and remineralization of dental enamel. J Dent Res. 1979;58(B):896–902.

Newbrun E. Cariology. Baltimore/London: Williams & Wilkins; 1983. p. 232–45.

Silverstone LM, Poole DFG. Histologic and ultrastructural features of remineralized carious enamel. J Dent Res. 1969;48:766–70.

Thylstrup A, Fejerskov O. Textbook of cariology. Copenhagen: Munsksgaard; 1986. p. 204–34.

Yassen GH, Platt JA, Hara AT. Bovine teeth as substitute for human teeth in dental research: a review of literature. J Oral Sci. 2011;53:273–82.

Dental Biofilms in Health and Disease

5

P.D. Marsh

Abstract

The mouth is colonised by a diverse range of microorganisms (the oral microbiota) that exist as biofilms on dental and mucosal surfaces. This microbiota is natural, enjoys a synergistic relationship with their host and confers benefits that are important to the well-being of that individual. On occasions, however, this synergistic relationship breaks down, and disease can occur (dysbiosis). In people who regularly consume fermentable carbohydrates, their dental biofilms spend longer periods at a low pH, and this selects for bacteria with a phenotype that is adapted for growth under these conditions, such as mutans streptococci, bifidobacteria and lactobacilli. Numerous clinical studies of people of various ages and in different countries have found increased proportions of these acidogenic and acid-tolerating bacteria in biofilms overlaying caries lesions compared to sound enamel. However, this relationship is not absolute, and other bacteria can be implicated. An 'Ecological Plaque Hypothesis' has been proposed to explain the relationship between the microbiota and the host in health and disease. A key feature of this hypothesis is that caries can be prevented not just by targeting the causative bacteria but also by interfering with the factors that cause the dysbiosis.

5.1 Introduction

Humans are made up of approximately 10^{14} cells, of which only 10 % are mammalian. The majority are the microorganisms that comprise the human microbiota and which are found naturally on all environmentally exposed surfaces of the body. The host and its microbiota have co-evolved to have a symbiotic or mutualistic relationship (Chow et al., 2010). The resident microorganisms

P.D. Marsh
Department of Oral Biology, School of Dentistry, University of Leeds, St James's University Hospital, Leeds, UK
e-mail: p.d.marsh@leeds.ac.uk

M. Goldberg (ed.), *Understanding Dental Caries*, DOI 10.1007/978-3-319-30552-3_5

gain a secure, warm, nutritious habitat from the host and, in return, deliver essential functions for the normal development of the host. For example, the resident microbiota plays a role in nutrition and metabolism, in differentiation of the host mucosa, in immune development and function and in preventing colonisation by exogenous and often pathogenic microbes (Relman 2012).

5.2 Resident Microbiota of the Mouth

The mouth is similar to other habitats in the body in having a natural resident microbiota with a characteristic composition. The infant is exposed from birth to a wide range of microorganisms, derived mainly from the mother, but only a subset are able to establish successfully in the mouth. The biological and physical properties of each habitat determine which microorganisms can colonise and grow, and dictate which will be major or minor components of the resident microbiota of a site. This results in different oral surfaces having distinct but characteristic microbiotas. These microbial communities are in a dynamic equilibrium with their environment, and this fact is of crucial importance to understanding the relationship between the host and the resident microbiota in health and disease. There can be significant reassortment and rearrangement of the composition and metabolic activity of these microbial consortia in response to changes in the biology of the mouth (e.g. eruption of teeth, flow of saliva, integrity of the host defences) and in the lifestyle of the individual (e.g. smoking, diet, medication) (Crielaard et al. 2011; Sampaio-Maia and Monteiro-Silva 2014).

The primary sources of nutrients for the resident oral microbiota are provided by the host, i.e. endogenous nutrients such as the proteins and glycoproteins in saliva. These complex host molecules have to be catabolised in a concerted and sequential manner by interacting bacterial consortia resulting in the establishment of numerous nutritional interdependencies (food webs) among the microorganisms (Wright et al. 2013). These co-dependencies make a major contribution to the stability of the oral microbiota at a site over time. The diet, in general, has little impact on the oral microbiota, except in the case of frequency of intake of fermentable sugars, which plays a fundamental role in perturbing this natural stability, and predisposes a site to caries (Sheiham and James 2015).

Traditionally, the oral microbiota has been characterised using sophisticated but laborious culture techniques, involving dispersal of the biofilms followed by serial dilution, plating and incubation on a range of selective and non-selective agar plates, usually under strictly anaerobic conditions. However, comparisons of the number of cells visualised by microscopy from a sample with the total viable counts demonstrated that, at best, only about 50–70 % of the oral microbiota could be cultured. Recent advances in technology have resulted in the development of culture-independent molecular approaches that have enabled the detection of far more taxa and a better description of the microbial richness of the oral microbiota. Just over 700 bacterial species have been isolated from the human oral cavity, with 49 % of these officially named, 17 % unnamed (but can be cultured) and 34 % as currently unculturable phylotypes.

The composition of the oral microbiota can remain stable over time (microbial homeostasis) (Marsh 1989). This is not due to any biological indifference among the members of the biofilm community; the relationship is not passive but highly dynamic. As mentioned earlier, biofilm composition will shift in response to changes in local environment and lifestyle. Such changes can perturb biofilm composition and activity and predispose a site to disease.

5.3 Benefits of the Oral Microbiota

As at other sites in the body, the microbiota of the mouth provides important benefits to the host. There is active communication between the resident oral microbiota and host cells ('cross-talk'). Some resident bacteria, especially streptococci, downregulate potentially damaging pro-inflammatory host responses to components of the normal oral microbiota, such as the Gram-negative commensals, while the host retains the ability to respond to genuine microbial insults (Devine et al. 2015).

The resident oral microbiota contributes to the host defences by preventing the establishment of the many exogenous microorganisms the host comes into contact with on a regular basis. This 'colonisation resistance' is because the natural oral microbiota is better adapted at attaching to oral surfaces, is more efficient at metabolising the available nutrients for growth and can produce inhibitory factors and create hostile environments that restrict colonisation by potential microbial invaders (Van der Waaij et al. 1971).

Resident oral bacteria also contribute to the general health of their host by regulating gastrointestinal and cardiovascular systems via the metabolism of dietary nitrate (Kapil et al. 2013). Approximately 25% of ingested nitrate is secreted in saliva, from where it is reduced to nitrite by oral bacteria. Nitrite regulates blood flow, blood pressure, gastric integrity and tissue protection against ischemic injury. Nitrite is converted to nitric oxide in the acidified stomach, and this has antimicrobial properties and contributes to defence against enteropathogens and in the regulation of gastric mucosal blood flow and mucus formation.

These findings confirm the importance of the natural resident oral microbiota for both oral and general health, which has implications for treatment strategies by oral care professionals.

5.4 Dental Biofilms

The oral microbiota grows on surfaces in the mouth as structurally and functionally organised communities of interacting species, termed biofilms (Zijnge et al. 2010). Microorganisms display an altered phenotype when growing on a surface as a biofilm. The properties of these biofilm communities are more than the sum of the component organisms. A clinically relevant feature of biofilms is that they display an enhanced tolerance to antimicrobial agents.

The composition of these biofilms differs at distinct surfaces on teeth due to variations in the prevailing conditions. Bacteria found in occlusal fissures are mainly Gram-positive and facultatively anaerobic (especially streptococci) and metabolise host and dietary sugars; the site is heavily influenced by the properties of saliva. In contrast, the biofilms from the healthy gingival crevice contain many Gram-negative and obligately anaerobic species that have a proteolytic style of metabolism, and the community is influenced more by gingival crevicular fluid, GCF (Marsh and Martin 2009). The composition of the microbiota of approximal surfaces lies in between that seen in fissures and the gingival crevice. There are large numbers of streptococci and obligately anaerobic bacteria, but *Actinomyces* are one of the most prevalent groups of organisms. This site distribution is further evidence that the composition and metabolism of the oral microbiota at a site are sensitive to, and responsive to, the oral environment and that there is a dynamic relationship between them both.

5.5 Dental Plaque Formation

The development of dental plaque can be subdivided into several stages. As a bacterium approaches the tooth surface, a number of specific and non-specific interactions occur between the substratum and the cell, and these determine whether successful attachment and colonisation will take place.

1. *Acquired pellicle formation.* As soon as a tooth is cleaned, molecules from the environment, especially salivary proteins and glycoproteins, are adsorbed onto the enamel surface, forming a conditioning film, termed the acquired enamel pellicle (Hannig and Joiner 2006; Lindh et al. 2014). The major constituents of this pellicle are salivary glycoproteins, phosphoproteins and lipids, and include statherin, proline-rich peptides (PRPs) and host defence components. Several enzymes of host and bacterial origin are located in an active form in the pellicle,

including amylase, lysozyme, carbonic anhydrases, fructosyltransferases (FTFs) and glucosyltransferases (GTFs) (Hannig et al. 2005). Bacterial glucans have also been detected in pellicle.

2. *Reversible attachment.* The earliest colonising bacteria interact with the molecules in this conditioning film, so that in this way, pellicle plays a critical role in biofilm formation. Long-range but relatively weak physicochemical forces between the charged molecules on the bacterial surface and the charge in the molecules in the pellicle can hold a cell reversibly near the tooth surface (Busscher et al. 2008).
3. *Permanent attachment.* These weak physicochemical interactions become stronger if molecules on the microbial cell surface (adhesins) engage in specific, short-range interactions with complementary receptors in the acquired pellicle (Nobbs et al. 2009, 2011). These interactions are strong and make the attachment more permanent. The initial colonisers are mainly streptococci, especially members of the mitis group of streptococci (e.g. *S. sanguinis*, *S. oralis* and *S. mitis*); *Actinomyces* species are also commonly isolated, as are haemophili and *Neisseria*.

   The surfaces of bacteria are richly decorated with these adhesins, some of which are proteins while others are lectins. Examples include antigen I/II on mutans streptococci that binds to glucan, collagen or immunoglobulins in pellicle, etc., while adhesins on *S. gordonii* bind to α-amylase, and those on *A. naeslundii* and *F. nucleatum* interact with statherin. Some adhesins are located on bacterial surface appendages, such as pili (Nobbs et al. 2009, 2011).
4. *Microbial succession.* Once attached, these pioneer populations start to divide and form a confluent layer. Over time, the plaque microbiota becomes more diverse; there is a shift away from the initial preponderance of streptococci to a biofilm with increasing proportions of *Actinomyces* and other Gram-positive bacilli. Some organisms that were unable to colonise the pellicle-coated tooth surfaces are able to attach to already-adherent pioneer species by further adhesin–receptor interactions (coaggregation/co-adhesion) (Kolenbrander et al. 2006). In addition, the metabolism of the pioneer community alters the local environment and makes conditions more suited to the growth of some fastidious bacteria. For example, early bacterial colonisers utilise oxygen and make conditions more suitable for the growth of obligately anaerobic bacteria. Similarly, the metabolism of pioneer species produces end products of metabolism (e.g. peptides) and fermentation products (lactate, butyrate, acetate) that can be used by other organisms as primary nutrient sources (i.e. in this way, food chains develop) (Wright et al. 2013). Thus, the composition of the plaque microbiota changes over time due to a series of complex interactions and becomes more diverse; the process is termed microbial succession.
5. *Maturation of the biofilm and matrix formation.* The microbial diversity of plaque biofilms increases over time due to further phases of microbial succession and growth. A key feature of the maturation of dental plaque is the synthesis of an extracellular matrix of polymers, which includes soluble and insoluble glucans, fructans, proteins and extracellular DNA (eDNA) (Jakubovics et al. 2013). The glucans and fructans are synthesised by glucosyltransferases and fructosyltransferases, respectively (Fig. 5.1). Fructans are short-lived in plaque and act as extracellular nutrient storage compounds for use by other plaque bacteria, while many glucans are insoluble and provide structural integrity to the biofilm. Extracellular DNA can be released from cells as a result of lysis, but in some situations, it can also be actively secreted. eDNA also contributes to the structural integrity of the biofilm as well as being involved in conventional gene transfer (Jakubovics et al. 2013; Okshevsky and Meyer 2015).

   A matrix is a common feature of all biofilms and is biologically active, retaining water, nutrients and enzymes within the biofilm (Flemming and Wingender 2011; Koo et al. 2013). The chemistry of the matrix can also help exclude or restrict the penetration of

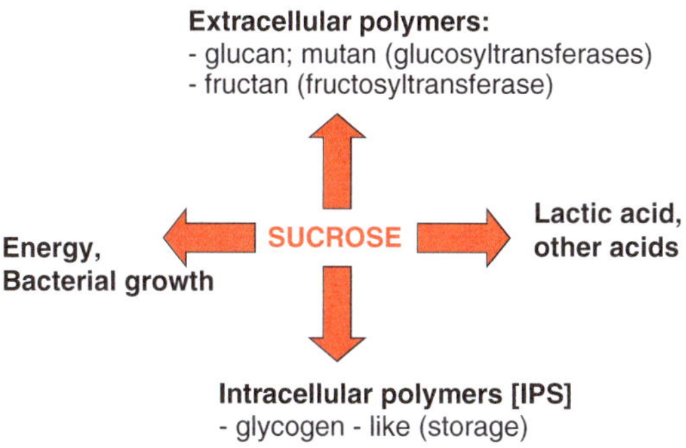

Fig. 5.1 Metabolic fate of sucrose. Sucrose can be metabolised to acids; energy is also generated during glycolysis which is needed for bacterial growth. Sucrose can also be converted to intracellular polymers (which can be catabolised to acid in the absence of dietary sugars) or extracellular polysaccharides (which contribute to the plaque matrix)

other types of molecules, especially charged antimicrobial agents, while enabling some uncharged small molecules to penetrate deep into the biofilm. Gradients develop in factors that are critical to microbial growth, due to bacterial metabolism and diffusion restrictions, so that sites close together may be vastly different in the concentration of essential nutrients and toxic products of metabolism, as well as in terms of pH and oxygen tension, etc. Such vertical and horizontal stratification creates local environmental heterogeneity resulting in a mosaic of microhabitats or microenvironments and explains how organisms with apparently contradictory growth requirements (e.g. in terms of nutritional, atmospheric or pH requirements) coexist in plaque at the same site.

Multispecies biofilms create opportunities for numerous interactions among the constitutive species that are physically close to one another (Fig. 5.2). These include examples of conventional antagonistic and synergistic biochemical interactions, as well as gene transfer via plasmids and cell–cell signalling mediated by small diffusible molecules that enable similar bacteria to communicate with each other and coordinate their activities. Gram-positive bacteria communicate using small peptides, while both Gram-positive and Gram-negative species can use different molecules, such as autoinducer-2 (Jakubovics et al. 2014; Wright et al. 2013).

As plaque matures, the microbiota becomes more diverse. A small sample of plaque may contain up to 100 distinct species, but the bacterial composition will vary at distinct anatomical sites due to differences in the prevailing biological conditions on each surface.

6. *Detachment from surfaces.* Bacteria may be able to 'sense' adverse changes in environmental conditions, and these may act as cues to induce the genes involved in active detachment.

5.6 Microbiology of Caries

Despite dental biofilms being natural and contributing to the well-being of the host, on occasions, this symbiotic relationship can break down and disease occurs (dysbiosis) (Marsh et al. 2015b).

Fissures are the most caries-prone sites of the dentition. Early cross-sectional and longitudinal studies of fissures reported a strong relationship between increased proportions of mutans streptococci (mainly *Streptococcus mutans* and *S. sobrinus*) in the biofilm and the detection of a caries lesion (Loesche 1986). However, this relationship was not absolute, and there were lesions from which these organisms could not be detected in the overlying biofilm and cases of mutans streptococci persisting in the absence of a lesion.

Similarly, early cross-sectional studies of approximal surfaces found a positive correlation between elevated mutans streptococci levels and lesion development, although a less clear-cut association was found in some longitudinal studies (Marsh and Martin 2009; Marsh et al. 2015b). Again, at some sites, mutans streptococci could be found in high numbers before the radiographic detection of demineralisation, while some lesions developed in the apparent absence of these bacteria. Mutans streptococci could also be present at some sites for prolonged periods in high numbers without any evidence of caries.

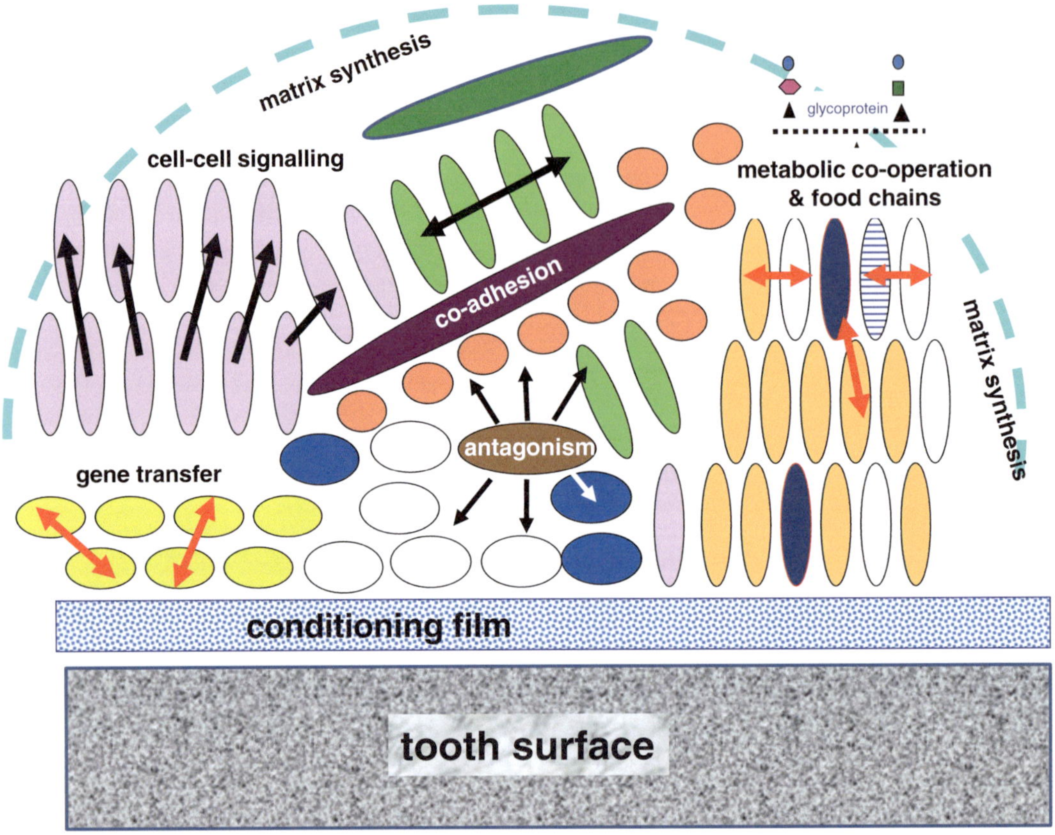

Fig. 5.2 A schematic representation of the interactions within a microbial biofilm such as dental plaque. The primary bacterial colonisers attach to the conditioning film (acquired pellicle) on the tooth surface by adhesin–receptor interactions; later, colonisers attach to the primary colonising bacteria (co-adhesion). As the biofilm develops, numerous interactions can occur among the component species. Synergistic interactions involve metabolic co-operation to catabolise endogenous nutrients (e.g. salivary glycoproteins), the development of food chains, cell–cell signalling, gene transfer and synthesis of an extracellular matrix. Antagonism can occur, for example, by the production of inhibitory molecules, which enable some species to outcompete others

When appropriate culture media have been used, recent studies have found associations between other groups of bacteria and caries, especially bifidobacteria (Mantzourani et al. 2009a, b).

Contemporary studies of dental biofilms now use either culture-independent molecular approaches or a combination of culture and molecular techniques to analyse the microbiota. A recent study of severe early childhood caries of different tooth surfaces at various stages of caries formation using a combination of anaerobic culture and molecular-based techniques found that disease was associated with a diverse microbiota, including some previously uncultivated species. The species most closely associated with this severe form of caries included *S. mutans*, *Scardovia wiggsiae*, *Veillonella parvula*, *Streptococcus cristatus* and *Actinomyces gerencseriae* (Tanner et al. 2011). Similar findings had been reported in a previous study of early childhood caries using culture-independent approaches but with the limitation that samples of dental biofilms had been pooled prior to analysis. *S. sanguinis* was associated with sound enamel, while *A. gerencseriae*, *Bifidobacterium* spp., *S. mutans*, *S. salivarius*, *S. constellatus*, *S. parasanguinis*, *L. fermentum* and *Veillonella* spp. were associated with caries (Becker et al. 2002). The data suggested that some *Actinomyces* spp. may be significant in caries initiation while *Bifidobacterium* spp. may play a role in more advanced lesions. Likewise, in a molecular-based study of pooled plaque of caries in primary and permanent teeth in children, a number of species in addition to *S. mutans* were shown to play a role in caries progression; these bacteria included members of the genera *Veillonella*, *Lactobacillus*, *Bifidobacterium*, *Propionibacterium*, *Actinomyces* and *Atopobium*, plus low-pH non-*S. mutans* streptococci (Aas et al. 2008).

Collectively, the data from numerous surveys of various tooth surfaces, of different patient age groups from numerous countries and populations with different dietary habits, etc., have shown a strong positive association between increased levels of mutans streptococci and the initiation of demineralisation. However, not every study identified all of the bacteria present in the clinical samples, and some focussed only on organisms already implicated in disease, e.g. mutans streptococci and lactobacilli.

While several bacterial species may contribute to demineralisation, a number of others may reduce the impact of acid production either by utilising the lactate produced from sugar metabolism (e.g. *Veillonella* spp.) or by producing alkali from saliva components (*S. salivarius*, *S. sanguinis*, *A. naeslundii*) (Marsh et al. 2015b). Thus, caries is a complex microbiological process as it is the outcome of a number of interactions between acid-producing and acid-utilising or acid-neutralising species in a structurally organised biofilm.

5.7 Cariogenic Features of Dental Biofilm Bacteria

In order for bacteria to play a role in caries, they must possess certain caries-promoting characteristics (Marsh et al. 2015b), which centre around the metabolism of fermentable dietary sugars, especially sucrose (Fig. 5.1), and include:

- The ability to rapidly transport fermentable sugars when competing with other plaque bacteria and the conversion of such sugars to acid and the generation of a low pH. Most saccharolytic bacteria in dental plaque, including mutans streptococci, possess several sugar transport systems, including high-affinity phosphoenolpyruvate: sugar phosphotransferase (PEP-PTS) systems, which are able to scavenge sugars even when they are present in the oral environment only in low concentrations. These sugars are converted to acids (and predominantly lactic acid) by glycolysis; caries-associated bacteria can generate a low pH (e.g. less than pH 5.0) in a few minutes.
- The ability to maintain sugar metabolism and remain viable under extreme environmental conditions, such as at a low pH. Many plaque bacteria can make acid from sugar metabolism, but far fewer are able to tolerate acidic conditions for prolonged periods. Mutans streptococci, lactobacilli and bifidobacteria not only remain viable at a low pH but manage to continue to grow and metabolise, i.e. they are both acidogenic and aciduric (acid tolerant). This ability relies on a series of biochemical properties: (i) the activity of proton-translocating ATPase (proton exclusion inside to outside of bacterial cells); (ii) alkali production, due to the activity of bacterial ureases, arginine deiminase and other alkali-producing systems; (iii) proton impermeability of bacterial cell membrane; and (iv) the production of stress proteins (protection of cellular structural and functional proteins from acid denaturation) (Takahashi and Yamada 1999).
- The production of extracellular (EPS) and intracellular polysaccharides (IPS). EPS include glucans and fructans, both of which contribute to the biofilm matrix. IPS are glycogen-like storage compounds that can be used for energy production and converted to acid when free sugars are not available in the mouth.

Mutans streptococci are known to have all these properties (Table 5.1) and are well equipped to act as cariogenic bacteria (Loesche 1986). However, these properties are not specific to mutans streptococci in the same way that the

Table 5.1 Cariogenic characteristics of some oral bacteria

Bacterium	Cariogenic property				
	Sugar transport (rate)	Acid production (rate)	Acid tolerance	Polymer production	
				Extracellular	Intracellular
Mutans streptococci[a]	Multiple systems (Very rapid)	<pH 4.0 (Very rapid)	High Grows at pH 5.5 and below	Soluble and insoluble polysaccharides (glucans and fructan)	Yes[b]
Lactobacilli[c]	Little known of systems (Rapid)	<pH 4.0 (Rapid)	Very high Growth at pH 5.0	Heteropolysaccharide Glucan	No
Actinomyces species[d]	Little known of systems (Medium)	pH 4.5–5.0 (Medium)	Medium	Heteropolysaccharide Fructan	Yes
Streptococcus sanguinis	Multiple systems (Medium)	pH 4.5–4.9 (Medium)	Poor	Soluble and insoluble polysaccharides	Yes

[a]*Streptococcus mutans* and *Streptococcus sobrinus*
[b]*Streptococcus sobrinus* does not make much intracellular polysaccharide
[c]Little is known about most *Lactobacillus* species
[d]Little is known about many *Actinomyces* species; most data are on *A. naeslundii*

possession of some virulence factors (e.g. cholera toxin for *Vibrio cholerae*, pertussis toxin for *Bordetella pertussis*) helps to define certain classical medical pathogens. Indeed, the acidogenic and aciduric profile of bacterial species lies along a continuum, with evidence of considerable overlap (Table 5.1). Some strains of non-mutans streptococcal species, e.g. *S. mitis*, *S. gordonii*, *S. anginosus* and *S. oralis*, can be as acidogenic and acid tolerating as some examples of mutans streptococci (de Soet et al. 2000; van Houte 1994; van Ruyven et al. 2000). Therefore, it is not surprising that there is a lack of total specificity in the microbial aetiology of dental caries.

5.8 Theories to Explain the Association of Dental Plaque Biofilms to Caries

The 'Specific Plaque Hypothesis' was proposed initially, in which disease was attributed to only a very small number of species out of the many present in the biofilm (Loesche 1976, 1979). This was a major advance in that it enabled attention to be focussed on a limited subset of bacteria in subsequent clinical studies. Mutans streptococci, primarily *S. mutans* and *S. sobrinus*, were present more often and in higher proportions from sites with caries, while lactobacilli were isolated commonly from advanced lesions. A consistent observation, however, was that caries could occur on occasions in the apparent absence of these bacteria while these organisms could persist at healthy sites. Over time, it became clear that other bacteria within these diverse biofilms could also generate a low pH from sugars, while others could ameliorate the potentially damaging effect of lactic acid by (a) utilising them as a nutrient source and converting them to weaker acids or (b) generating alkali from the metabolism of arginine or urea in saliva. This resulted in the 'non-specific plaque hypothesis' being proposed, in which disease is the outcome of the net biochemical activity of the biofilm, including both acid-producing and acid-utilising species; although generally applied to periodontal disease, it was also applicable to understanding the microbial aetiology of dental caries (Theilade 1986). However, if the microbial aetiology was not totally specific, it was also not totally random, and there was agreement on the phenotype of the bacteria involved (acid pro-

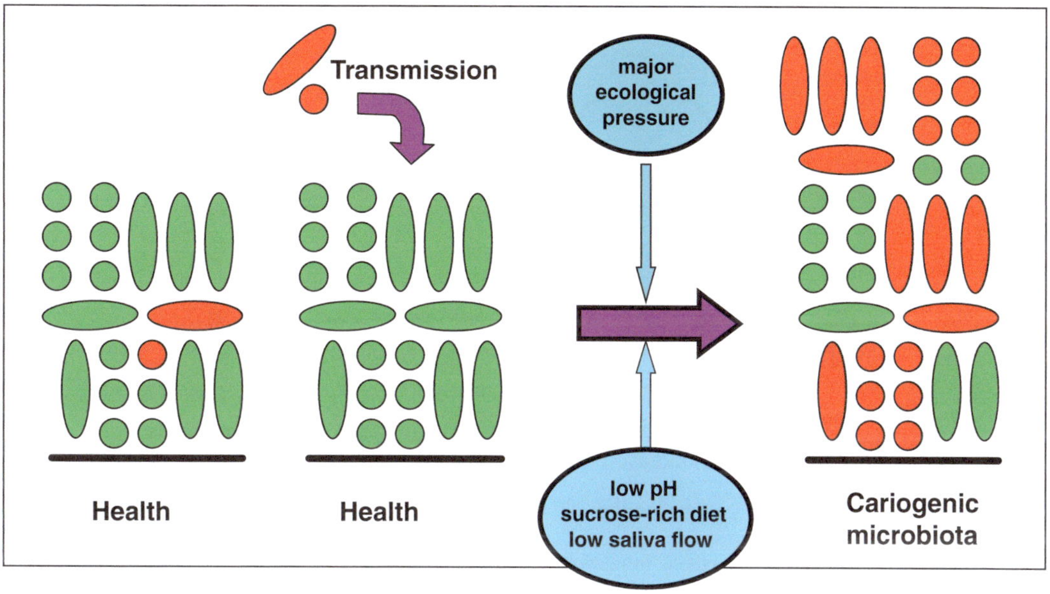

Fig. 5.3 Schematic representation of dysbiosis in dental caries. Teeth are colonised naturally by oral bacteria, and these form multispecies biofilms. The majority of these bacteria are beneficial to the physiology of the host (green cells). Biofilms taken from sites with caries have increased numbers of cariogenic bacteria (red cells). These cariogenic bacteria may be present in low numbers in health or transmitted between sites/subjects in low numbers; both situations will be compatible with dental health. In health, the cariogenic bacteria are uncompetitive with the beneficial species and remain in low proportions. A major change to the ecology of the mouth can alter this relationship. An increased exposure to fermentable sugars in the diet leads to regular conditions of low pH in the biofilm; these conditions will favour the growth of cariogenic bacteria at the expense of beneficial species. Similar events can occur if saliva flow is perturbed

ducing, acid tolerating) and on the critical role played by the host (e.g. in terms of diet and saliva flow).

In view of the findings summarised above, an alternative concept was proposed in order to accommodate the consistency of bacterial function in the absence of specificity in bacterial type and the essential requirement for a caries-conducive environment (e.g. sugar-rich diet and/or low saliva flow) to drive deleterious changes in the composition of the microbiota (Fig. 5.3). In the 'Ecological Plaque Hypothesis', micro-organisms that are implicated with caries can be present in biofilms on sound enamel, but at levels too low to be clinically relevant (Marsh 1994, 2003). Disease is a result of a deleterious shift in the balance of the resident microbiota driven by a change in local environmental conditions. Repeated conditions of low pH in plaque biofilms due to frequent sugar intake select for higher numbers of acid-tolerating bacteria while inhibiting the growth of beneficial organisms that preferentially grow at neutral pH (Fig. 5.4). Thus, the specificity in the aetiology resides in the similarity of the bacterial phenotype that is necessary for demineralisation. Implicit in this hypothesis is the concept that disease can be controlled not only by directly targeting the putative pathogens (e.g. inhibition of mutans streptococci by antimicrobial agents) but also by interfering with the factors that drive the deleterious shifts in the microbiota (e.g. lowering the acid challenge by reducing sugar intake frequency or by promoting snacks containing sugar substitutes).

This hypothesis has been further developed to recognise the ability of some bacteria to adapt to acid stress. The 'Extended Caries Ecological Hypothesis' divides the caries process into three reversible stages (Takahashi and Nyvad 2008). In early biofilms, when acid is produced mainly during main meals, the acids

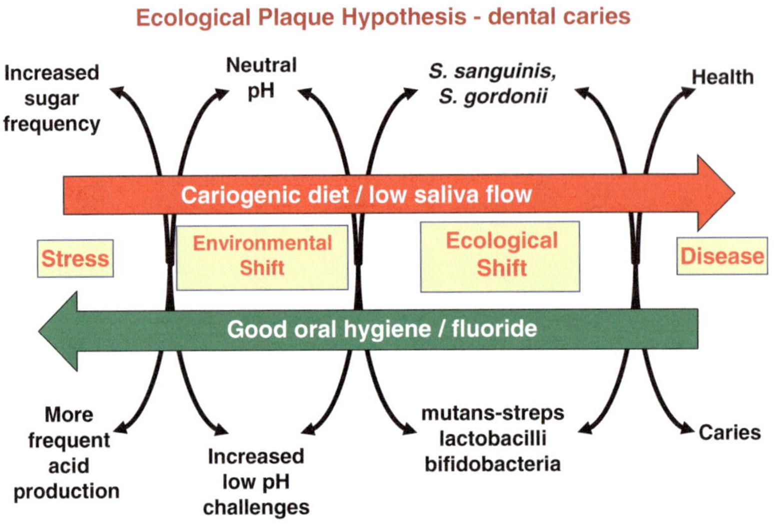

Fig. 5.4 The Ecological Plaque Hypothesis in relation to dental caries. Frequent exposure of dental plaque to fermentable sugars leads to regular and prolonged conditions of low pH within the biofilm. This environmental change favours the growth of acid-tolerating bacteria (such as mutans streptococci, lactobacilli and bifidobacteria) at the expense of the beneficial species associated with sound enamel and increases the risk of demineralisation. Caries is promoted in individuals who regularly consume fermentable carbohydrates and/or have an impaired saliva flow, while good oral hygiene and exposure to optimum levels of fluoride would reduce the risk of demineralisation. Disease could be prevented by not only targeting the cariogenic bacteria but also by interfering with the factors driving their selection

can be readily neutralised by saliva or by alkali production in the biofilm, and demineralisation and remineralisation are in equilibrium (the 'dynamic stability' stage). If sugar intake becomes more frequent, then the regular conditions of low pH encourage acid adaptation in some bacteria, which can result in increased acid production. Such conditions favour acidogenic and acid-tolerating strains of streptococci and *Actinomyces*, and the mineral equilibrium is shifted towards demineralisation (the 'acidogenic' stage). If these conditions persist, then the most efficient acidogenic and acid-tolerating bacteria are selected. This 'aciduric' stage further drives demineralisation and accelerates the progression of caries. As with the original Ecological Plaque Hypothesis, environmental acidification acts as the main driving force for enrichment of an acid-tolerating bacterial community (Marsh 2003; Takahashi and Nyvad 2008). Unless the factors that are driving the dysbiosis are identified and remedied, it is inevitable that the patient will suffer further episodes of disease.

5.9 Implications for Prevention and Control

It has been emphasised that the mouth is naturally colonised by diverse microbial communities that confer important benefits to the host. Caries is a consequence of perturbations to this symbiotic relationship, with persistent and regular acidification following sugar metabolism driving the selection of previously minor components of the biofilm. Therefore, oral care strategies should be focussed on maintaining the composition and activity of these biofilms at levels compatible with oral health rather than trying to eliminate them.

Effective plaque control will always be central to oral care practices, and the appropriate use of fluoride, but these approaches can be augmented by other practices. These include:

- The avoidance between main meals of snacks and drinks that contain fermentable sugars or the use of products that contain sugar substitutes.

- Stimulation of saliva flow, for example, by sugar-free gum.
- Inhibition of acid production. Many oral care products are formulated with agents that at high concentrations can kill oral bacteria, but which at lower concentrations (as occurs over time after brushing or mouthrinsing) are able to inhibit cariogenic traits such as sugar transport, acid production and extracellular polysaccharide production (Marsh et al. 2015a).

Such approaches will help to maintain the beneficial properties of the resident oral microbiota while restricting the opportunities for dysbiosis.

References

Aas JA, Griffen AL, Dardis SR, Lee AM, Olsen I, Dewhirst FE, Leys EJ, Paster BJ. Bacteria of dental caries in primary and permanent teeth in children and young adults. J Clin Microbiol. 2008;46:1407–17.

Becker MR, Paster BJ, Leys EJ, Moeschberger ML, Kenyon SG, Galvin JL, Boches SK, Dewhirst FE, Griffen AL. Molecular analysis of bacterial species associated with childhood caries. J Clin Microbiol. 2002;40:1001–9.

Busscher HJ, Norde W, van der Mei HC. Specific molecular recognition and nonspecific contributions to bacterial interaction forces. Appl Environ Microbiol. 2008;74:2559–64.

Chow J, Lee SM, Shen Y, Khosravi A, Mazmanian SK. Host-bacterial symbiosis in health and disease. Adv Immunol. 2010;107:243–74.

Crielaard W, Zaura E, Schuller AA, Huse SM, Montijn RC, Keijser BJ. Exploring the oral microbiota of children at various developmental stages of their dentition in the relation to their oral health. BMC Med Genomics. 2011;4:22.

de Soet JJ, Nyvad B, Kilian M. Strain-related acid production by oral streptococci. Caries Res. 2000;34:486–90.

Devine DA, Marsh PD, Meade J. Modulation of host responses by oral commensal bacteria. J Oral Microbiol. 2015;7:26941.

Flemming HC, Wingender J. The biofilm matrix. Nat Rev Microbiol. 2011;8:623–33.

Hannig M, Joiner A. The structure, function and properties of the acquired pellicle. Monogr Oral Sci. 2006;19:29–64.

Hannig C, Hannig M, Attin T. Enzymes in the acquired enamel pellicle. Eur J Oral Sci. 2005;113:2–13.

Jakubovics NS, Shields RC, Rajarajan N, Burgess JG. Life after death: the critical role of extracellular DNA in microbial biofilms. Lett Appl Microbiol. 2013;57:467–75.

Jakubovics NS, Yassin SA, Rickard AH. Community interactions of oral streptococci. Adv Appl Microbiol. 2014;87:43–110.

Kapil V, Haydar SM, Pearl V, Lundberg JO, Weitzberg E, Ahluwalia A. Physiological role for nitrate-reducing oral bacteria in blood pressure control. Free Radic Biol Med. 2013;55:93–100.

Kolenbrander PE, Palmer Jr RJ, Rickard AH, Jakubovics NS, Chalmers NI, Diaz PI. Bacterial interactions and successions during plaque development. Periodontol 2000. 2006;42:47–79.

Koo H, Falsetta ML, Klein MI. The exopolysaccharide matrix: a virulence determinant of cariogenic biofilm. J Dent Res. 2013;92:1065–73.

Lindh L, Aroonsang W, Sotres J, Arnebrant T. Salivary pellicles. Monogr Oral Sci. 2014;24:30–9.

Loesche WJ. Chemotherapy of dental plaque infections. Oral Sci Rev. 1976;9:63–107.

Loesche WJ. Clinical and microbiological aspects of chemotherapeutic agents used according to the specific plaque hypothesis. J Dent Res. 1979;58:2404–12.

Loesche WJ. Role of *streptococcus mutans* in human dental decay. Microbiol Rev. 1986;50:353–80.

Mantzourani M, Fenlon M, Beighton D. Association between bifidobacteriaceae and the clinical severity of root caries lesions. Oral Microbiol Immunol. 2009a; 24:32–7.

Mantzourani M, Gilbert SC, Sulong HN, Sheehy EC, Tank S, Fenlon M, Beighton D. The isolation of bifidobacteria from occlusal carious lesions in children and adults. Caries Res. 2009b;43:308–13.

Marsh PD. Host defenses and microbial homeostasis: role of microbial interactions. J Dent Res. 1989;68: 1567–75.

Marsh PD. Microbial ecology of dental plaque and its significance in health and disease. Adv Dent Res. 1994;8:263–71.

Marsh PD. Are dental diseases examples of ecological catastrophes? Microbiology. 2003;149:279–94.

Marsh PD, Martin MV. Oral microbiology. 5th ed. Edinburgh: Churchill Livingstone; 2009.

Marsh PD, Head DA, Devine DA. Ecological approaches to oral biofilms: control without killing. Caries Res. 2015a;49:46–54.

Marsh PD, Takahashi N, Nyvad B. Biofilms in caries development. In: Fejerskov O, Nyvad B, Kidd E, editors. Dental caries: the disease and its clinical management. Oxford: Wiley Blackwell; 2015b. p. 107–31.

Nobbs AH, Lamont RJ, Jenkinson HF. Streptococcus adherence and colonization. Microbiol Mol Biol Rev. 2009;73:407–50.

Nobbs AH, Jenkinson HF, Jakubovics NS. Stick to your gums: mechanisms of oral microbial adherence. J Dent Res. 2011;90:1271–8.

Okshevsky M, Meyer RL. The role of extracellular DNA in the establishment, maintenance and perpetuation of bacterial biofilms. Crit Rev Microbiol. 2015;41: 341–52.

Relman DA. The human microbiome: ecosystem resilience and health. Nutr Rev. 2012;70 Suppl 1:S2–9.

Sampaio-Maia B, Monteiro-Silva F. Acquisition and maturation of oral microbiome throughout childhood: an update. Dent Res J. 2014;11:291–301.

Sheiham A, James WP. Diet and dental caries: the pivotal role of free sugars reemphasized. J Dent Res. 2015;94:1341–7.

Takahashi N, Nyvad B. Caries ecology revisited: microbial dynamics and the caries process. Caries Res. 2008;42:409–18.

Takahashi N, Yamada T. Acid-induced acid tolerance and acidogenicity of non-mutans streptococci. Oral Microbiol Immunol. 1999;14:43–8.

Tanner AC, Kent Jr RL, Holgerson PL, Hughes CV, Loo CY, Kanasi E, Chalmers NI, Johansson I. Microbiota of severe early childhood caries before and after therapy. J Dent Res. 2011;90:1298–305.

Theilade E. The non-specific theory in microbial etiology of inflammatory periodontal diseases. J Clin Periodontol. 1986;13:905–11.

Van der Waaij D, Berghuis de Vries JM, Lekker-Kerk van der Wees JEC. Colonisation resistance of the digestive tract in conventional and antibiotic-treated mice. J Hygiene. 1971;69:405–11.

van Houte J. Role of micro-organisms in caries etiology. J Dent Res. 1994;73:672–81.

van Ruyven FO, Lingstrom P, van Houte J, Kent R. Relationship among mutans streptococci, "low pH" bacteria, and iodophilic polysaccharide-producing bacteria in dental plaque and early enamel caries in humans. J Dent Res. 2000;79:778–84.

Wright CJ, Burns LH, Jack AA, Back CR, Dutton LC, Nobbs AH, Lamont RJ, Jenkinson HF. Microbial interactions in building of communities. Mol Oral Microbiol. 2013;28:83–101.

Zijnge V, van Leeuwen MB, Degener JE, Abbas F, Thurnheer T, Gmur R, Harmsen HJ. Oral biofilm architecture on natural teeth. PLoS One. 2010; 5:e9321.

New Caries Diagnostic Methods

6

Klaus W. Neuhaus and Adrian Lussi

Abstract

Several noninvasive physicochemical methods have been developed during the last two decades to detect, measure, and monitor early caries lesions. Among these, the laser-induced fluorescence method is probably the best-tested technology. Many methods that are presented in this chapter are based on simple physical facts of the caries process. Demineralized enamel is more porous than sound enamel. Transmitted light is scattered in this region, and measuring the differences between reflected light of carious and sound enamel renders both qualitative and quantitative ways to detect lesions. Fluorescence is another phenomenon that can be measured for caries diagnostic purposes. For caries and caries-causing bacteria, characteristic fluorescence can be caused by specific wavelengths. This chapter focuses on (laser-)light-induced caries detection methods.

6.1 Introduction

Apart from visual-tactile inspection and bitewing radiographs, several additional technologies and methods have been developed for lesion detection. The main reasons for employing additional methods are:

- Early lesion detection and detection of hidden occlusal lesions
- Objective and quantitative lesion assessment (for monitoring purposes)
- Visualization of the caries process
- Avoidance of potentially harmful ionizing radiation

While in the early developmental stages of additional caries detection measures mainly pen-type devices were used for local caries assessment, there is a clear tendency nowadays toward camera-type systems. The reason might be that more and more dental offices are digitized, that they are using intraoral cameras anyway, and that data storage is not a problem anymore.

The main drawback of most of these methods is the relatively small body of clinical evidence compared to a large quantity of in vitro studies. The best clinically validated method is laser fluorescence. In the following sections, basic

K.W. Neuhaus (✉) • A. Lussi
Department of Prevenive, Restorative and Pediatric Dentistry, School of Dental Medicine, University of Bern, Bern, Switzerland
e-mail: klaus.neuhaus@zmk.unibe.ch

M. Goldberg (ed.), *Understanding Dental Caries*, DOI 10.1007/978-3-319-30552-3_6

principles of additional caries detection devices will be explained, and, whenever available, valid clinical data will be reported.

6.2 Laser-Induced Fluorescence Methods

The most common laser fluorescence (LF)-based caries detection device is the DIAGNOdent (KaVo, Biberach, Germany), which comes as a pen-type device (LFpen) (Lussi et al. 1999, 2001, 2006a). The design of the tip allows for assessments of occlusal or smooth surfaces including approximal surfaces (Fig. 6.1). It is a laser-based instrument that emits light at 655 nm from a fiber-optic bundle and is able to capture the fluorescence emitted by oral bacterial metabolites (fluorophores) present in the caries lesions; this yields a quantitative measurement of caries development. In the case of 655 nm, the fluorescing objects have been identified as bacterial protoporphyrins (König et al. 1998; Buchalla et al. 2008). This device is based on the principle that carious tissue fluoresces more than sound tissue. A photodetector quantifies the emitted fluorescence that passes through the filter and displays a real-time and a maximum value. When a critically increased pore volume is exceeded, the amount of backscattered fluorescence – theoretically – is proportional to the amount of bacterial infection, pore volume, and lesion depth. The measurements of the DIAGNOdent render values between 0 (minimum fluorescence) and 99 (maximum fluorescence). Changes in emitted fluorescence register as an increase in the digital number displayed on a monitor, thus making quantitative caries monitoring possible. Two controlled clinical trials showed that the diagnostic accuracy of LFpen was comparable to bitewing radiography in occlusal (Huth et al. 2008) and in approximal lesions (Novaes et al. 2009; Huth et al. 2010). For occlusal lesions on the enamel caries detection threshold, clinical evidence suggests a sensitivity of 0.88 and a specificity of 0.85. On the dentine threshold, the calculated values were 0.67 and 0.79, respectively (Huth et al. 2008). For approximal lesions, the sensitivity and specificity values were 0.86 and 0.7 (enamel threshold) and 0.6 and 0.84 (dentine threshold), respectively (Huth et al. 2010). However, the method is likely to produce more false-positive estimates because it is also sensitive for some filling materials, to some prophylaxis pastes, and to calculus (Bader and Shugars 2004; Lussi and Reich 2005; Lussi et al. 2006b). Therefore, there is little advantage of using LFpen for approximal lesion detection at composite margins (Rodrigues et al. 2010a) and no advantage at approximal amalgam margins (Neuhaus et al. 2012). Furthermore, in root caries detection LF is a not reliable method as well (Karlsson et al. 2009). LF devices have been also studied in other clinical situations, e.g., for the detection of residual caries during excavation (Lennon et al. 2002),

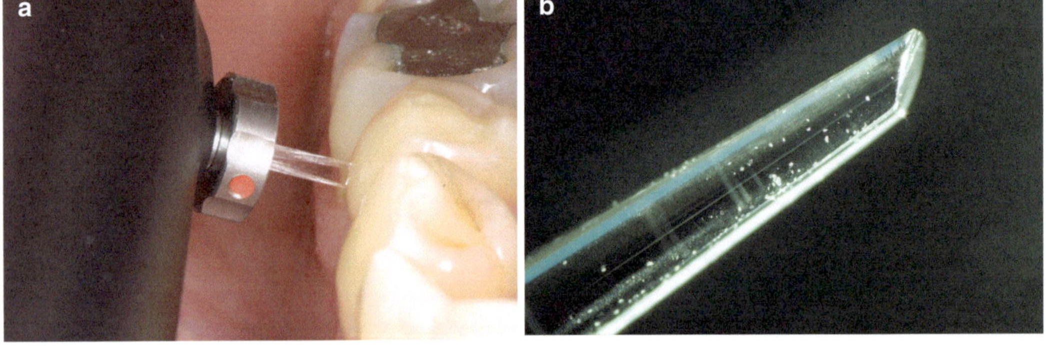

Fig. 6.1 (**a**) The DIAGNOdent pen (KaVo) can be inserted in the approximal space to detect caries below the contact area. It should be inserted from both the buccal and the lingual aspect. (**b**) The sapphire tip of the DIAGNOdent pen directs the laser light toward the tooth surface and captures the fluorescence signal

caries around orthodontic brackets (Aljehani et al. 2004), and caries under sealants (Diniz et al. 2008; Rodrigues et al. 2010b).

Slightly different from laser-induced fluorescence, another device using red LED light fluorescence has been marketed for caries detection purposes (Midwest Caries I.D., Dentsply, USA). The caries detection is semiquantitative, i.e., a green light signals healthy teeth, while red light indicates the presence of caries. The velocity of accompanying beeping noises indicates the severity of the caries process. There is no clinical study at hand that supports the use of this caries detection device. However, limited in vitro evidence shows that it may be useful for occlusal caries detection (Rodrigues et al. 2011), but has no validity for detection of approximal lesions (Neuhaus et al. 2015) (Fig. 6.1).

More recently, camera-based devices (VistaProof and VistaCam iX, both Dürr, Germany) and system were marketed and tested in vitro (Jablonski-Momeni et al. 2011) and in vivo (Diniz et al. 2012; Jablonski-Momeni et al. 2013, 2014). The clinical diagnostic accuracy was reported to be 0.46 for enamel lesions and 0.91 for dentine lesions. However, the reported sensitivity value at the dentine threshold was 0.26 (specificity being 0.98), while at the enamel threshold sensitivity was found to be 0.92 (specificity 0.41). It was concluded that the device could support the treatment decision in combination with meticulous visual-tactile inspection (Jablonski-Momeni et al. 2014). The advantage of such a camera-based system however is the possibility to quantify the caries process and to store the captured images in order to monitor lesions and allow a comparison at later recall appointments. Thus, invasive treatment could be postponed and only be performed when a lesion clearly shows to be progressive.

6.3 Quantitative Light-Induced Fluorescence (QLF)

Excitation of dentine with blue light (370 nm) causes it to fluoresce in the green-yellow spectrum. The method that uses this particular wavelength is known as quantitative light-induced fluorescence. The fluorescence is observed through a yellow filter ($\lambda \geq 540$ nm) to cut out the excitation light. An incipient enamel lesion can be observed because of an increase of light scattering relative to the surrounding enamel. Two effects thus occur: 1) because less excitation light reaches the dentine, less fluorescence is produced underneath the lesion; and 2) less fluorescent light is observed because it is scattered through the lesion. Consequently, the contrast between the surrounding sound enamel and the lesion is enhanced. An incipient lesion can be seen as a dark spot on a light green background. In addition to green fluorescence from dentine, the fluorescence of bacterial porphyrins is visible in red (Neuhaus et al. 2009).

The QLF method was originally developed for intraoral quantification of mineral loss in enamel lesions. A color microvideo CCD camera and computed image analysis were assembled and used (Inspektor Research Systems, the Netherlands) (de Josselin de Jong et al. 1995). The software subtracts the digital fluorescence images of the enamel. Three lesion quantities are thus being calculated: fluorescence loss (mean ΔF or $\Delta Fmax$), area of the lesion (in mm^2), and their product (ΔQ).

In order to enhance the application in clinical studies at different locations, a smaller, portable system for intraoral use was developed. Data is collected, stored, and analyzed by custom-made software. The portable QLF device was validated against chemical analysis and microradiography for the assessment of mineral changes in enamel and compared with results from laser-light measurements (Pitts and Longbottom 1987). It was concluded that QLF was a valid method for quantification of incipient enamel lesions. However, accurate assessments were limited to a depth of about 400 µm. Thus, the QLF method could be regarded as sensitive enough to measure remineralization in early enamel lesions. Moreover, attempts to establish suitable cutoffs for dentin lesions were made (Longbottom and Pitts 1990).

The in vivo reliability of QLF is excellent for the quantification of smooth-surface caries, with intraclass correlation coefficients for interexaminer reproducibility of $r = 0.95–0.99$ (Lagerweij et al. 1999; Tranaeus et al. 2002). The QLF method has been applied in a number of clinical trials. The QLF method has been applied to test the natural behavior of white spot lesions after removal of orthodontic brackets (van der Veen et al. 2007; Mattousch et al. 2007), for the evaluation of preventative measures in patients at high caries risk (Al-Khateeb et al. 1998), and for comparing different prophylactic means in clinical studies (Tranaeus et al. 2001; Karlsson et al. 2007). In a clinical trial with 34 fifteen-year-old students with non-cavitated occlusal surfaces, QLF was more sensitive than meticulous visual inspection and yielded double the number of carious sites (Kuhnisch et al. 2007). Recently, the QLF method was used as a gold standard in 39 children at nursery schools to compare the effect of a remineralizing agent (CPP-ACP) with toothbrushing with a fluoridated toothpaste (Sitthisettapong et al. 2015). Although QLF is a sensitive and accurate method to assess and monitor enamel lesions, its time-consuming image processing and analysis and its costs are the biggest obstacles for wide use in private dental practice.

An intraoral QLF camera system was lately marketed that offers the choice between white light mode and fluorescent light mode (Soprolife, Acteon, France). The fluorescence images are not quantitative but allow qualitative discrimination between autofluorescence and bacterial fluorescence. Effort to translate the images into a clinically relevant classification system has recently been made (Rechmann et al. 2012). It was shown that the Soprolife camera with the blue fluorescence mode yielded a sensitivity at dentine threshold of 0.95 and a specificity of 0.55 in vitro (Rechmann et al. 2012). It must be kept in mind that such a low specificity means a high fraction of false-positive findings, i.e., many teeth would have received unnecessary invasive treatments. Consequently, such a camera-based system should never be a stand-alone device for decision-making. Despite of the limited clinical value in caries diagnostics, with regard to periodontal diseases the same device was shown to provide reliable information about the presence of microbial plaque and gingival inflammation (Rechmann et al. 2016) (Fig. 6.2).

6.4 Fiber-Optic Transillumination (FOTI)

The method of tooth transillumination with an appropriate intense light source is widely accepted by dental practitioners for caries detection in anterior teeth. For this purpose, FOTI is simple and quickly to apply, and dentists usually have polymerization lamps at hand which might also be used.

Fibre-optic transillumination (FOTI) uses the principle of light scattering to increase contrast between sound and carious enamel. The light source is applied at an accessible smooth surface of a tooth. Light transmission is then observed from either the opposing side in front teeth or from the occlusal aspect in premolars or molars. Carious enamel appears dark in FOTI, because it is demineralized and porous, and light is scattered more than in healthy and sound enamel. Dentine caries appears as an orange or brown shadow from underneath the enamel. This observation helps to discriminate between lesions that are restricted to enamel and those reaching into dentin. More recently high-intensity LED light sources have become available that are inexpensive and have the potential to be widespread in dental offices. Most of the early FOTI research concentrated on the detection of proximal lesions and the performance with respect to this has been reviewed by (Vaarkamp et al. 2000). It was concluded that the specificity of both FOTI and bitewing radiography was high but that the sensitivity of FOTI was significantly lower than bitewing radiography. FOTI could therefore be used as a complementary method in the caries diagnostic process. In digital FOTI (DIFOTI), a CCD sensor replaces the human eye (Schneiderman

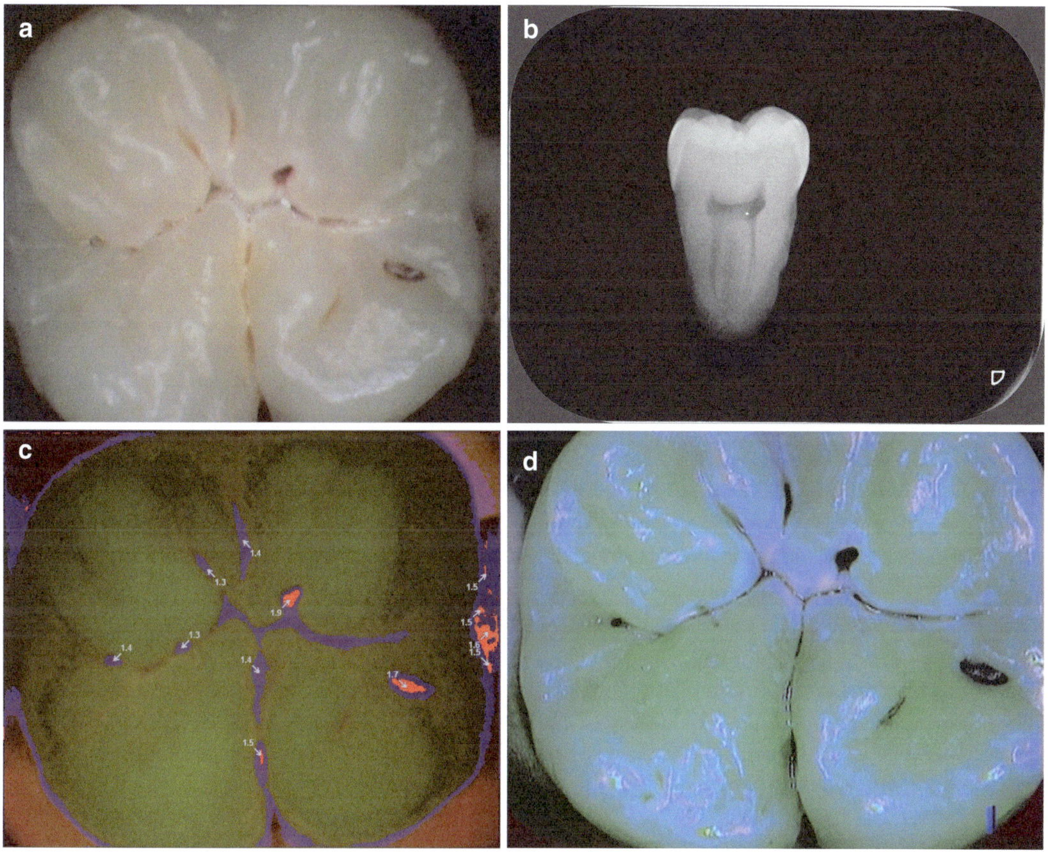

Fig. 6.2 (**a**) Occlusal surface, clinical view. (**b**) Radiograph shows initial dentine caries. (**c**) VistaProof camera (Dürr) indicates three spots that need some kind of invasive treatment (*red areas*). (**d**) Soprolife camera (Acteon) indicates a carious process in the main fissure (*light red areas*)

et al. 1997; Young and Featherstone 2005). It was reported that compared to bitewing radiography DIFOTI performs significantly better in enamel lesions, but specificity in dentine lesions was significantly lower (Astvaldsdottir et al. 2012). Intra- and interobserver agreement were reported to be similar between DIFOTI and both digital and film radiography (Astvaldsdottir et al. 2012). It should be kept in mind that up to now no clinical trial has been conducted using DIFOTI as a sole diagnostic method. Regarding other applications of FOTI, it should me mentioned that especially for detecting enamel cracks FOTI is a very helpful method (Ellis 2001). (DI) FOTI may support *instantaneous* decision-making in the dental office, but for monitoring lesions or assessing the effect of preventative measures, it is not suitable.

6.5 Near-Infrared Transillumination

A new camera-based device (DIAGNOcam, KaVo, Biberach, Germany) uses near-infrared light transillumination (NILT) for caries detection in posterior teeth. This method can be understood as further development of the DIFOTI and uses invisible long-wave light (λ ~780 nm) instead of visible light. Another modification

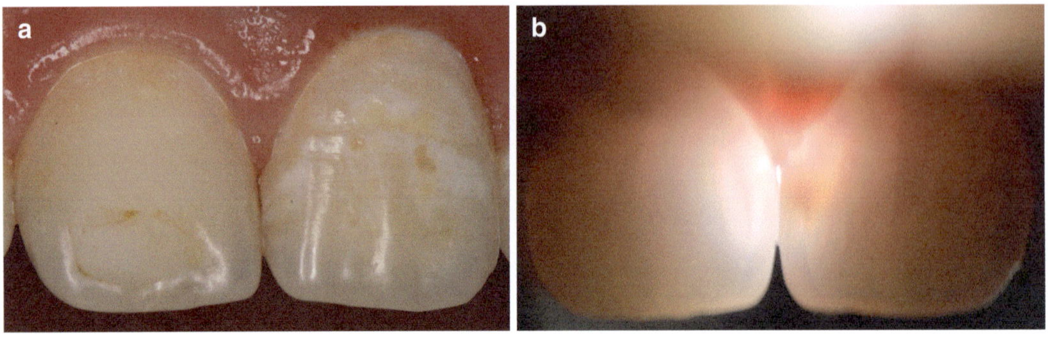

Fig. 6.3 FOTI can be easily applied on front teeth (**a**) and displays caries nicely (**b**)

is that the illuminating light enters the body at the alveolar process, far below the interproximal space. Both modifications improved considerably the quality of diagnostic imaging of interproximal sites from the occlusal aspect (Fig. 6.3a, b). The device has most recently been marketed, and an ongoing clinical validation study showed that NILT-based treatment decisions to excavate caries were in most cases the same as those by conventional bitewing radiographs (Kühnisch et al. 2015). Caries depth into dentine cannot be reliably visualized with NILT. Dentine affection is displayed only sporadically, but deep dentine lesions become regularly visible in NILT (Kühnisch et al. 2015). Therefore, the shape of the shadow in enamel has to be taken into account when assessing lesion depth (Söchtig et al. 2014). Only shadows that touch the enamel-dentine border with a broad base can be regarded as established dentine lesions. With respect to early caries lesions restricted to the enamel, there seems to be a learning curve with this technology, because the clinical performance of NILT was reported to be moderate for enamel lesions and not better than bitewing radiography (Jost et al. 2015). Next to handling issues, the projection of anatomic surface features such as steep slopes or grooves could be misinterpreted as enamel caries.

The NILT technology is not capable to detect proximal cavities, nor can it display secondary caries at cervical restoration margins. Additionally, in children the visibility of the crowns might be severely hampered by physiological root resorption, which disrupts the path of incoming light. Furthermore, enamel lesions that are infiltrated or treated with self assembling peptides are visible to the same degree after the treatment as before. The NILT method could, however, be used for screening purposes. In questionable patients further diagnostic measures such as radiography can then be applied in a more tailored way. Thus, especially younger patients could be prevented from too often applied ionizing radiation (Fig. 6.4).

Conclusions

None of the mentioned methods is able to detect cavities. The methods display lesion depth or degree of bacterial infection, which in turn helps in decision-making. However, none of the additional methods should be regarded as a stand-alone diagnostic tool. Instead, they ought to be used as a second opinion device in the decision-making process. Meticulous visual inspection still remains – in most cases – the first choice for caries diagnostics, but for caries monitoring additional measures are more suitable. Especially camera-based systems make it easier to follow up lesions over time. Modern physicochemical noninvasive caries detection devices allow for reducing the frequency of taking bitewing radiographs. Finally, no single diagnostic aid replaces clinical decision-making that is based on understanding the concepts of caries risk and lesion activity, detection, and diagnosis to determine the best treatment for each individual patient.

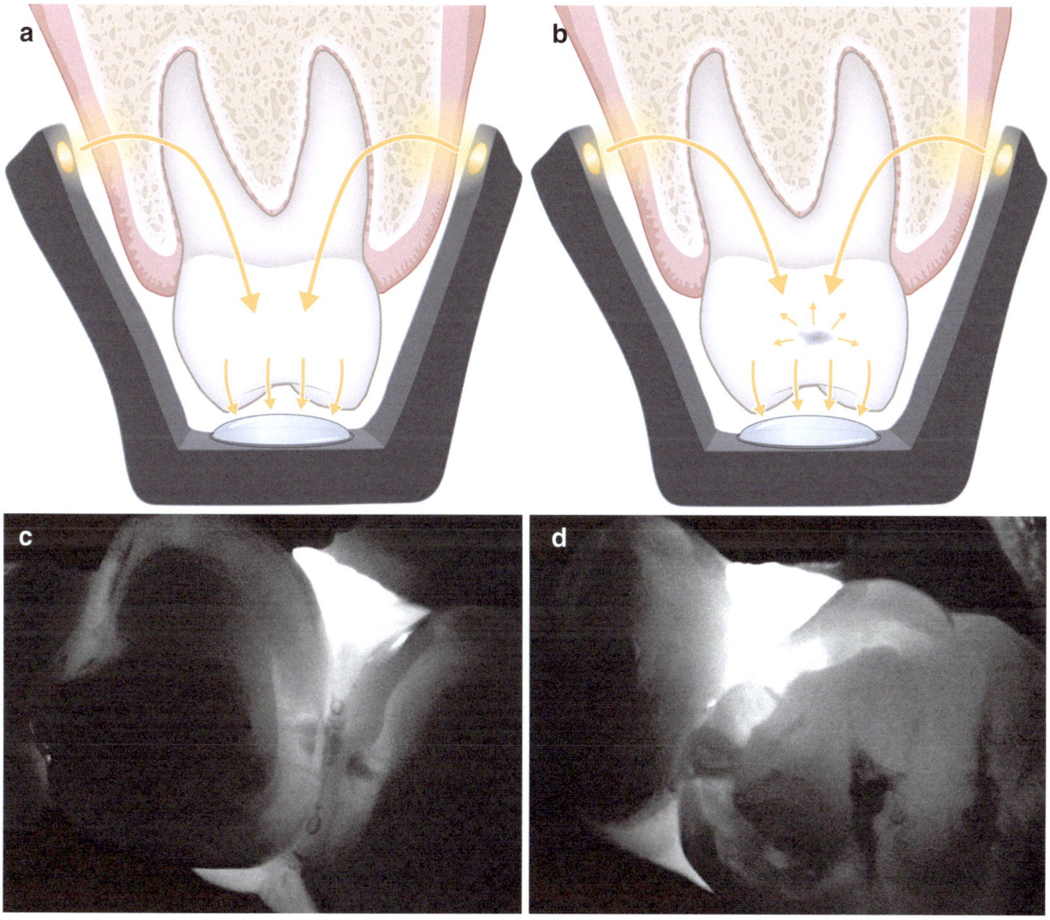

Fig. 6.4 (**a**) Light enters through the alveolar mucosa and the alveolar bone. The roots act as light conductors. (**b**) If an approximal lesion is present, it might be displayed as a dark shadow. (**c**) Enamel caries; the shadow does not reach the enamel-dentine border. (**d**) Dentine caries; unfortunately, dentine caries becomes visible only in deep lesions

References

Aljehani A, Tranaeus S, Forsberg CM, Angmar-Mansson B, Shi XQ. In vitro quantification of white spot enamel lesions adjacent to fixed orthodontic appliances using quantitative light-induced fluorescence and DIAGNOdent. Acta Odontol Scand. 2004;62:313–8.

Al-Khateeb S, Forsberg CM, De Josselin De Jong E, Angmar-Mansson B. A longitudinal laser fluorescence study of white spot lesions in orthodontic patients. Am J Orthod Dentofacial Orthop. 1998;113:595–602.

Astvaldsdottir A, Ahlund K, Holbrook WP, de Verdier B, Tranaeus S. Approximal caries detection by DIFOTI: in vitro comparison of diagnostic accuracy/efficacy with film and digital radiography. Int J Dent. 2012;2012:326401.

Bader JD, Shugars DA. A systematic review of the performance of a laser fluorescence device for detecting caries. J Am Dent Assoc. 2004;135:1413–26.

Buchalla W, Attin T, Niedmann Y, Niedmann PD. Porphyrins are the cause of red fluorescence of carious dentine: verified by gradient reversed-phase HPLC (abstract). Caries Res. 2008;42:223.

Diniz MB, Rodrigues JA, Hug I, Cordeiro RC, Lussi A. The influence of pit and fissure sealants on infrared fluorescence measurements. Caries Res. 2008;42: 328–33.

Diniz MB, Boldieri T, Rodrigues JA, Santos-Pinto L, Lussi A, CORDEIRO RC. The performance of conventional and fluorescence-based methods for occlusal caries detection: an in vivo study with histologic validation. J Am Dent Assoc. 2012;143:339–50.

Ellis SG. Incomplete tooth fracture – proposal for a new definition. Br Dent J. 2001;190:424–8.

Huth KC, Neuhaus KW, Gygax M, Bücher K, Crispin A, Paschos E, Hickel R, Lussi A. Clinical performance of a new laser fluorescence device for detection of occlusal caries lesions at permanent molars. J Dent. 2008;36(1):1033–40.

Huth KC, Lussi A, Gygax M, Thum M, Crispin A, Paschos E, Hickel R, Neuhaus KW. In vivo performance of a laser fluorescence device for the approximal detection of caries in permanent molars. J Dent. 2010;38:1019–26.

Jablonski-Momeni A, Schipper HM, Rosen SM, Heinzel-Gutenbrunner M, Roggendorf MJ, Stoll R, Stachniss V, Pieper K. Performance of a fluorescence camera for detection of occlusal caries in vitro. Odontology. 2011;99:55–61.

Jablonski-Momeni A, Liebegall F, Stoll R, Heinzel-Gutenbrunner M, Pieper K. Performance of a new fluorescence camera for detection of occlusal caries in vitro. Lasers Med Sci. 2013;28:101–9.

Jablonski-Momeni A, Heinzel-Gutenbrunner M, Klein SM. In vivo performance of the VistaProof fluorescence-based camera for detection of occlusal lesions. Clin Oral Investig. 2014;18:1757–62.

Jong De Josselin De E, Sundstrom F, Westerling H, Tranaeus S, Ten Bosch JJ, Angmar-Mansson B. A new method for in vivo quantification of changes in initial enamel caries with laser fluorescence. Caries Res. 1995;29:2–7.

Jost FN, Kühnisch J, Lussi A, Neuhaus KW. Reproducibility of near-infrared light transillumination for approximal enamel caries: a clinical controlled trial. Clin Oral Investig. 2015;19:1752.

Karlsson L, Lindgren LE, Trollsas K, Angmar-Mansson B, Tranaeus S. Effect of supplementary amine fluoride gel in caries-active adolescents. A clinical QLF study. Acta Odontol Scand. 2007;65:284–91.

Karlsson L, Johansson E, Tranaeus S. Validity and reliability of laser-induced fluorescence measurements on carious root surfaces in vitro. Caries Res. 2009;43:397–404.

König K, Flemming G, Hibst R. Laser-induced autofluorescence spectroscopy of dental caries. Cell Mol Biol (Noisy-le-Grand). 1998;44:1293–300.

Kühnisch J, Ifland S, Tranaeus S, Hickel R, Stosser L, Heinrich-Weltzien R. In vivo detection of non-cavitated caries lesions on occlusal surfaces by visual inspection and quantitative light-induced fluorescence. Acta Odontol Scand. 2007;65:183–8.

Kühnisch J, Söchtig F, Pitchika V, Laubender R, Neuhaus KW, Lussi A, Hickel R. In vivo validation of near-infrared light transillumination for interproximal dentin caries detection. Clin Oral Investig. 2015. DOI: 10.1007/s00784-015-1559-4.

Lagerweij M, Van Der Veen M, Ando M, Lukantsova L, Stookey G. The validity and repeatability of three light-induced fluorescence systems: an in vitro study. Caries Res. 1999;33:220–6.

Lennon AM, Buchalla W, Switalski L, Stookey GK. Residual caries detection using visible fluorescence. Caries Res. 2002;36:315–9.

Longbottom C, Pitts NB. Initial comparison between endoscopic and conventional methods of caries diagnosis. Quintessence Int. 1990;21:531–40.

Lussi A, Reich E. The influence of toothpastes and prophylaxis pastes on fluorescence measurements for caries detection in vitro. Eur J Oral Sci. 2005;113:141–4.

Lussi A, Imwinkelried S, Pitts N, Longbottom C, Reich E. Performance and reproducibility of a laser fluorescence system for detection of occlusal caries in vitro. Caries Res. 1999;33:261–6.

Lussi A, Megert B, Longbottom C, Reich E, Francescut P. Clinical performance of a laser fluorescence device for detection of occlusal caries lesions. Eur J Oral Sci. 2001;109:14–9.

Lussi A, Hack A, Hug I, Heckenberger H, Megert B, Stich H. Detection of approximal caries with a new laser fluorescence device. Caries Res. 2006a;40:97–103.

Lussi A, Zimmerli B, Hellwig E, Jaeggi T. Influence of the condition of the adjacent tooth surface on fluorescence measurements for the detection of approximal caries. Eur J Oral Sci. 2006b;114:478–82.

Mattousch TJ, Van Der Veen MH, Zentner A. Caries lesions after orthodontic treatment followed by quantitative light-induced fluorescence: a 2-year follow-up. Eur J Orthod. 2007;29:294–8.

Neuhaus KW, Longbottom C, Ellwood R, Lussi A. Novel lesion detection aids. Monogr Oral Sci. 2009;21: 52–62.

Neuhaus KW, Rodrigues JA, Seemann R, Lussi A. Detection of proximal secondary caries at cervical class II-amalgam restoration margins in vitro. J Dent. 2012;40:493–9.

Neuhaus KW, Ciucchi P, Rodrigues JA, Hug I, Emerich M, Lussi A. Diagnostic performance of a new red light LED device for approximal caries detection. Lasers Med Sci. 2015;30:1443–7.

Novaes TF, Matos R, Braga MM, Imparato JC, Raggio DP, Mendes FM. Performance of a pen-type laser fluorescence device and conventional methods in detecting approximal caries lesions in primary teeth – in vivo study. Caries Res. 2009;43:36–42.

Pitts NB, Longbottom C. The use of endoscopically viewed filtered fluorescence for the clinical diagnosis of carious lesions in dental enamel. Med Sci Res. 1987;15:535–6.

Rechmann P, Charland D, Rechmann BM, Featherstone JD. Performance of laser fluorescence devices and visual examination for the detection of occlusal caries in permanent molars. J Biomed Opt. 2012;17:036006.

Rechmann P, Liou SW, Rechmann BM, Featherstone JD. Performance of a light fluorescence device for the detection of microbial plaque and gingival inflammation. Clin Oral Investig. 2016;20(1):151–9.

Rodrigues JA, Neuhaus KW, Hug I, Stich H, Seemann R, Lussi A. In vitro detection of secondary caries associated with composite restorations on approximal surfaces using laser fluorescence. Oper Dent. 2010a; 35:564–71.

Rodrigues JA, Diniz MB, Hug I, Cordeiro RC, Lussi A. Relationship between DIAGNOdent values and sealant penetration depth on occlusal fissures. Clin Oral Investig. 2010b;14:707–11.

Rodrigues JA, Hug I, Neuhaus KW, Lussi A. Light-emitting diode and laser fluorescence-based devices in detecting occlusal caries. J Biomed Opt. 2011;16: 107003.

Schneiderman A, Elbaum M, Shultz T, Keem S, Greenebaum M, Driller J. Assessment of dental caries with Digital Imaging Fiber-Optic TransIllumination (DIFOTI): in vitro study. Caries Res. 1997;31:103–10.

Sitthisettapong T, Doi T, Nishida Y, Kambara M, Phantumvanit P. Effect of CPP-ACP paste on enamel carious lesion of primary upper anterior teeth assessed by quantitative light-induced fluorescence: a one-year clinical trial. Caries Res. 2015;49:434–41.

Söchtig F, Hickel R, Kühnisch J. Caries detection and diagnostics with near-infrared light transillumination: clinical experiences. Quintessence Int. 2014;45:531–8.

Tranaeus S, Al-Khateeb S, Bjorkman S, Twetman S, Angmar-Mansson B. Application of quantitative light-induced fluorescence to monitor incipient lesions in caries-active children. A comparative study of remineralisation by fluoride varnish and professional cleaning. Eur J Oral Sci. 2001;109:71–5.

Tranaeus S, Shi XQ, Lindgren LE, Trollsas K, Angmar-Mansson B. In vivo repeatability and reproducibility of the quantitative light-induced fluorescence method. Caries Res. 2002;36:3–9.

Vaarkamp J, Ten Bosch JJ, Verdonschot EH, Bronkhoorst EM. The real performance of bitewing radiography and fiber-optic transillumination in approximal caries diagnosis. J Dent Res. 2000;79:1747–51.

van der Veen MH, Mattousch T, Boersma JG. Longitudinal development of caries lesions after orthodontic treatment evaluated by quantitative light-induced fluorescence. Am J Orthod Dentofacial Orthop. 2007;131:223–8.

Young DA, Featherstone JD. Digital imaging fiber-optic trans-illumination, F-speed radiographic film and depth of approximal lesions. J Am Dent Assoc. 2005;136:1682–7.

From the Initial Carious Lesion of Enamel to the Early Development of Coronal Dentin Carious Lesion

7

Michel Goldberg

Abstract

Once the initial carious decay crosses the whole enamel thickness, diffusion occurs at the dentinoenamel junction, mostly in the mantle dentin direction where the dentinal carious decay displays an early development. After the collapse of the non-sustained enamel surface, a cavity starts to be formed, containing residual food debris (zone of degradation), above a zone of bacterial invasion. The demineralized dentin layer displays an infected zone, where dentinal tubules are enlarged. They are filled with active bacteria. Intertubular dentin is demineralized, removable manually by sharp curettes and forming the soft carious dentin. The affected zone is located beneath. Intertubular dentin is gradually recovering from the demineralization process. The lumens of tubules display normal diameter, and the peritubular dentin gradually reappears. In the sclerotic zone, either reprecipitation of non-apatitic mineral contributes to fill partially the lumen of the tubules or apatitic-like structures seal more or less homogeneously the lumen of tubules (intratubular mineralization). The subjacent layer contains lipid-loaded odontoblast processes. These cells contribute to the formation of reactionary dentin. They are implicated in slowing down the speed of diffusion of the carious lesion in the crown.

7.1 Dentin Caries: The Different Layers

7.1.1 Non-carious Dentin

Structurally, the dentin located in the crown includes an outer layer, identified as mantle dentin. In the root, the Hopewell-Smith translucent zone and Tome's granular layer form two outer layers, located at the periphery of the circumpulpal human dentin. Dentin includes between 20.000 and

M. Goldberg
University Paris Descartes, Sorbonne, Paris Cité and INSERM UMR-S1124, 45 rue des Saints Pères, Cedex 06, 75270 Paris, France
e-mail: mgoldod@gmail.com

M. Goldberg (ed.), *Understanding Dental Caries*, DOI 10.1007/978-3-319-30552-3_7

Table 7.1 Global dentin composition (Zavgorodnuy et al. 2008)

Dentin composition	Apatite crystals (mineral)	Organic matrix (type I collagen and non-collagenous proteins)	Water (free and bound)
	50 %	30 %	20 %

38.000 tubules/mm^2, depending on the zone that is observed and the scoring method used.

Dentin combines inter- and peritubular structures, containing odontoblast processes and some liquid phase present either as free or bound water, or also as lymph serum. Table 7.1 summarizes the dentin composition, although major differences are detectable between the outer and inner dentin zones and between the crown and root parts of the teeth. Around tubules, the peritubular dentin reinforces the resistance to axial and lateral pressures, whereas intertubular dentin forms a continuous network. Crystallites in the intertubular dentin display a needlelike structure, whereas in the peritubular dentin isodiametric, rhombohedric crystals form a dense mineralized ring.

7.1.2 Extracellular Organic Matrix

The intertubular dentin matrix is mainly composed of type I collagen fibrils which are associated to non-collagenous proteins and proteoglycans, forming a three-dimensional organic network associated in a mineral phase constituted mostly by hydroxyapatite crystallites.

Dentin Composition Ninety percent of the sound dentin is composed by type I collagen fibrils and 10 % appear as non-collagenous proteins (NCPs). They are located in dentin as components of the matrix extracellular molecules (ECM). NCPs include the family of SIBLINGs, which are phosphorylated proteins implicated in dentin mineralization (osteopontin, dentin sialoprotein (DSP) 1, bone sialoprotein (BSP), MEPE). Other molecules characterized as non-phosphorylated ECM proteins (osteocalcin, osteonectin) act as promotor or inhibitors of mineralization. Some molecules take origin in the serum (α_2HS glycoproteins, albumin). Proteoglycans or SLRPs, including decorin, biglycan, lumican, and fibromodulin, play role in the formation of dentin complexes. Phospholipids, a series of small proteases, and ECM enzymes are also located within the ECM (Goldberg et al. 2011).

During the carious decay, NCP are the main targets for acidic or enzymes degradation. Type I collagen is more resistant. Collagenases, gelatinases, and some MMPs (matrix metalloproteinases) contribute to collagen degradation. The cross-links between collagen fibrils better resist bacterial attacks. All the molecules listed in the previous paragraphs provide substrates implicated in dentin degradation during the carious decay. For example, this is namely the case for MMP2, an enzyme modulating BSP, and detected by immunohistochemistry in association with the full-length molecule associated to the caries-affected dentinal tubules (Boushell et al. 2011). However, the degradation is not uniform and depends specifically on the dentin layer and the site of exposure to bacteria.

7.2 Size of the Hydroxyapatite Crystallites in the Intertubular Dentin

The size of needlelike apatite crystals is approximately 5 nm × 30 nm × 100 nm [length and width of the sound dentin intertubular crystals (109.6 ± 19.9 nm and 6.2 ± 1.2 nm)]. It contains less calcium (calcium deficient) and more carbonate (carbonate-rich hydroxyapatite) and therefore is more soluble than stoichiometric apatite (Zavgorodnuy et al. 2008). In sound dentin, the length of crystallites is 109 nm ± 19.9 nm, whereas in the transparent zone, crystals located in the middle dentin display 51 ± 13.0 nm as mean length and near the DEJ after demineralization 37.8 ± 20.1 nm (Zavgorodnuy et al. 2008).

7.3 White and Brown Spots

When the carious enamel lesion reaches the dentinoenamel junction (DEJ), a brownish discoloration in dentin suggests that the dentin

Table 7.2

Zone of degradation: food debris (Vegetal and animal: meat, muscle). Degradation front of demineralized dentin Outer carious dentin infected (Fig. 7.2)	*Zone of bacterial invasion* (Soft carious dentin) Inner carious dentin (Fig. 7.3)	*Zone of demineralization* (*Infected* soft carious dentin) enlarged tubules (*Affected* tubules + mineral reprecipitations) intratubular non-apatitic precipitation Whitlockite, calcium phosphate, non-occluding the lumen of tubules (Fig. 7.4)	*Zone of dentin sclerosis* (transparent dentin): Intratubular needlelike apatitic ghostlike mineral occluding the lumens of tubules (Figs. 7.5 and 7.6)	*Zone of fatty degeneration*
Carious cavity: degraded dentin unremineralizable	Carious cavity: >Enlarged tubules > intertubular dentin demineralized >No peritubular dentin Discolored layer	Carious cavity: *Infected*: active bacteria inside tubules. *Affected*: gradient of peritubular dentin + increase of intertubular dentin mineralization Transparent layer	Sclerotic dentin Occlusion of the lumens of tubules by: Reprecipitation in non-apatitic and hydroxyapatite mineral forms Subtransparent layer	"Sound" dentin with lipidic inclusions. Reactionary dentin (Fig. 7.7)

respond with the formation of translucent dentin. There is no spreading of dentin caries along the DEJ but penetration of the lesion may be observed within dentin, at least in non-cavitated occlusal lesions with an apparently intact enamel surface (Bjorndal and Thylstrup 1995). Lateral spread along the DEJ was found in lesions with micro-cavitation or cavitation, therefore when soft and infected dentin was present (Ekstrand et al. 1998).

In the carious dentin, five zones have been identified (Newbrun 1983; Yamada et al. 1983). A simplified classification of the different carious layers allows distinguishing between the caries-infected dentin layers, which cannot be remineralized, located in the outer caries layer, and the caries-affected layers. These layers are both superficial and partially demineralized, but they may also be remineralizable. The inner caries layer, which is sclerotic (transparent), displays a subtransparent highly mineralizable sclerotic layer, located between the carious lesion and the normal dentin (Mazzoni et al. 2015).

Table 7.2 summarizes the different zones and events occurring during the development of carious events (Fig. 7.1):

1. *Zone of decomposed dentin* where food debris accumulates beneath enamel broken roof. Plant cell wall or degraded meat fibrils taking origin from the nutriments. This is the zone of complete dentin dissolution, where demineralization and proteolysis occur (Fig. 7.2a).
2. *Zone of bacterial invasion* limiting the soft carious dentin surface. At the dentin surface, bacteria are grouped and they synthesize a soft dental plaque. The acid pH and chelating properties of the bacteria colonies contribute to dissolve the outer surface of dentin (Figs. 7.2a–d and 7.3b, c).
3. *Zone of demineralization*. Dentin decalcification is seen below the most superficial layers. Intertubular crystallites partially mineralized decrease in size as the carious lesion progresses. Two different layers are identified: *3a*, a well-demineralized dentin layer, where the intertubular dentin is largely demineralized, peritubular dentin has melt, and the diameter of the dentinal tubules is enlarged. This *soft carious dentin* has a leather-like consistence and appears well (but not fully) demineralized. This infected dentin may be eliminated manually with curettes (Figs. 7.3

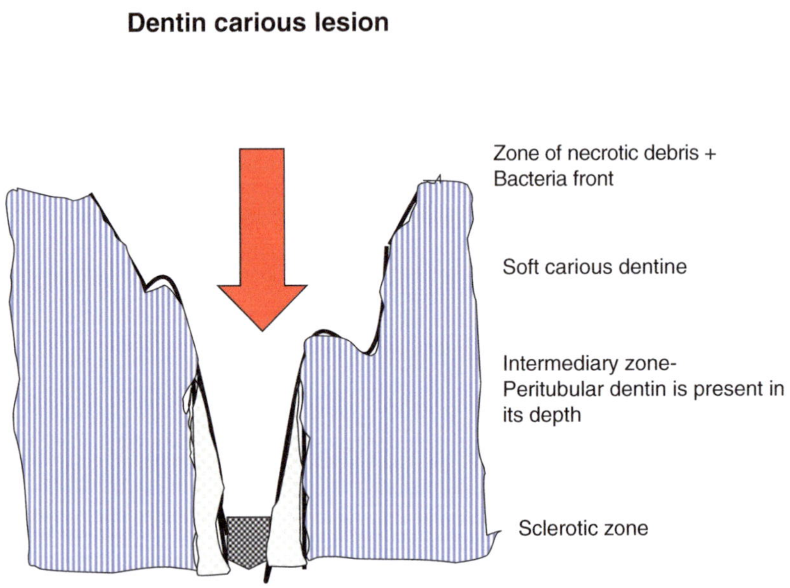

Fig. 7.1 Schematic diagram of a dentin carious lesion. Beneath the zone of necrotic debris, a soft carious dentin is found, followed by the intermediary zone. Peritubular dentin has been dissolved, but reappears in the depth of the lesion. The sclerotic dentin where tubules are occluded by intratubular mineralization formed the sclerotic zone

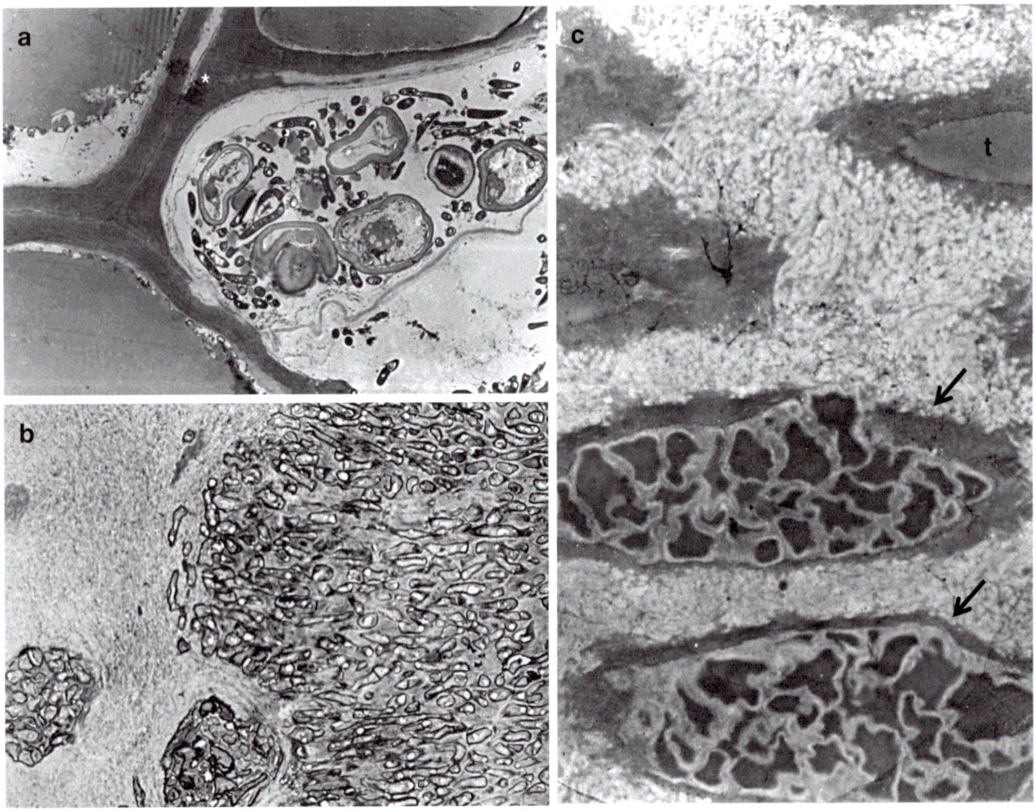

Fig. 7.2 (**a**) Food debris (here a cell wall residual inclusion, *white asterisk*) accumulate in the carious cavity where dentin is decomposed. They are associated with bacteria. (**b**) Accumulation of bacteria that are destroying frontally the soft carious dentin surface. Inside the decayed dentin, tubules filled with bacteria are enlarged. (**c**) In the soft carious dentin, some tubules are empty, whereas others are filled with bacteria (*arrows*), which contribute to tubules enlargement, to the diffusion of acids and crystals demineralization

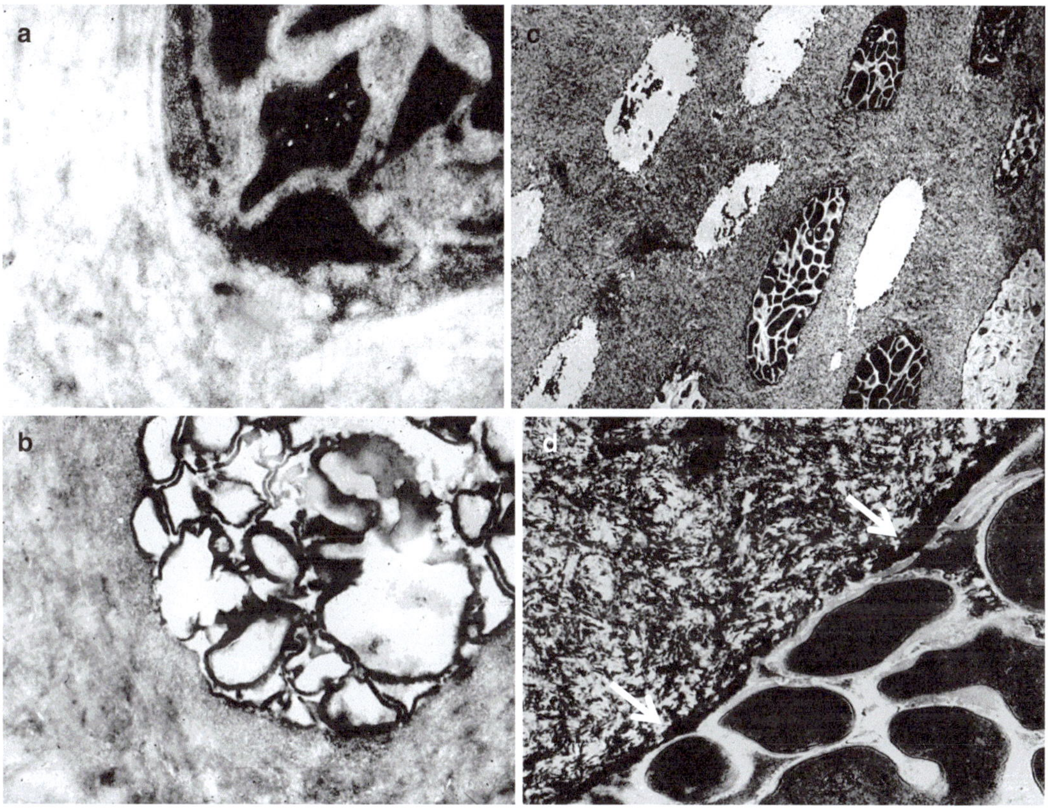

Fig. 7.3 Zone of bacterial invasion. (**a**) Dentinal tubule containing bacteria, (**b**) residual bacteria walls within a tubule. The inactivated bacteria do not contain any internal structure. (**c**) Concomitant presence of empty dentinal tubules, slightly enlarged, and tubules containing active bacteria colonies contribute to the lumen enlargement and demineralization of intertubular dentin. (**d**) Cariogenic bacteria destroy remnants of the peritubular dentin (*white arrows*)

and 7.4a). *3b*: In deeper areas, the degree of mineralization is increased. In the demineralized dentin, the peritubular dentin reappears gradually, forming mineralized spots near the surface, and as a continuous and with an increasing thickness afterward. This dentin layer has an increased mineral content. It is referred in the literature as affected dentin, containing a "peritubular matrix, peritubular dentin, peritubular translucent zone and tubulo-fibrillar complex" (Takuma 1960) (Fig. 7.4a–c).

4. *Zone of dentin sclerosis*. In the "*transparent dentin*," the intratubular mineral phase is chemically similar to intertubular dentin. However, in the transparent zone, dentin crystallites are 53 % smaller in length and 12 % smaller in width than in sound intertubular dentin. After demineralization intertubular dentin crystals are 65 % smaller in length and 32 % smaller in width compared with the sound intertubular dentin. Therefore, the dissolution and reprecipitation mechanism is a key factor to understand the formation of the sclerotic inner carious layer (Zavgorodnuy et al. 2008) (Figs. 7.5 and 7.6).

Reprecipitation of mineral in another crystallo-chemical form (non-apatitic crystals) occludes partially of totally the lumen of the tubules. Concomitantly, we observed (a) tubules invaded by bacteria, (b) tubules partially filled by mineral reprecipitation, and (c) tubules totally filled by ghostlike elongated structures resembling crystal-ghost (a membrane-like envelope) hydroxyapatite-like crystallites. Altogether, this heterogeneous

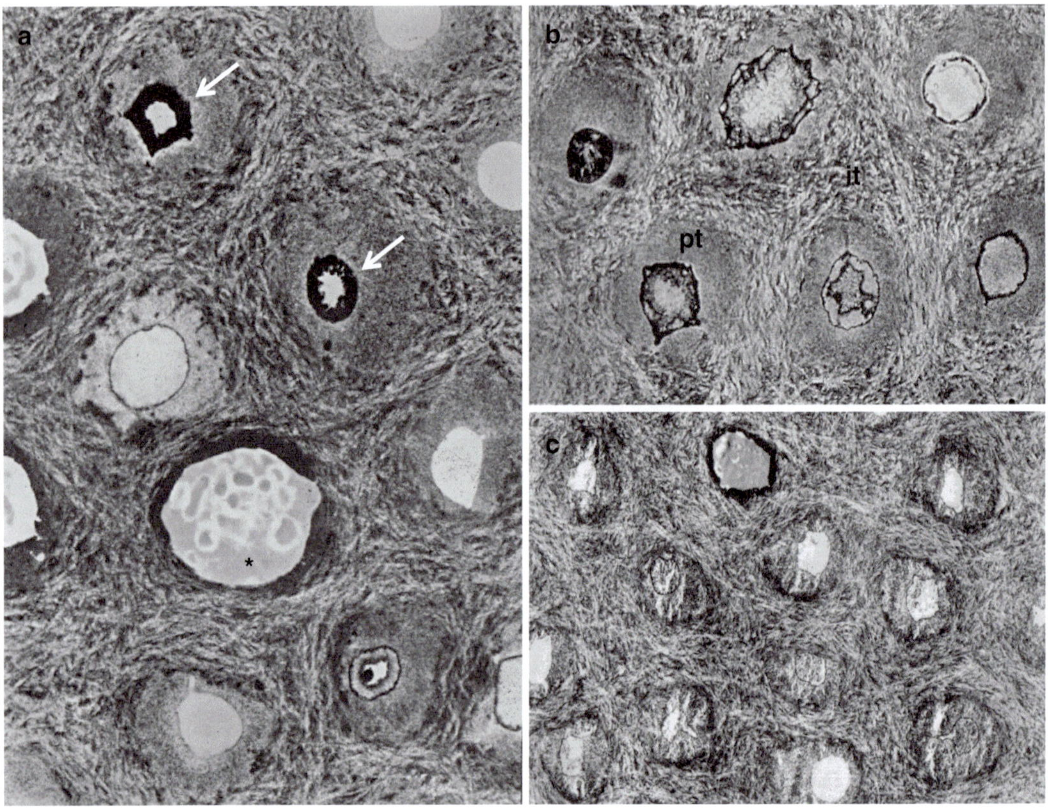

Fig. 7.4 Intermediary area between the demineralized zone and the dentinal sclerosis zone. (**a**) Some tubules are filled with bacteria (*asterisk*), whereas reprecipitation is occurring in some others (*white arrows*). (**b**) Intertubular (*it*) forms a continuous network, while peritubular (*pt*) forms a continuous ring around tubules. Inside the lumens of the tubules reprecipitation in non-apatitic forms occlude the lumens. (**c**) The formation of intratubular mineralizations contributes to dentin sclerosis

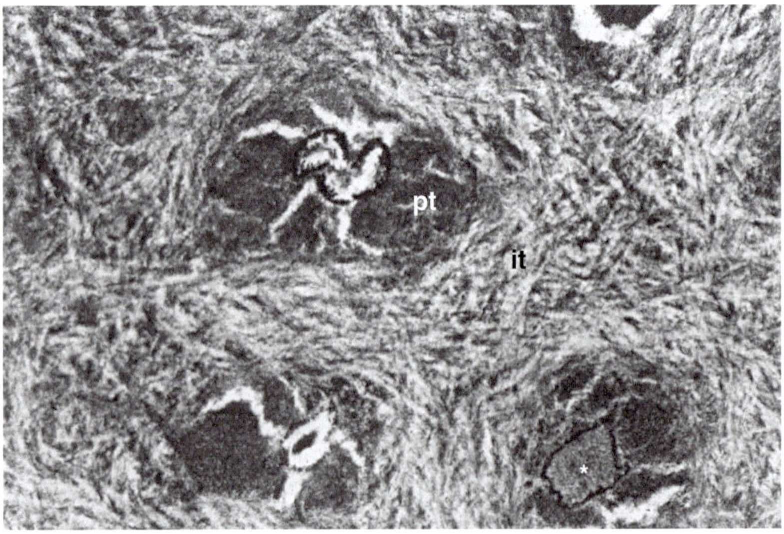

Fig. 7.5 Zone of dentin sclerosis. Intertubular (*it*) and peritubular (*pt*) dentin displays high degree of mineralization. Inside the lumen, intratubular mineralization (*asterisk*) contributes to dentin sclerosis

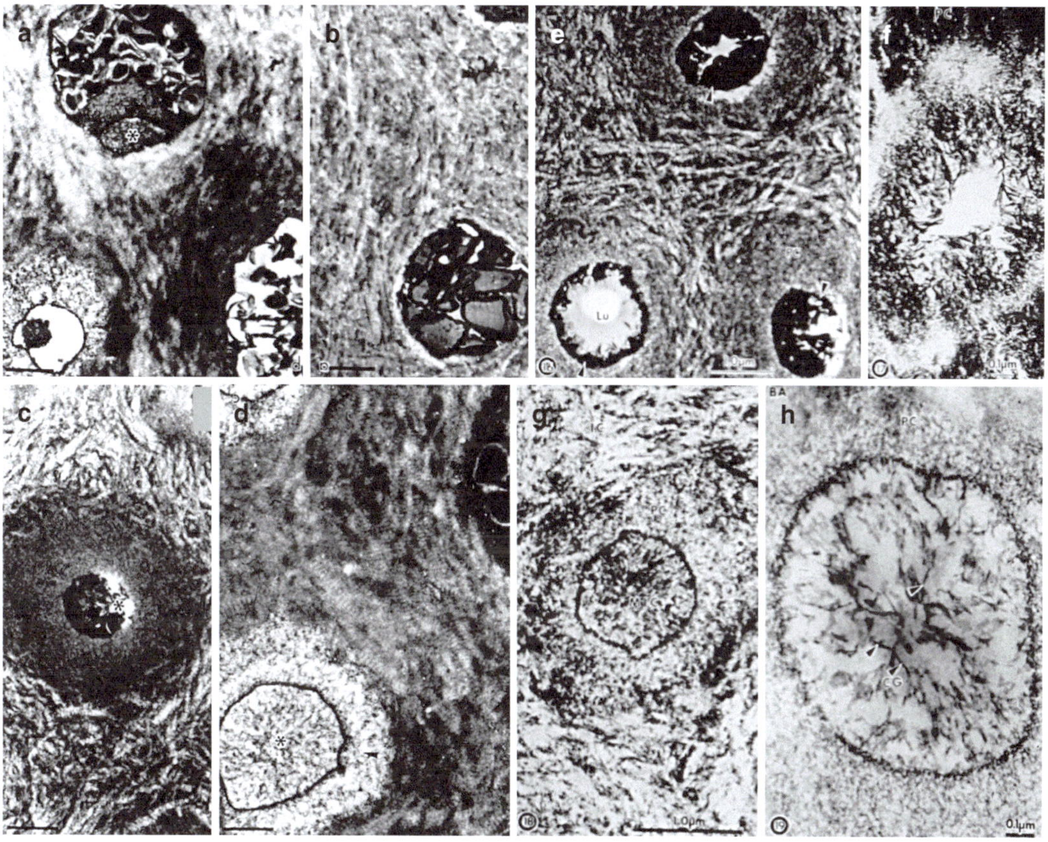

Fig. 7.6 In (**a**, **b**), demineralized dentin display bacteria in the lumen of tubules. In (**c**, **d**), non-apatitic mineralizations (reprecipitations) contribute to dentin sclerosis. This is more accentuated in (**e**), but the closure is only partial, whereas in (**f–h**), needlelike apatitic structures are implicated in the gradual closure of the tubules

material fills the lumen of tubules. This persistent mineralization constitutes an intratubular occluding structure. Sclerotic dentin is similar to the translucent zone. Occlusion of dentinal tubules may be due to the reprecipitation of crystalline material. Arrested or slow-advancing carious lesions are filled by such mineralization, which constitute an efficient barrier of permeability against acidic exotoxin diffusion issued from bacteria. Occlusion of the tubule by a mineral phase induces the formation of two types of crystals: platelike hydroxyapatite crystals and large isodiametric rhombohedral crystals, which do not occlude completely the tubule. In addition to apatitic crystals, the second group of crystals has been identified as Mg-substituted β-TCP large crystals (whitlockite) by electron diffraction and also as calcium phosphate appearing as crystallites or forming an amorphous phase. They may result from reprecipitation of ions dissolved during the carious destruction.

5. *Zone of fatty degeneration*. Beneath the sclerotic zone, odontoblasts are still alive. Long processes extend along tubules, and some of them contain inclusions stained as fatty acids or lipid-like structures by specific dyes. This may eventually precede the formation of sclerotic dentin. In a more inner zone, odontoblasts are functional and contribute to the formation of reactionary dentin. Wounded odontoblasts lost their polarity and secrete around the cells what is structurally recognized to be an osteodentin. Odontoblast-like cells look as osteocytes and are located in osteoplasties, resembling a bone-like

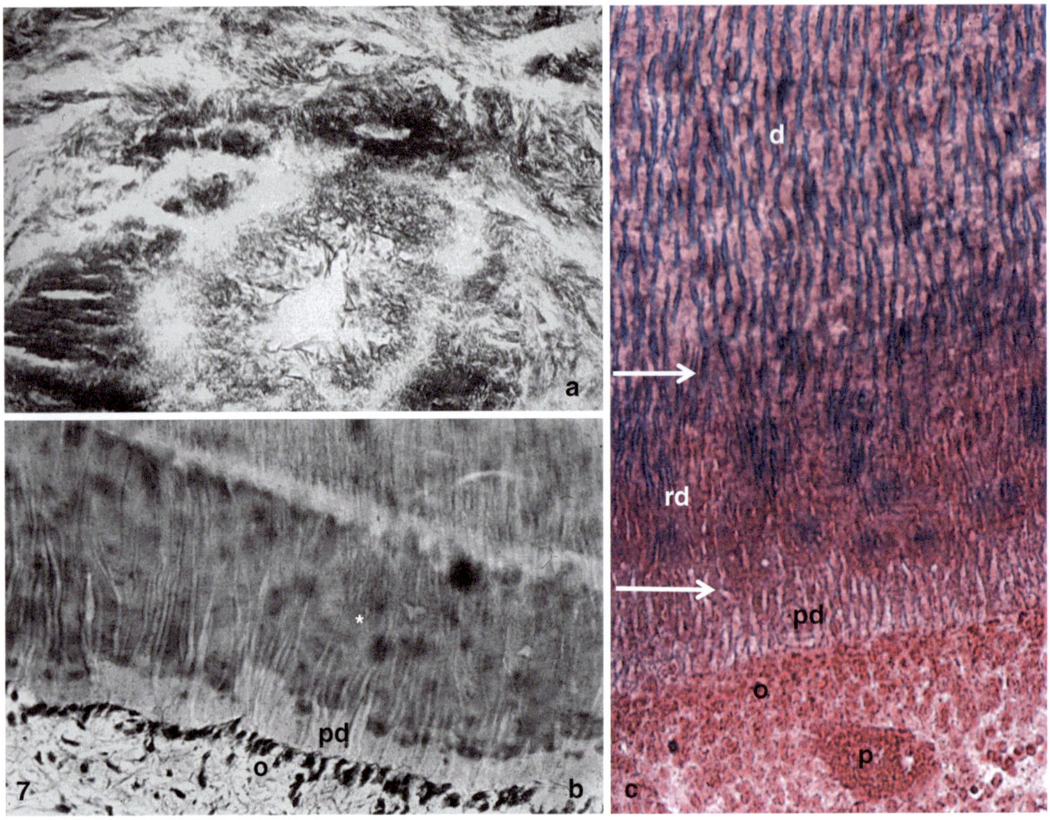

Fig. 7.7 (**a**) Intertubular and peritubular dentin are mineralized, while intratubular mineralization is in progress and needlelike structures are implicated in the closure of the tubule lumen. (**b**) Beneath the carious lesion, reactionary dentin (*white asterisk*) is formed and produced by odontoblasts (*o*). The predentin (*pd*) and the reactionary dentin (*rd*) are of the orthodentin type. (**c**) Stains all evidences calcospherites in the reactionary dentin layer (*rd*), of the osteodentin type. *d* dentin; *o* odontoblasts; *p* pulp

structure. Reactionary dentin forms along the primary or secondary dentin. This dentin constitutes a physiopathological answer to the dentin carious pathology (Fig. 7.7).

Inside the dental pulp, pulp cells are contributing to the formation of pulp stone, to the detriment of pulp space. These pulp stone may be adherent to the pulp wall or isolated inside the pulp as pulpolithes.

At the chair side, dental practitioners have tried to establish a clear-cut clinical difference between the infected and affected dentins. In this outer carious layer, enlarged tubules contain bacteria, and no remineralization can be expected. Using discoloration and bacteria invasion, the affected inner dentin displays reparative potential and reversible remineralization may occur. According to Fusayama (1979), a brief staining with 0.5 % solution of basic fuchsine in propylene glycol stains the superficial carious zone, whereas the inner carious layer does not take the fuchsine stain. Using the Mallory-Azan stain evidence in the superficial outer layer that the collagen fibrils are irreversibly denatured, the cross-links being markedly decreased. In contrast, in the inner part, collagen denaturation is reversible. Correlations between the stainability of the carious lesion and the molecular changes might be expected and used at the chair side.

References

Bjorndal L, Thylstrup A. A structural analysis of approximal enamel caries lesions and subjacent dentin reactions. Eur J Oral Sci. 1995;103:25–31.

Boushell LW, Nagoka H, Nagoka H, Yamauchi M. Increased matrix metalloproteinase-2 and bone SialoProtein response to human coronal caries. Caries Research. 2011;45:453–9.

Ekstrand KR, Ricketts DN, Kidd EA. Do occlusal carious lesions spread laterally at the enamel-dentin junction? A histopathological study. Clin Oral Investig. 1998;2:15–20.

Fusayama T. Two layers of carious dentin. Diagnosis and treatment. Oper Dent. 1979;45:63–70.

Goldberg M, Kulkarni AB, Young M, Boskey A. Dentin: structure, composition and mineralization. The role of dentin ECM in dentin formation and mineralization. Front BioSci (Elite Ed). 2011;3:711–35.

Mazzoni A, Tjäderhane L, Checchi V, Di Lenarda R, Salo T, Tay FR, Pashley DH, Breschi L. Role of dentin MMPs in caries progression and bond stability. J Dent Res. 2015;94(2):241–251.

Newbrun E. Cariology. Baltimore/London: Williams & Wilkins; 1983. p. 245–51.

Takuma S. Electron microscopy of the structure around the dentinal tubule. J Dent Res. 1960;39:973–81.

Yamada T, Nakamura K, Iwaku M, Fusayama T. The extent of odontoblast process in normal and carious human dentin. J Dent Res. 1983;62:798–802.

Zavgorodnuy AV, Rohanizadeh R, Swain MV. Ultrastructure of dentine carious lesions. Arch Oral Biol. 2008;53:124–32.

Part II

The Carious Dentin

The Dentinoenamel Junction

8

Michel Goldberg

Abstract

The dentinoenamel junction (DEJ) is the border where five different structures meet: the cervical enamel, two superficial outer dentin layers (Tomes' granular and Hopewell-Smith hyaline layers), located over the inner circumpulpal dentin, and cementum (afibrillar acellular cementum and fibrillar cellular cementum). The DEJ is a complex scalloped structure associating at least two calcified tissues and preventing the propagation of cracks from enamel to dentin. It constitutes a biomimetic model of a structure uniting dissimilar materials. Its composition includes type I collagen, phosphorylated (SIBLINGs) and non-phosphorylated proteins (e.g., small leucine-rich proteoglycans (SLRPs), and some extracellular matrix molecules taking origin from the blood serum. Enzymes, metalloproteinases, and lipoproteins participate in its formation. Altogether they contribute to the DEJ mineralization, human enamel rod presenting anisotropic and nanotribological properties. Gradient of mineralization influences abfraction formation (Cuy et al. Arch Oral Biol 47:281–91, 2002; He and Swani J Dent 35:431–7, 2007; Imbeni et al. Nat Mater 4:229–32, 2005). The mechanical properties of the cervical zone of the teeth are functions of microstructural orientation of the mineral and organic matrix.

8.1 Cervical Cemento-Dentinal Formation

During initial tooth formation, four layers of the enamel organ (the outer and inner enamel layers associated with the stellate reticulum and stratum intermedium) contribute to the construction of the crown. Building the limits of the coronal part of the tooth, the outer and inner enamel layers merge in the cervical zone and form the so-called epithelial Hertwig's root sheath. During the

M. Goldberg
University Paris Descartes, Sorbonne, Paris Cité and INSERM UMR-S1124, 45 rue des Saints Pères, Cedex 06, 75270 Paris, France
e-mail: mgoldod@gmail.com

M. Goldberg (ed.), *Understanding Dental Caries*, DOI 10.1007/978-3-319-30552-3_8

initial root shaping, the epithelial cells influence the recruitment and cytodifferentiation of pulp stem cells, which migrate from the neural crest toward the dental mesenchyme. Later, stem cells move from the central embryonic pulp toward the pulp periphery, where they differentiated into pre-odontoblasts, and then become polarizing odontoblasts. Odontoblasts initiate the synthesis and secretion of predentin, which represent an early stage of dentinogenesis. Predentin matures and some extracellular matrix components are added, contributing to dentin formation and mineralization. At this stage of crown formation, maturing enamel covers primary dentin.

Near the outer dentin surface, the inner layer of the Hertwig's epithelial sheath synthetizes and secretes an acellular afibrillar cementum covering the rudiments of the roots. As an alternative possibility, it was also reported that the cells issued from the dental sac or from the dental follicle migrate through the enlarged intercellular spaces. They migrate between the cells of the disintegrated Hertwig's sheath, cross through the periodontal ligament, and migrate toward the forming root, where they contribute to the acellular cervical cementum formation. At that stage, the initial root elongates but is not yet associated with tooth eruption. During primary eruption, the lengthening of the root occurs in close association with the onset of tooth development.

Therefore, the cervical region involves a complex imbrication of tissues and cells. In the cervical zone, at the enamel margin, two outer dentin layers are found. Depending on the species studied, the Tomes' granular layer and the Hopewell-Smith hyaline zone are involved. The structure formed is also named intermediate cementum layer. Either cementum covers the cemento-dentinal junction of human teeth, or enamel and dentin are contiguous, end-to-end, or there is a gap between enamel and cementum, the dentin outer layer being naked, uncovered by cementum.

According to some authors, the growth of enamel crystals starts from the underlying calcified dentin, promoting the formation of enamel crystals (Arsenault and Robinson 1989). An opposite point of view was developed by Diekwisch et al. (2001). They put emphasis on the fact that enamel crystal formation is totally independent from the dentin crystals. Enamel crystal formation starts near the DEJ; some distance away from the mineralizing dentin, but seem to be not associated to the formation of dentin crystals. These diverging views still need to be elucidated or reconciled, perhaps depending on the species examined (Diekwisch et al, 1995, Baldassarri et al. 2008, Weber et al. 1974, and Hayashi 1992).

8.2 Biomechanical Aspects of the Cervical Zone

8.2.1 Structural Aspects of Cervical Enamel and Dentin

8.2.1.1 Enamel

In the cervical region, the prisms appear to be directed horizontally, passing from the amelodentinal junction to the surface of the tooth, and covered by a thin aprismatic enamel layer. In a few cases, this enamel layer is partially covered in the cervical region by a thin border of aprismatic afibrillar cementum. The tissue nonspecific alkaline phosphatase (TNAP) and blood circulation act as a major source of osteopontin (VandenBos et al. 1999) and they regulate its formation (Fig. 8.1).

Non-carious cervical lesions refer to the loss of tooth structure at the cemento-enamel junction, and they are unrelated to bacterial action (see Chapter 2 of this book). Horizontal scratch marks are characteristics of the abrasion processes. Shallow, grooved, and wedge-shaped cervical lesions were identified. Corrosion induces a smoother appearance. Enamel displays a honeycomb structure, whereas dentin exhibits an undulating or rippled surface. In vitro study notes fracture and chipping of enamel in the cervical region (Nguyen et al. 2008). The AFM nanoindentation was used to probe the mechanical and tribological properties of enamel rods. Microhardness and elastic properties are significantly higher in the head region of the rod rather than in the tail region (Jeng et al. 2011).

Enamel, dentin, and cementum are coupled at the DEJ. The DEJ is a complex structure associating

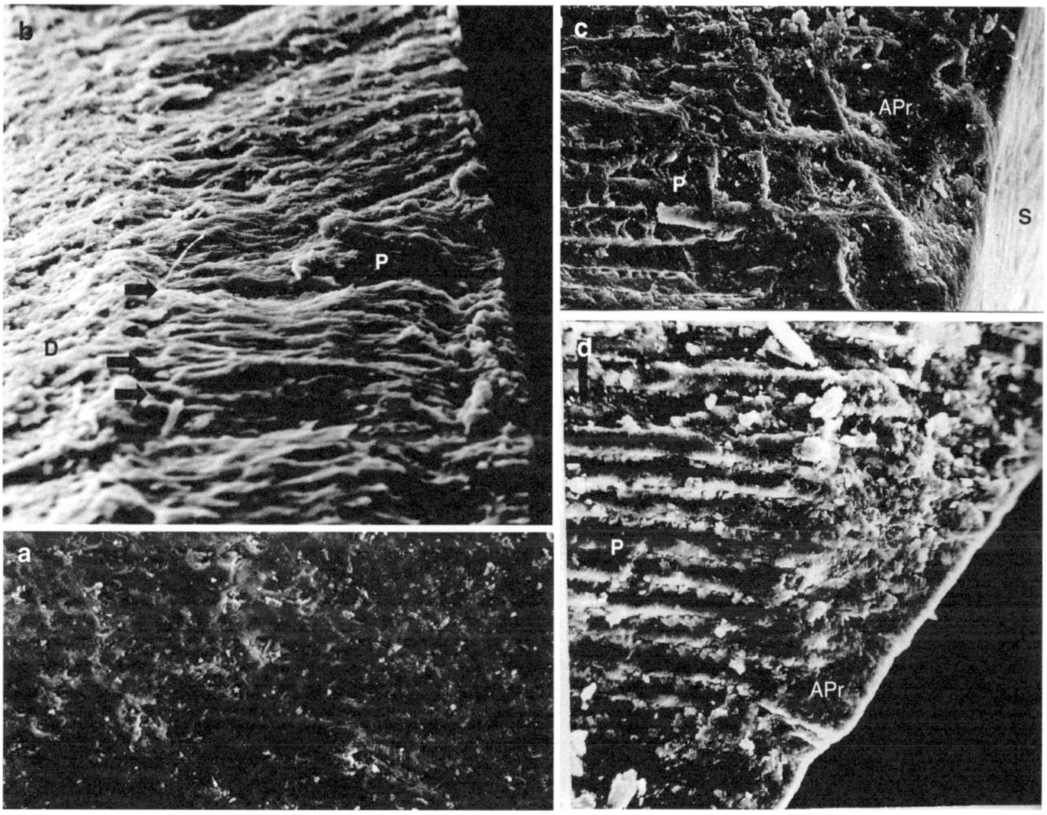

Fig. 8.1 (**a**) Enamel surface near the enamel-cementum junction. Prints or depressions of the proximal zone of ameloblasts form alignments (*asterisk*). (**b**) In the cervical zone, prisms (*P*) are aligned and parallel. The dentinoenamel junction (*black arrows*) separates the cervical enamel from dentin (*D*). In (**c**), the prismatic enamel (*P*) is covered by a thin layer of aprismatic enamel (*Apr*), ending at the enamel surface (*S*). In (**d**), in older enamel, the same distribution is visible

two calcified tissues, preventing the propagation of cracks from enamel to dentin. It is a scalloped structure with convexities toward dentin and concavities toward enamel (Shimizu & Macho 2007, Brauer et al. 2010, Beniash et al 2006) (Figs. 8.2 and 8.3).

8.2.1.2 Dentin

In the superficial part of the outer dentin, two different layers have been identified. The thin (8–15 μm thick) Tomes' granular layer is composed by calcospheritic (oval or round) structures. This zone contains a few minute tubules. The thin curved tubules are scarce and bent around the calcospheritic structures. Between the calcospherites, interglobular spaces are hypomineralized.

The subjacent layer (Hopewell-Smith hyaline layer, 8–15 μm thick) displays a small number of tubules. These tubules are straight, aligned, and at right angles to the tooth surface. The bulk of inner dentin, located around the dental pulp, is implicated in circumpulpal dentin formation. Usually, cells are alive and tubules are filled with odontoblast processes and their lateral branching. The zone of sclerotic dentin is thinner in these areas compared with normal dentin, and the changes occurring near the dentin surface are due to abrasion, abfraction, erosion, and wedge-shaped lesions. The carious decay contributes to the occlusion of the tubules by intratubular mineralizations (whitlockite crystallites, tricalcium phosphate) (Goldberg 2014; Tay and Pashley 2004) (Figs. 8.3 and 8.4).

AFM-based nanoindentations found the DEJ to only be 11.8 μm across. Micro-Raman indicated a DEJ width of 7.0 μm, while dynamic

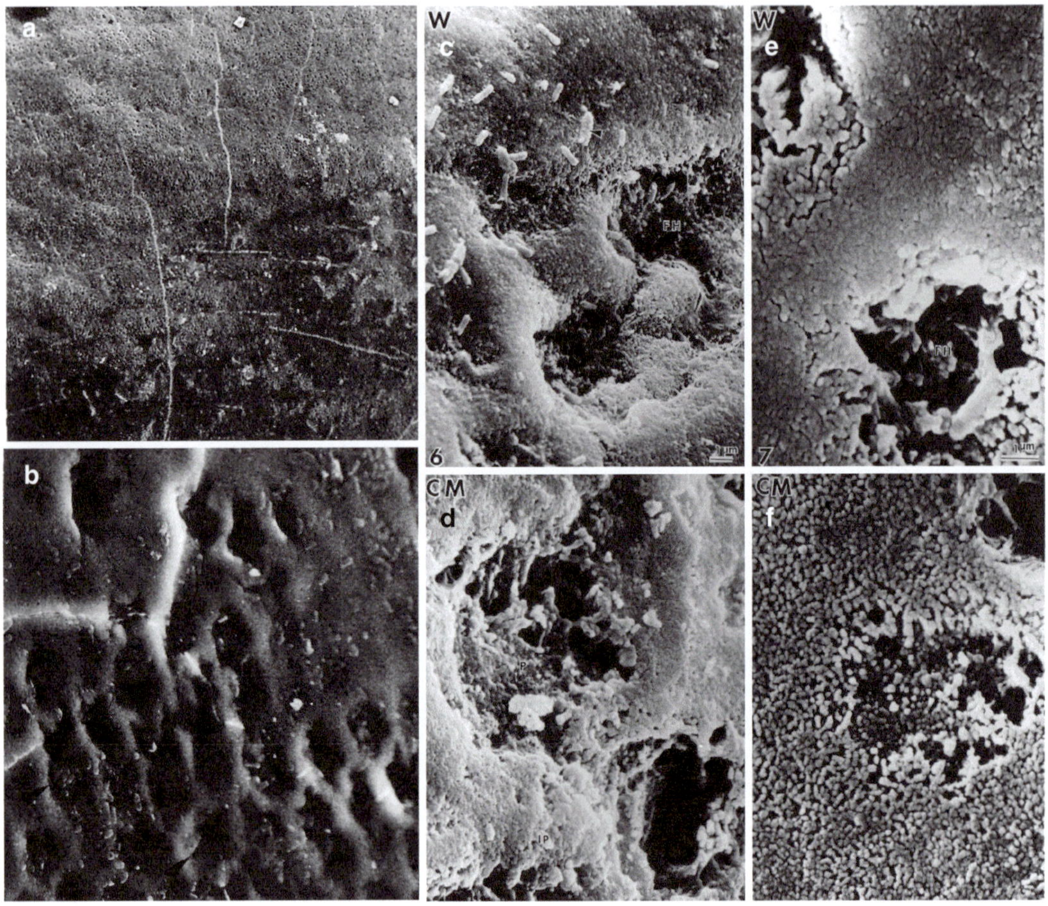

Fig. 8.2 (a) Water-treated enamel surface. (b) Enamel surface after water treatment. (c) Water treatment (d) enamel surface treated with chloroform-methanol. (e) Water treatment revealed the end of rods. (f) Chloroform-methanol treatment of enamel surface. The distal ending of rods displays large porosities, whereas in the interrod enamel, inter-crystallite porosities appear after the removal of extracellular lipids

modulus mapping indicated it was less than 1 μm across. The variations based on enamel-dentin phase intermixing suggest that DEJ is a biomimetic model for interfaces joining dissimilar materials (Marshall et al. 2003).

8.2.1.3 Cervical Lesions

Cracks generated in enamel stop at the DEJ, preventing catastrophic failure of the tooth. The major emerging question concerns the effects of organic matrix and water on the structural organization and how tooth microhardness and fracture toughness are affected. The removal of organic matrix resulted in 23 % increase in microhardness and 46 % decrease in fracture toughness. In contrast, water does not seem to influence these parameters. Moreover, the removal of organic matrix weakened the DEJ, leading to the formation of longer and more numerous cracks. Delamination of dentin and enamel along the DEJ suggests a strong physical bond between dentin and enamel crystals at the interface.

Retzius lines in the human cervical enamel display a staircase configuration. The Retzius lines have a curvilinear configuration, and

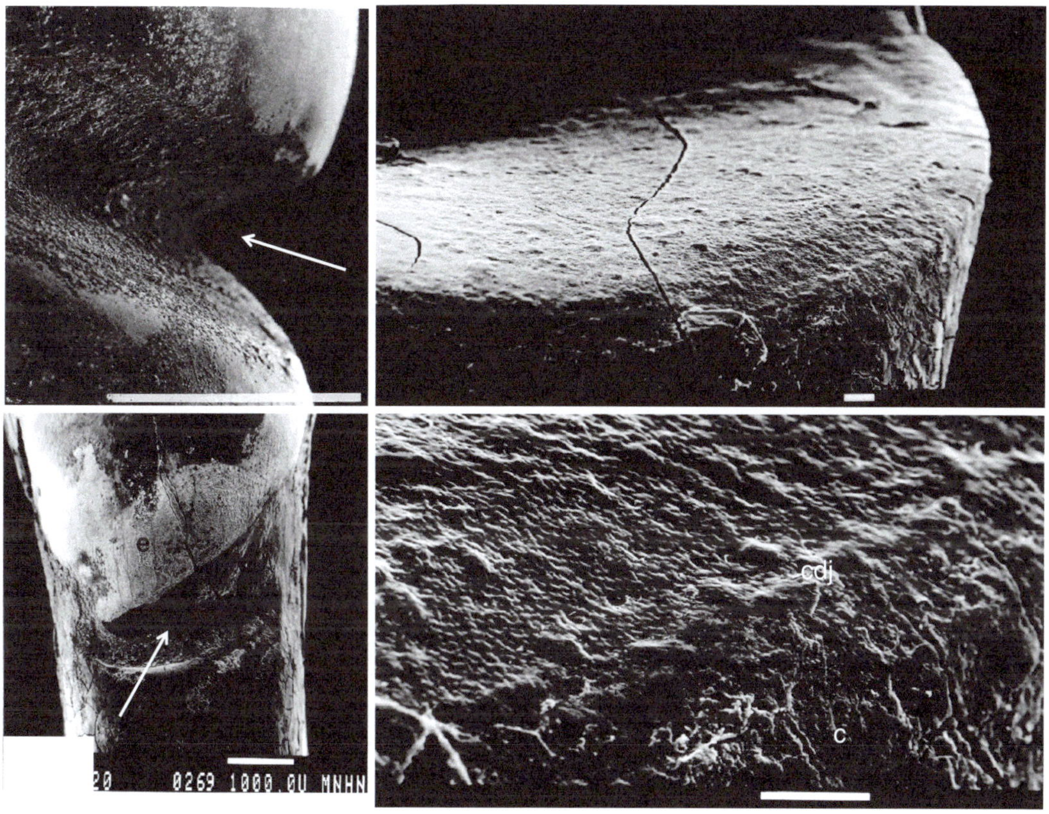

Fig. 8.3 Cervical erosion (*arrows*); *C* cementum, *cdj* cemento-dentinal junction

crystallites are deficient in composition. Finally, direct contact is occurring between lattice fringes of dentin and enamel crystals, fusion being observed between enamel and dentin crystals. The DEJ is weak in mechanical and/or chemical attacks (Fig. 8.3).

8.2.2 Mechanical and Tribological Properties of the DEJ

The DEJ is a complex structure and poorly defined, bridging enamel to the bulk dentin. This structure constitutes a biomimetic model of a structure uniting dissimilar materials. Cracks cannot traverse the DEJ and/or produce cracks in dentin. The fracture toughness values for enamel were evaluated as 0.6–0.9 MPa.m1/2 (Marshall et al. 2001) (Figs. 8.3 and 8.4).

Many reports suggest that abfraction lesion formation is caused by the physical overloading of enamel (Rees and Hammadeh 2004). In the crowns of human teeth, beneath enamel, a 200–300 μm zone of resilient (less mineralized and elastic) dentin has been found in the DEJ (Zaslansky et al. 2006). The strain distribution in the 200 μm thick zone in dentin beneath the DEJ is a structural adaptation for transferring and minimizing stress (Wang and Weiner 1997). Root dentin is highly anisotropic in fracture behavior. Coronal dentin has a typical brittle fracture behavior along peritubular dentin, and this should be taken into consideration that dentin is not homogeneous with respect to fracture properties (Wang 2005).

Peritubular dentin located at some distance from the DEJ gradually thickens with increasing depth in the bulk dentin. A significant reduced stiffness of

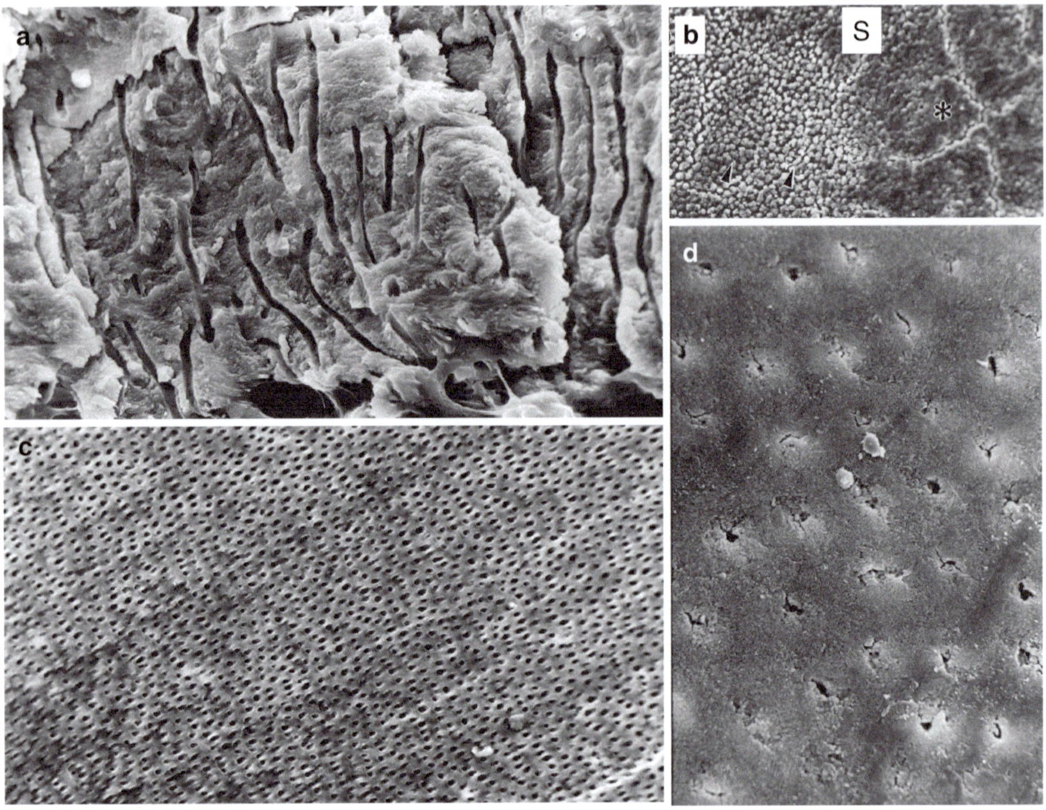

Fig. 8.4 (**a**) Outer globular Tomes' granular structure. (**b**) Cementum covering the root surface (*S*). *Left part of the figure*: acid-etched enamel. (**c**) Circumpulpal dentin. (**d**) Sclerotic dentin

the superficial zone has been reported compared to bulk dentin. In mid-buccal regions of teeth, the average was 3.5GPa, compared with the 9.7 GPa in the mid-lingual regions. It was concluded that the superficial layer behaves as a stress-relieving layer between enamel and bulk dentin.

Microhardness and elastic modulus are higher in the head region of enamel rods. They decrease from the enamel surface toward the DEJ. Head and tail area are questionable structures, and many ultrastructural studies deny the reality of this organization. The mechanical and nanotribological properties of enamel rods depend on HAp orientation inside each rod. The wear rate increases with an increasing distance from the outer enamel surface along the longitudinal axis of the enamel rod reaching the DEJ (Jeng et al. 2011).

The DEJ exhibits a scalloped appearance. The scalloped model has higher maximum tensile stresses than the straight model, but axial pressures would push the two tissue apart, leading to delamination of the DEJ during loading (mastication). There is a direct correlation between prism decussation and scallop magnitude. The scallops are linked with the response to high bite forces. *Exaptation* is used for a function other than what is developed by natural selection.

The posterior teeth showed larger scallops compared to anterior teeth. Molars subjected to higher masticatory loads showed larger and more pronounced scallops (Simmer et al. 2011; Ivancik et al. 2011).

8.2.3 Specific Composition of the DEJ

The enamel layer has a rich content in enamel proteins (amelogenins, enamelin, tuftelin, and other molecules). The proteins are characterized

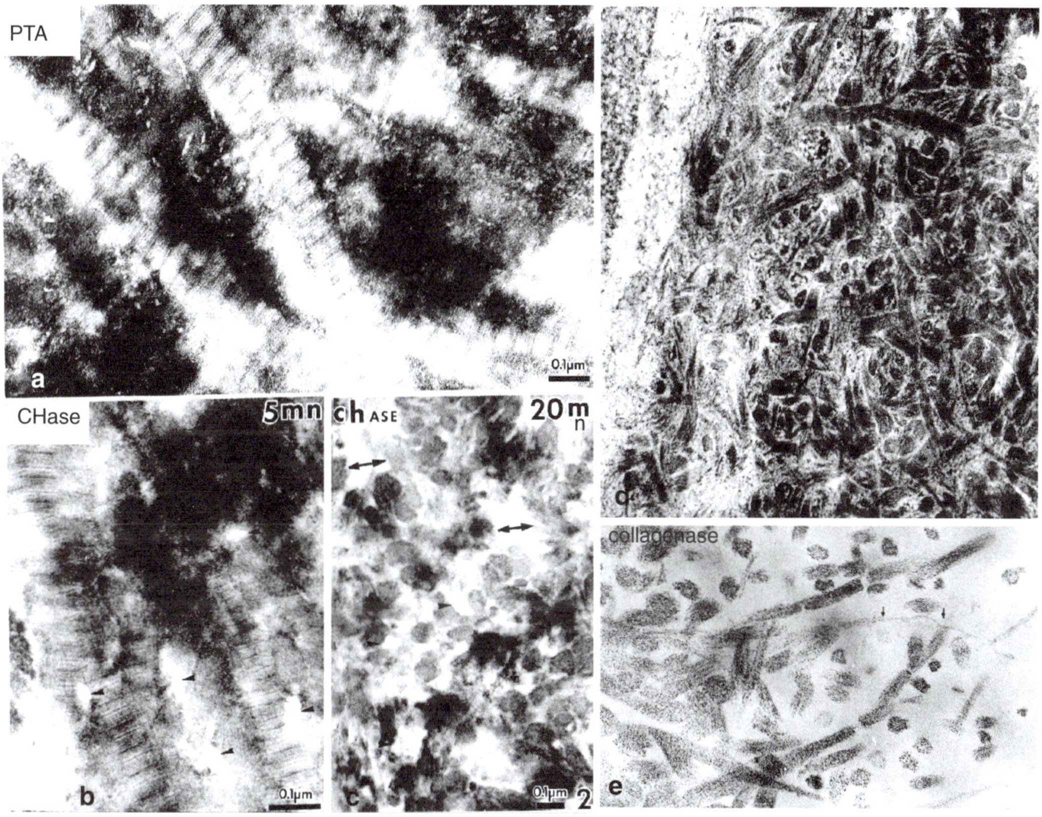

Fig. 8.5 (**a**) Phosphotungstic acid-stained circumpulpal dentin. At the surface of the collagen fibrils (characterized by their periodic banding), PTA (glycoprotein-stained) electro-dense underlines the collagen profile. Electro-dense staining is present in the intercollagen spaces. These phosphorylated glycoproteins (SIBLINGs) contribute to dentin mineralization. (**b, c**) Chondroitinase acting for 5 min (**b**) or 20 min (**c**) removes gradually intercollagen fibrils glycosaminoglycans, without destruction of the collagen fibrils. (**d**) In circumpulpal dentin, a dense network of collagen fibrils forms the intertubular dentin, whereas along the tubule (left part of the figure), collagen fibrils are less numerous and display less density. (**e**) Section treatment with a bacterial collagenase removes a large part of the collagen fibrils. Thin fibrils are cut in ¼ and ¾ (*small arrows*), contributing to gelatinase A and B formation

by the presence of high serine, glutamic acid, and glycine content. Components rich in proline and histidine are lost during enamel development and maturation (Glimcher et al. 1964).

These extracellular matrix proteins contribute to initiate the formation of the large and elongated enamel crystallites. By contrast, the ECM dentin molecules are composed by 90 % collagen, namely, type I collagen (Lin et al. 1993). The dentinoenamel junction is a fibril-reinforced bond, which is mineralized to a moderate degree.

Other types of collagen are scarce (type III and V collagens), but actually present. Deposition of dentin crystallites occurs (1) within the collagen gap regions (due to the quarter stagger structure of collagen fibrils), (2) along the collagen fibrils network, and (3) bridging inter-collagen spaces. The nucleation and crystal growth of dentin crystals are promoted and developed by a series of non-collagenous proteins, namely, phosphorylated proteins (SIBLINGs) (Fig. 8.5a, b). Five of them play crucial roles in the mineralization process: the dentin phosphoprotein, dentin matrix protein-1, bone sialoprotein, osteopontin, and MEPE.

Dentin sialoprotein and dentin phosphoprotein have distinct functions related to tooth formation and DEJ formation. Dentin proteins expressed by presecretory ameloblasts contribute to the unique properties of the dentinoenamel junction. These results support the notion that the dentin proteins expressed by presecretory ameloblasts contribute to the unique properties of the dentinoenamel junction (Paine et al. 2005).

Non-phosphorylated molecules such as γ-carboxyglutamic acid (GLA-rich, osteocalcin) are also found in the developing enamel proteins. They are inhibitors of mineralization.

Proteins issued from the serum, proteoglycans (small leucine-rich proteoglycans (SLRPs)), nucleating enzymes (tissue nonspecific alkaline phosphatases – TNAP), and a series of proteases (MMPs and ADAMs) act either as nucleators or inhibitors of dentin mineralization.

The dentinoenamel junction is not a simple inert interface between two mineralized structures. A less simplistic view suggests that the dentinoenamel junctional complex should also include the inner aprismatic enamel and the mantle dentin. At early stages of enamel formation, fibroblast growth factor (FGF)-2 is stored in and released from the inner aprismatic enamel, possibly under the control of matrix metalloproteinase (MMP)-3 (DenBesten et al. 1989). The concentration peak for MMP-2 and MMP-9 observed in the mantle dentin coincided with a very low labeling for TIMP-1 and TIMP-2 (Fig. 8.5e). This distribution favors the cross talk between mineralizing epithelial and connective structures and as a consequence the translocation of enamel proteins toward odontoblasts and pulp cells. Vice versa, it facilitates the translocation of dentin proteins toward secretory ameloblasts and cells of the enamel organ (Goldberg et al. 2002). Finally, in X-linked hypophosphatemic rickets, large interglobular spaces in the circumpulpal dentin were the major defect induced by the gene alteration, whereas the mantle dentin was constantly unaffected. Altogether, these data plead for the recognition of the dentinoenamel junctional complex as a specific entity bearing its own biological characteristics.

8.2.4 Enzymes

Host MMP-2 may be involved in caries progression and BSP in MMP-2 modulation. Enamelysin (MMP-20)-deficient mouse incisors display delamination of the enamel layer. At early stages of tooth morphogenesis of KO mice (MMP-20 KO mice), the mantle dentin is hypomineralized at the onset of enamel mineralization. Later no difference is found, so the mineralization of mantle dentin is simply postponed but not arrested.

A KLK4-null mouse has a normal thickness and pattern of enamel rods but contains residual enamel proteins. Enamel is less mineralized, and fractures are just above the DEJ. The breakage of enamel is apparently related to the progressive hypomineralization of enamel with depth.

The relationship between deep, middle, and peripheral coronal dentin supports that deep dentin exhibits significantly lower resistance to the initiation and growth of fatigue crack growth compared with the middle and peripheral dentin.

Different types of dentin are observed in human teeth. The primary dentin is formed before any occlusal contact. Secondary dentin is formed during the whole life and constitutes an answer to physiological aging. This dentin corresponds to the gradual narrowing of the pulp chamber. Sclerotic dentin and transparent dentin refer to tertiary dentin. These structures result from caries or irritation processes. Aging, abrasion, and diseases processes are implicated in what has been named reactionary dentin formation. In addition to the peripheral dentin layers (Tomes' granular layer and Hopewell-Smith hyaline layer), the circumpulpal dentin varies between the lingual and labial zones, where dentin is mostly tubular, and the mesial or distal pulp surfaces (proximal dentin surfaces) are mostly formed by fibrodentin structures (Fig. 8.5e).

8.2.5 Abfraction Lesion Formation

In order to understand the microfracture and deformation and the microcrack-microstructure interactions, the influence (effect) of enamel rod orientation was checked by propagating cracks in the occlusal surface. The cracks propagating toward the DEJ were arrested and unable to penetrate dentin. The mechanical properties of teeth are functions of microstructural orientations (Xu et al. 1998).

References

Arsenault AL, Robinson BW. The dentino-enamel junction: a structural and microanalytical study of early mineralization. Calcif Tissue Int. 1989;45:111–21.

Baldassarri M, Margolis HC, Beniash E. Compositional determinants of mechanical properties of enamel. J Dent Res. 2008;87:645–9.

Beniash E, Skobe Z, Bartlett JD. Formation of the dentino-enamel interface in Enamelysin (MMP-20)-deficient mouse incisors. Eur J Oral Sci. 2006;114 suppl 1:24–9.

Brauer DS, Marshall GW, Marshall SJ. Variations in human DEJ scallop size with tooth type. J Dent. 2010;38:597–601.

Cuy J, Mann AB, Livi KJ, Teaford MF, Welhs TP. Nanoindentation mapping of the mechanical properties of human molar tooth enamel. Arch Oral Biol. 2002;47:281–91.

DenBesten PK, Heffernan LM, Treadwell BV, Awbrey BJ. The presence and possible functions of the matrix metalloproteinase collagenase activator protein in developing enamel matrix. Biochem J. 1989;264:917–20.

Diekwisch TG. The developmental biology of cementum. Int J Dev Biol. 2001;45(5–6):695–706.

Diekwisch TGH, Berman BJ, Gentner S, Slavkin HC. Initial enamel crystals are not spatially associated with mineralized dentine. Cell Tissue Res. 1995;279:149–67.

Glimcher MJ, Friberg UA, Levine PT. The isolation and amino acid composition of the enamel proteins of erupted bovine teeth. Biochem J. 1964;93:202–10.

Goldberg M. Pulp anatomy and characterization of pulp cells. The dental pulp; chapter 2. Springer; Heidelberg 2014.

Goldberg M, Septier D, Bourd K, Hall R, Jeanny J-C, Jonet L, Colin S, Tager T, Chaussain-Miller C, Garabédian M, George A, Goldberg H, Menashi S. The dentino-enamel junction revisited. Connect Tissue Res. 2002;43:482–9.

Hayashi Y. High resolution electron microscopy in dentino-enamel junction. J Electron Microsc (Tokyo). 1992;41:387–91.

He LH, Swani MV. Enamel – a "metallic-like" deformable biocomposite. J Dent. 2007;35:431–7.

Imbeni V, Kruzic JJ, Marshall GW, Marshall SJ, Ritchie RQ. The dentin-enamel junction and the fracture of human teeth. Nat Mater. 2005;4:229–32.

Ivancik J, Neerchal NK, Romberg E, Arola D. The reduction of fatigue crack growth resistance of dentin with depth. J Dent Res. 2011;90:1031–6.

Jeng Y-R, Lin T-T, Hsu H-M, Chang H-J, Shieh D-B. Human enamel rod present anisotropic nanotribological properties. J Mech Behav Biomed Mater. 2011;4:515–22.

Lin CP, Douglas WH, Erlandsen SL. Scanning electron microscopy of type I collagen at the dentin-enamel junction of human teeth. J Histochem Cytochem. 1993;41:381–8.

Marshall GW, Balooch M, Gallagher RR, Gansky SA, Marshall SJ. Mechanical properties of the dentinoenamel junction: AFM studies and microhardness, elastic modulus, and fracture. J Biomed Mater Res. 2001;54:87–95.

Marshall SJ, Balooch M, Habelitz S, Balooch G, Gallagher R, Marshall GW. The dentin-enamel junction- a natural, multilevel interface. J Eur Ceramic Soc. 2003;23: 2897–904.

Nguyen C, Ranjitkar S, Kaidonis JA, Townsend GC. A quantitative assessment of non-carious cervical lesions in extracted human teeth. Aust Dent J. 2008;53:46–51.

Paine ML, Luo W, Wang H-J, Bringas Jr P, Ngan AYW, Miklus VG, Zhu D-H, MacDougall M, White SN, Snead ML. Dentin sialoprotein and dentin phosphoprotein overexpression during amelogenesis. J Biol Chem. 2005;36:31991–8.

Rees JS, Hammadeh M. Undermining of enamel as a mechanism of abfraction lesion formation: a finite element study. Eur J Oral Sci. 2004;112:347–52.

Shimizu D, Macho GA. Functional significance of the microstructural detail of the primate dentino-enamel junction: a possible example of exaptation. J Hum Evol. 2007;52:103–11.

Simmer JP, Hu Y, Richerdson AS, Bartlett JD, Hu J. C-C. Why does enamel in KLK4-null mice break above the dentino-enamel junction? Cells. Tissues Organs. 2011;194:211–5.

Tay FR, Pashley DH. Resin bonding to cervical sclerotic dentin: a review. J Dent. 2004;32:173–96.

Vandenbos T, Bronkers ALJJ, Goldberg HA, Beertsen W. Blood circulation as source for osteopontin in acellular extrinsic fiber cementum and other mineralizing tissues. J Dent Res. 1999;78:1688–95.

Wang R. Anisotropic fracture in bovine root and coronal dentin. Dent Mater. 2005;21:429–36.

Wang RZ, Weiner S. Strain-structure relations in human teeth using Moiré fringes. J Biomechanics. 1997;31: 135–41.

Weber DF, Eisenmann DR, Glick PL. Light and electron microscopic studies of Retzius lines in human cervical enamel. Am J Anat. 1974;141:91–103.

Xu HH, Smith DT, Jahanmir S, Romberg E, Kelly JR, Thompson VP, Rekow ED. Indentation damage and mechanical properties of human enamel and dentin. J Dent Res. 1998;77:472–80.

Zaslansky P, Friesem AA, Weiner S. Structure and mechanical properties of the soft zone separating bulk dentin and enamel in crowns of human teeth: insight into tooth function. J Struct Biol. 2006;153:188–99.

Superficial and Deep Carious Lesions

9

Michel Goldberg

Abstract

Carious lesions start at the dentin surface and are oriented toward deeper regions. Their evolution is rapid or slow. They may be active or arrested, depending on the food intake, the oral mouth hygiene, and nature of the dental plaque. Near the dentinoenamel junction (DEJ), tubules filled with bacteria spread along the enlarged DEJ and start to destroy the mantle dentin. In the coronal part, the carious decay degrades the mantle dentin. In the root, in contrast, the two outer layers (the Hopewell-Smith hyaline and Tomes' granular layers) are corroded by bacteria diffusing acids and/or toxic components along the dentin canaliculi. Differences in invasion are due to the number and diameter of dentin tubules, which interfere with the diffusion of the carious lesion (active or arrested lesions). Tubule density and diameter expand from the surface to the middle dentin and reach the maximum diameter near the inner pulp. The wounded odontoblasts and the cells of the so-called Hoehl's layer beneath the calcio-traumatic line form reactionary dentin. This dentin is similar to the tubular or atubular dentin (similar to orthodentin, but sometimes osteodentin-like formation). Reparative dentine results from the differentiation and secretion of mesenchymal stem cells taking origin among pulp cells (atubular, osteodentin-like structures). Calcospherite (or lamellar pulp stones) structures formed within the pulp are in continuity with the blood vessels, or they may be isolated structures within the dental pulp.

9.1 Different Types of Carious Lesion

In human dentin, carious decay may be *rapidly progressing lesions*, also named active (infected), or *slowly progressing lesions* (arrested lesions) (Bjørndal 2002). In active lesions, dentin appears light yellowish brown, with a soft surface layer.

M. Goldberg
University Paris Descartes, Sorbonne, Paris Cité and INSERM UMR-S1124, 45 rue des Saints Pères, Cedex 06, 75270 Paris, France
e-mail: mgoldod@gmail.com

M. Goldberg (ed.), *Understanding Dental Caries*, DOI 10.1007/978-3-319-30552-3_9

Carious dentin may be arrested (deep brownish-black pigmentation). The degenerative changes interfere mostly with the sclerotic intracanalicular obliterations, combined with a bacteria-free zone. The possibility of a mixed lesion has also to be considered (Sarnat and Massler 1965).

The first dentin layer encountered in the crown is the mantle dentin. This layer is formed at early stages of coronal development. The backward movement of secretory ameloblasts leads to the formation of the aprismatic inner layer. The first 8–15 μm of the mantle dentin displays a small number of tubules. They are bent and thin, with lateral branchings. In some cases, they display calcospheritic configurations. Alcian blue staining reveals the existence of glycosaminoglycans, bound to proteins and therefore organized as proteoglycans (decorin, biglycan, fibromodulin, etc.). Along the dentinoenamel junction, a thin layer revealed by autometallography (0.5–0.8 μm wide, positively stained by cuprolinic blue) separated the two mineralized structures (Lormée et al. 1989). Therefore, diffusion and degradation of proteoglycans occur along the DEJ and enlarge the thin fissure between the inner enamel and dentin surface. After the occurrence of a limited destruction, (1) the initial carious lesion spreads laterally and (2) degrades the dentin surface, burying bacteria in the depth of the dentin through the lumen of the tubules, centripetally (Figs. 9.1, 9.2, 9.3, 9.4, and 9.5).

Caries may be superficial, located near the dentinoenamel junction (peripheral excavated and hard dentin), or located in the middle of the dentin layer (central demineralized dentin before the final excavation), or located in the inner part, near the pulp (central dentin after the final excavation) (Bjørndal et al. 1997). Therefore the lesion can be either superficial or degrade the deepest part of the coronal dentin. The density of

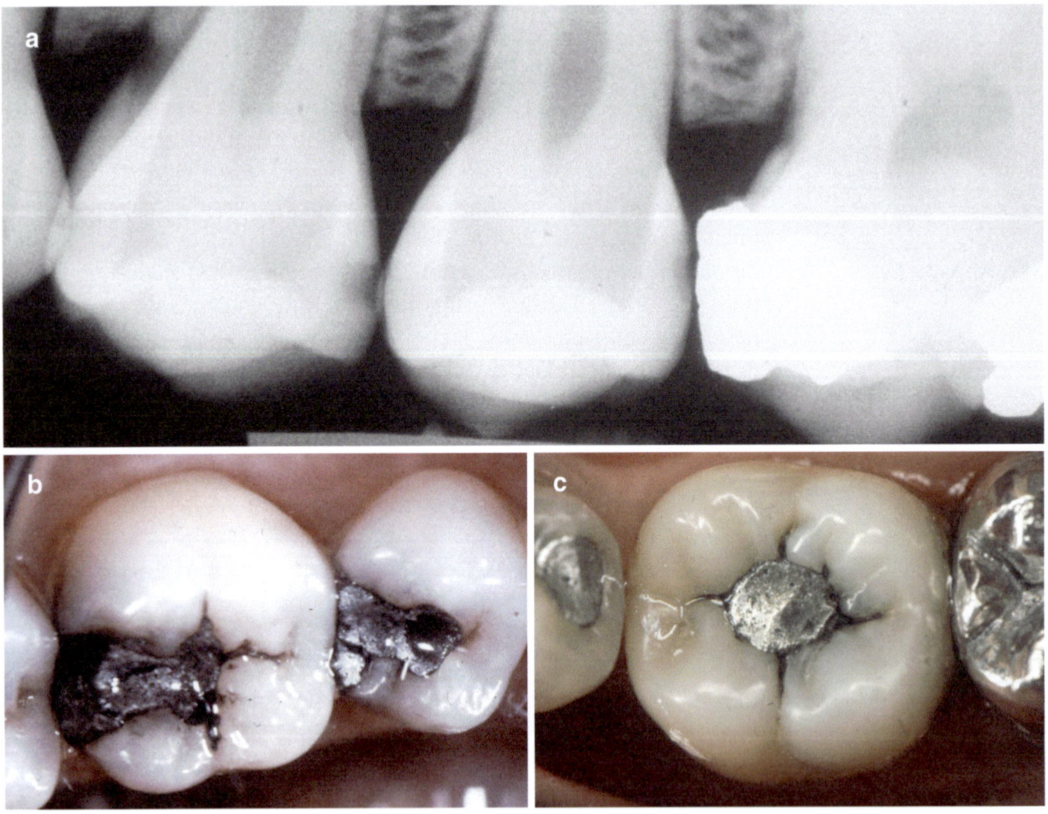

Fig. 9.1 (**a**) An X-ray figure showing proximal cavities in premolars. (**b**) An old silver amalgam restoration and fissures. (**c**) Occlusal restoration with caries-infiltrated fissures

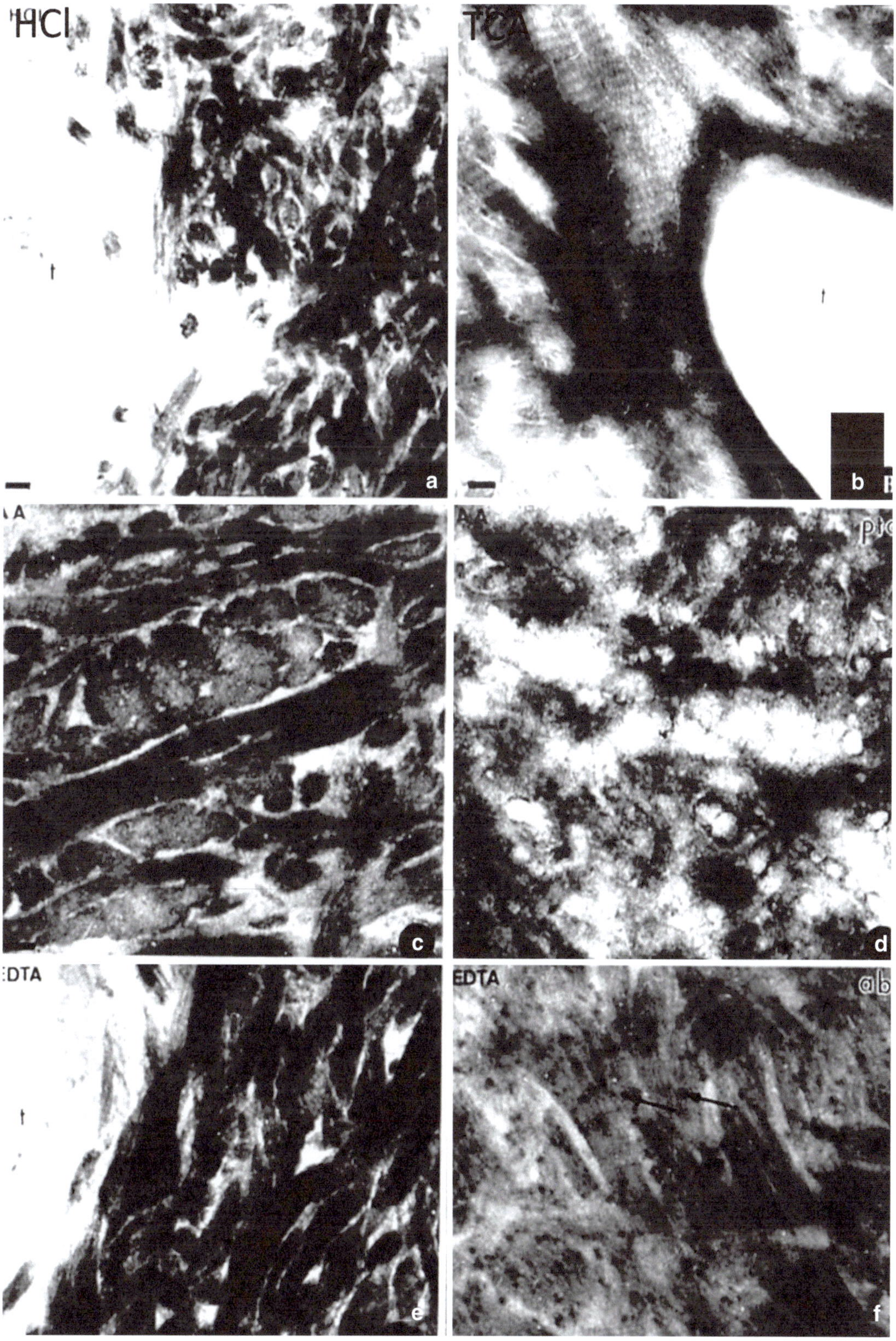

Fig. 9.2 After acid or chelator demineralization, intercollagenous spaces are widely open. After hydrochloric acid (*HCl*) (**a**), trichloroacetic acid (*TCA*) (**b**), acetic acid (*AA*) (**c, d**), or ethylendiamine tertracetic acid (*EDTA*) (**e**, **f**) demineralization, intercollagenous spaces are widely open

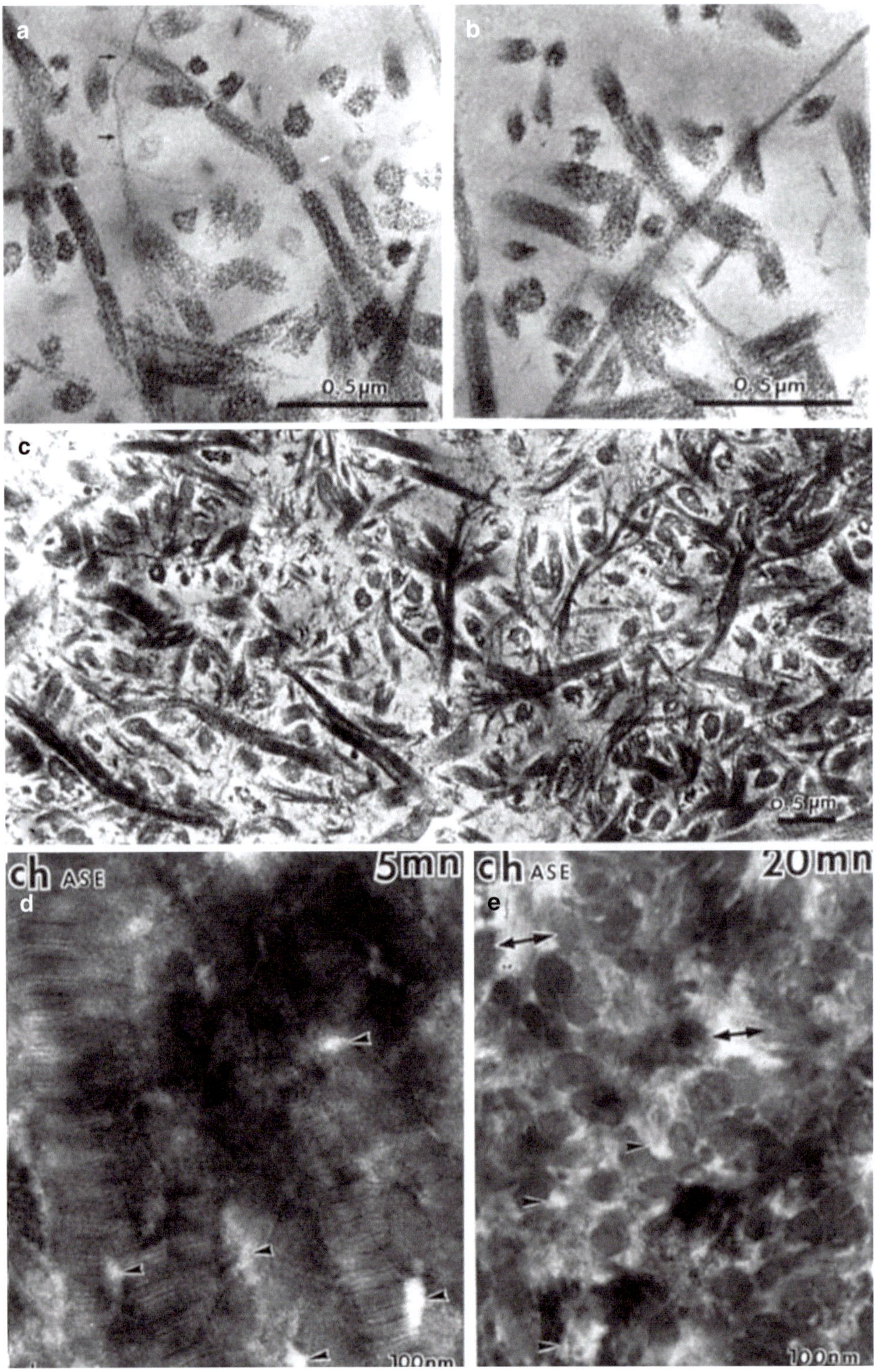

Fig. 9.3 (**a–c**) Collagen is broken in ¼ and ¾ peptides after action of a bacterial collagenase. (**d**, **e**) Effects of a chondroitinase A–C after 5 min (**d**) and 20 min (**e**). *Arrows*: collagen fibrils. *Arrowheads* and *double headed arrows*: intercollagen spaces enlarged after 20 min digestion by the enzyme

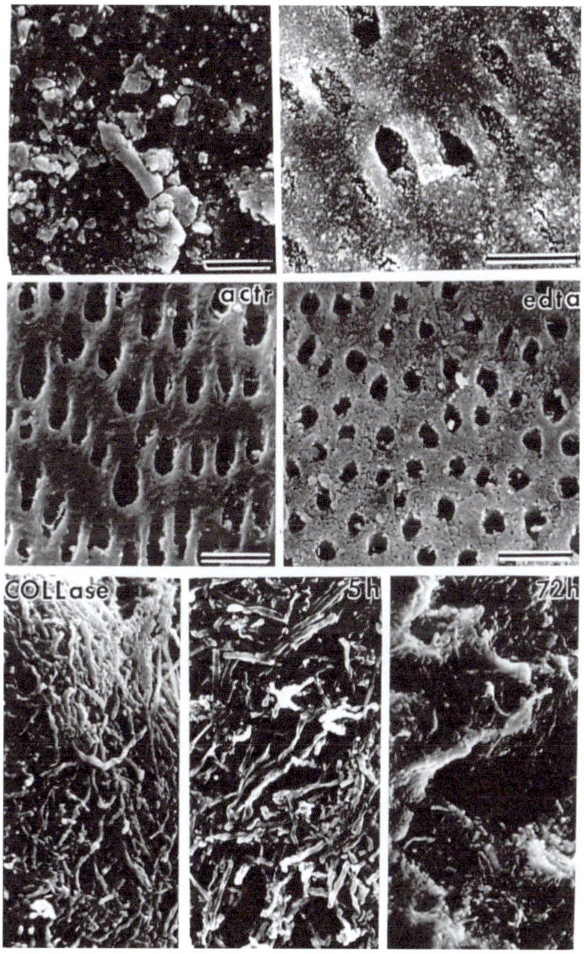

Fig. 9.4 Outer surface cleaning by orthophosphoric acid (*upper figures*), citric acid, and EDTA. *Lower figures*: action of a bacterial collagenase on carious dentin

the tubules (number of tubules/mm^2) and/or their diameter appears to be correlated to this anatomical distribution. The pulp chamber ceiling presents the higher tubule density. The rate of development of carious lesions is due, in part, to their tubule density; a high density implicates a rapid spread (Figs. 9.2, 9.3, and 9.4).

Tubule density in the middle layer of the crown was 18.243 ± 3.845 in human deciduous vs. human permanent dentin. In the deep layer, the mean value was 24.162 ± 5. 338. In the permanent dentin, the number of tubules per mm^2 was 21.343 ± 7.290 in the deep layer and 18.781 ± 5.855 in the middle layer (Schilke et al. 2000). Variations of tubule density have been noticed. It comes out that in the superficial dentin, the tubule density appears to be 17.433 ± 1.370, in the outer dentin 18.075 ± 2.415, in the intermediate layer 20.433 ± 2.568, and in the deep dentin 26.391 ± 6.605 (Koutsi et al. 1994). The mean numbers of tubules at any given age within coronal, cervical, and mid-rot dentin are quite similar (approximately 44.243, 42.360, and 39.010 mm^2, respectively) (Carrigan et al. 1984). However, significantly fewer dentinal tubules are found in apical dentin (approximately 8.190 mm^2). Differences reported between publications were striking, with a variation of 40.000–51.000

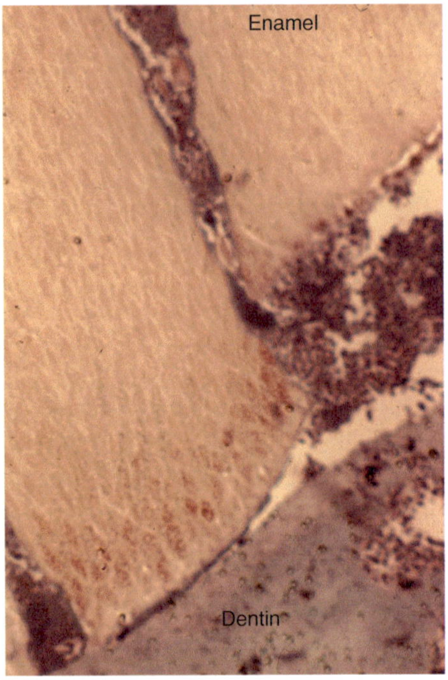

Fig. 9.5 Carious lesion penetrating up to the dentinoenamel junction (*DEJ*). This is followed by a lateral diffusion of bacteria destroying the superficial mantle dentin

tubules per mm^2. The number of dentinal tubules per mm^2 varies from 15.000 µm at the dentinoenamel junction to 45.000 µm near the pulp (Garberoglio and Brännström 1976). In general, the tubule density increases in relation with the dentin depth.

The diameter of the tubules was seen to vary depending the species and the location in space and time. In young people, the pulp chamber floor presents high tubule diameter, with a dimension of dentinal tubule openings decreasing with age (Kontakiotis et al. 2015). In deciduous dentin, the diameter of the tubules varied between the deep layer (2.82±0.28) and middle layer (2.55±0.16). In permanent dentin, the diameter varied between the deep layer (2.90±0.22) and the middle layer (2.65±0.19) (Schilke et al. 2000). The tubule diameter varies between the superficial 0.96, outer 1.08, intermediate 1.10, and deep layers 1.29 (Koutsi et al. 1994). The tubule diameter increases together with the dentin depth.

Human carious lesions imply collagen degradation. This is under the control of members of the metalloproteinase family (MMP-1, MMP-2, MMP-8, MMP-13, and MMP-14), human neutrophil elastase, and cysteine proteinases. MMP-2 and MMP-9, also named gelatinases A and B, cut the collagen fibers into two parts (1/4th and 3/4th) fragments. MMP-2 and MMP-9 can remove telopeptides from the ends of helical collagen, but only MMP-8 is a true collagenase that can cleave the collagen in 2 large fragments. Cathepsin K cleaves both helical and telopeptide regions. Expression in sound, caries-affected and caries-infected dentin. Cysteine cathepsins degrade type I collagen, laminin, fibronectin, and proteoglycans. Cathepsins B and L cleave the non-helical telopeptide extensions of collagens, whereas cathepsin K cleaves the collagen at the triple helical region. Caries stimulates MMP-2 expression in sound, caries-affected and caries-infected dentin. Cysteine cathepsins degrade

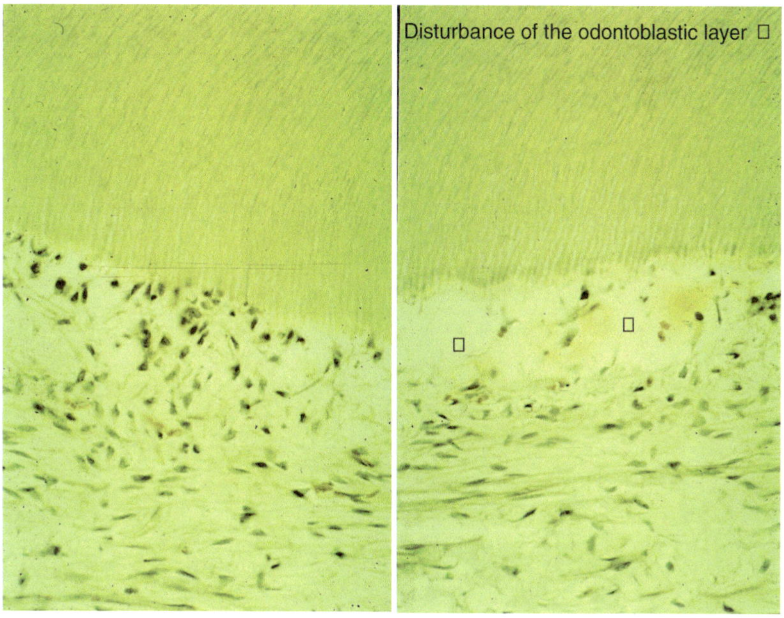

Fig. 9.6 Carious lesion: early disturbance on the odontoblastic layer

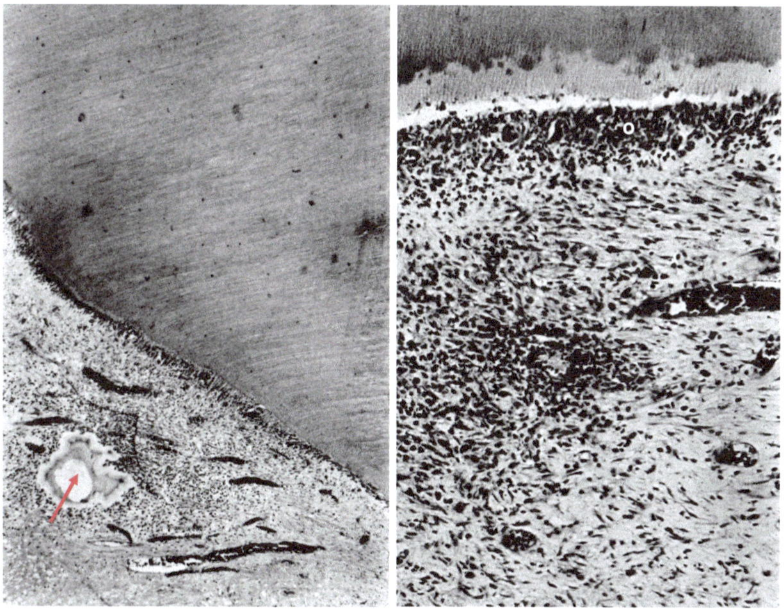

Fig. 9.7 Pulp lesion and accumulation of apoptotic cells beneath the carious lesion. *Red arrow*: empty space after local lysis in a pulp area

type I collagen, laminin, fibronectin, and proteoglycans. Cathepsins B and L cleave the non-helical telopeptides extensions of collagens, whereas cathepsin K cleaves the collagen at the triple helical region (Nascimento et al. 2011).

Dentin lesions may be classified in superficial lesion (depth up to 2–3 mm), deep lesion (depth up to 3–5 mm), and deep lesions (with pulp exposure) (Figs. 9.6, 9.7, 9.8, 9.9, and 9.10).

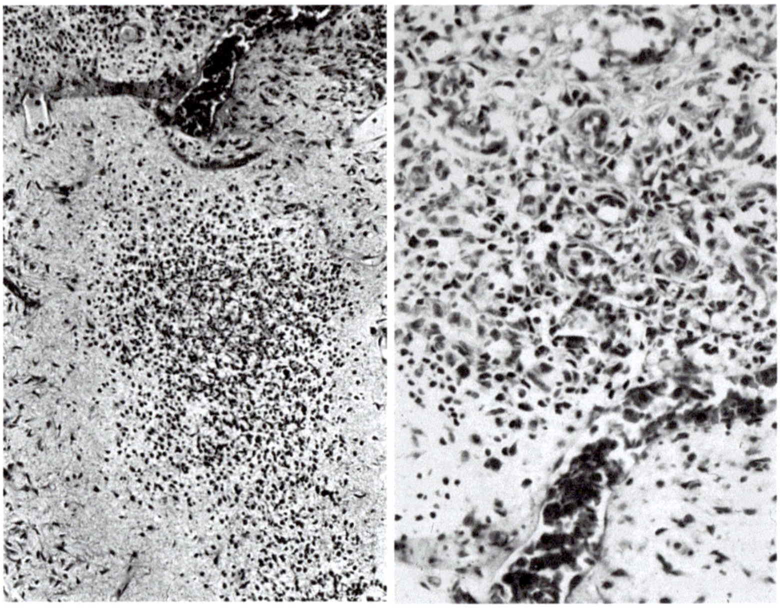

Fig. 9.8 Pulp apoptotic cells

Visualization of bacterial penetration by the Brown et Brenn's staining method.

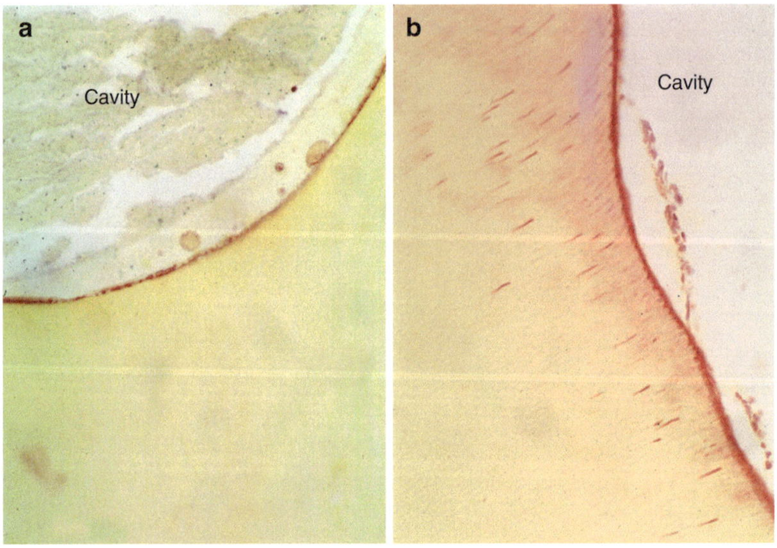

Fig. 9.9 (**a**) Dentin tubules beneath the cavity, (**b**) tubules invaded by bacteria in the bottom of a cavity

Dentin discs are divided into young and old, superficial and deep surfaces that display significant variations. It is quite different if it is an active carious process or not. Initial caries results from ion exchanges in both directions across the tooth surface. There is a continuous loss of mineral from the dental tissues, with a daily battle between progression and regression. Cavitation develops in 3–4 years.

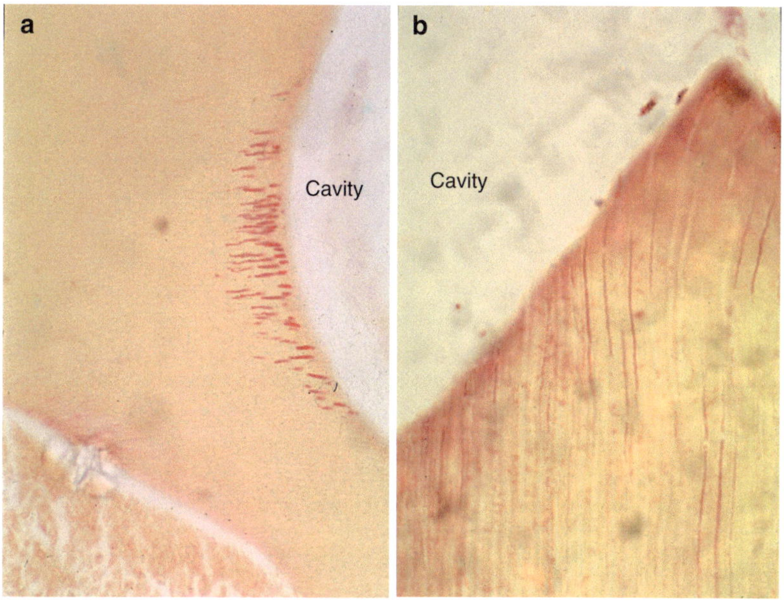

Fig. 9.10 (**a**) Dentinal tubules partially filled by bacteria; (**b**) invaded tubules

9.2 Reactionary and Reparative Dentin Formation

The formation of *reactionary dentin* accompanies the increased density of DSP, with a regular spatial distribution. DSP contribute to HAp nucleation on putative sites on the collagen scaffold. In response to bacterial invasion, there is also an increased activity of MMP-2, an upregulation of tissue inhibitor of metalloproteinase-2 (TIMP-2) and membrane type-1 matrix metalloproteinase (MT1-MMP). Next, modulation of odontoblastic dentinogenic enzyme repertoire was evidenced. In the odontoblast layer expression of Toll-like receptors was markedly altered in response to bacterial invasion. In carious teeth, TLR-2 and the gene encoding the corresponding adaptor protein MyD88 were downregulated, whereas genes encoding TLR-4 and adaptor proteins TRAM and Mal/TIRAP were upregulated. TLR-4 signaling mediated by binding of bacterial products has been linked to upregulation of MMP-2. Further, increased expression of genes encoding components of the TGF-β signaling pathway, namely, SMAD-2 and SMAD-4, may explain an increased synthesis of collagen by odontoblasts in caries (Charadram et al. 2012).

Reparative dentin (or tertiary dentinogenesis), also reported as atubular/fibrodentinogenesis, named in some publications fibrodentin/reparative dentinogenesis, is a slowly progressing lesion, strictly tubular (Bjørndal 2001). The formation of reparative dentin (tertiary dentin) is due to the precipitation of intratubular calcifications, the deposition of peritubular dentine, and the formation of tertiary dentine. This cascade of events depends on whether the dentine has been secreted by preexisting primary odontoblasts (reactionary dentin) or by newly differentiated secretory cells (reparative dentin), which have migrated to the region following death of primary odontoblasts. Collagen forms the bulk of reparative dentin. Non-collagenous proteins of the ECM play important roles in cytodifferentiation, secretion of ECM, and its mineralization. ECM and growth factors such as dentin phosphoproteins, dentin sialoprotein, TGFβ, insulin-like growth factor, fibroblast growth factor, and platelet-derived growth factor are synthetized and released by mesenchymal pulp cells (Sangwan et al. 2012) (Figs. 9.11, 9.12, 9.13, 9.14, 9.15, 9.16, and 9.17).

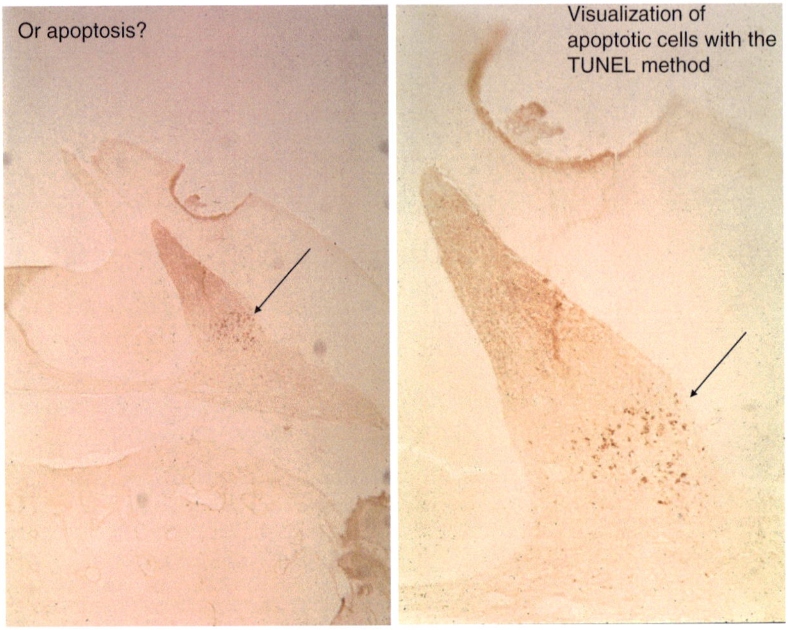

Fig. 9.11 Visualization of apopotic cells within the dental pulp using the TUNEL method. *Arrows*: Apoptotic pulp cells

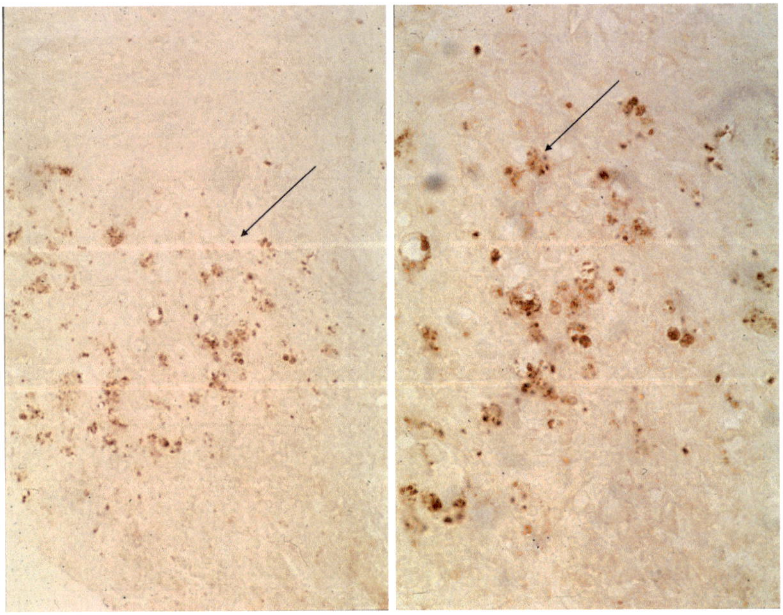

Fig. 9.12 Apoptotic pulp cells: TUNEL staining. *Arrows*: Apoptotic pulp cells

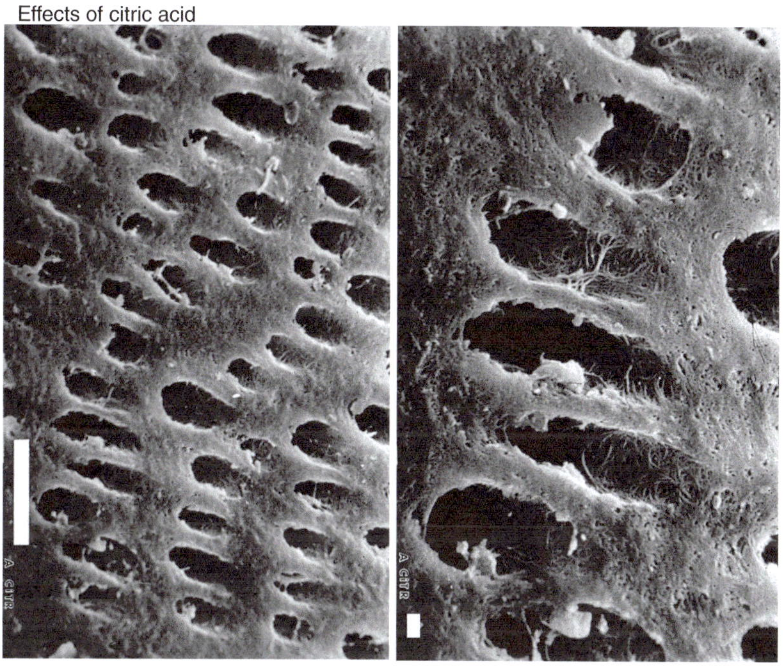

Fig. 9.13 Effects of citric acid on dentin slice

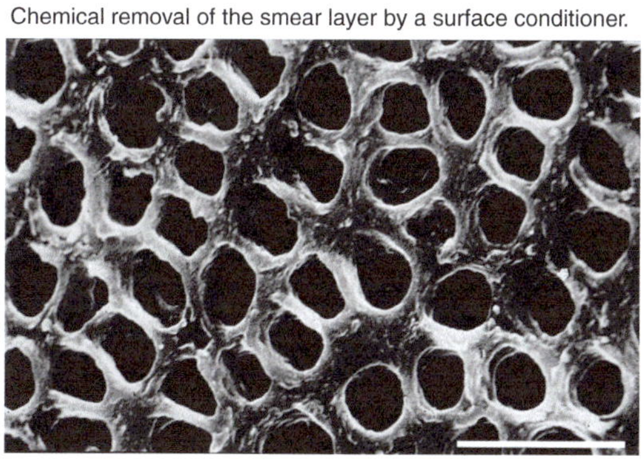

Fig. 9.14 Suppression of the smear layer after a surface conditioner

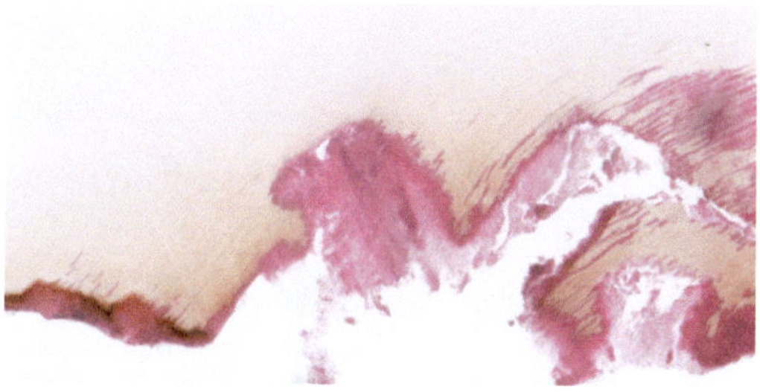

Fig. 9.15 Cervical carious lesion

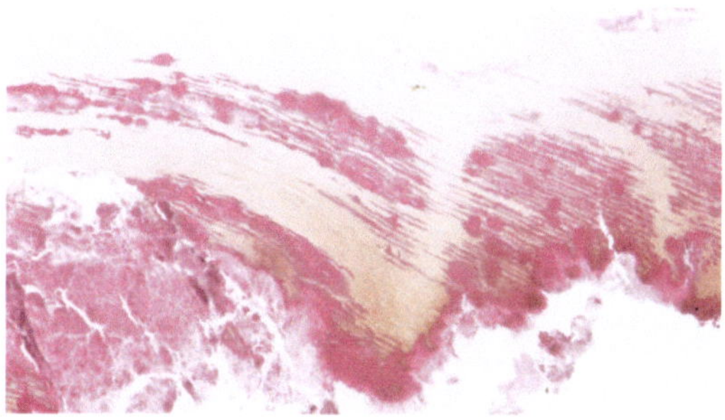

Fig. 9.16 Cervical carious lesion. Dentinal tubules are invaded by bacteria

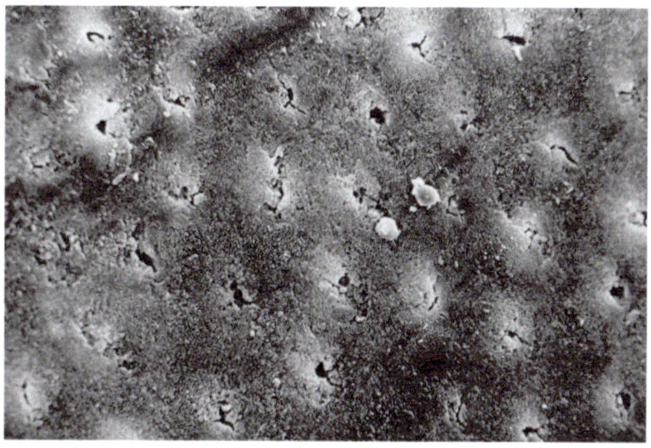

Fig. 9.17 Cleaned sclerotic dentin

References

Bjørndal L. Presence or absence of tertiary dentinogenesis in relation to caries progression. Adv Dent Res. 2001;15:80–3.

Bjørndal L. Dentin and pulp reactions to caries and operative treatment: biological variables affecting treatment outcome. Endodontic Topics. 2002;2:10–23.

Bjørndal L, Larsen T, Thylstrup A. A clinical and microbiological study of deep carious lesions during stepwise excavation using long treatment intervals. Caries Res. 1997;31:411–7.

Carrigan P, Morse JDR, Furst ML, Sinai IH. A scanning electron microscope evaluation of human dentinal tubules according to age and location. J Endod. 1984;10:359–63.

Charadram N, Farahani RM, Harty D, Rathsam C, Swain MV, Hunter N. Regulation of reactionary dentin formation by odontoblasts in response to polymicrobial invasion of dentin matrix. Bone. 2012;50: 265–75.

Garberoglio R, Brännström M. Scanning electron microscopic investigation of human dentinal tubules. Arch Oral Biol. 1976;21:355–62.

Kontakiotis EG, Tsatsoulis IN, Filippatos CG, Agrafioti A. A quantitative and symmetrical analysis of human dentinal tubules at pulp chamber ceiling and floor under scanning electron microscopy. Aust Endod J. 2015;41(1):29–34.

Koutsi V, Noonan RG, Horner JA, Simpson MD, Matthews WG, Pashley DH. The effect of dentin depth on the permeability and ultrastructure of primary molars. Pediatr Dent. 1994;16:29–35.

Lormée P, Lécolle S, Septier D, Le Denmat D, Goldberg M. Autometallography for histochemical visualization of rat polyanions with cuprolinic blue. J Histochem Cytochem. 1989;37:203–8.

Nascimento FD, Minciotti CL, Geraldeli S, Carrilho MR, Pashley DH, Tay FR, Nader HB, Salo T, Tjäderhane L, Tersariol IL. Cysteine cathepsins in human carious dentin. J Dent Res. 2011;90:506–11.

Sangwan P, Sangwan A, Duhan J, Rohilla A. Tertiary dentinogenesis with calcium hydroxide: a review of proposed mechanisms. Int Endod J. 2012;46:3–19.

Sarnat H, Massler M. Microstructure of active and arrested dentinal caries. J Dent Res. 1965;44:1389–401.

Schilke R, Lisson JA, Bauss O, Geurtsen W. Comparison of the number and diameter of dentinal tubules in human and bovine dentine by scanning electron microscopic investigation. Arch Oral Biol. 2000;45:355–61.

Cervical Sclerotic Dentin: Resin Bonding

10

Franklin R. Tay, Manar Abu Nawareg, Dalia Abuelenain, and David H. Pashley

Abstract

Many reports have indicated that resin bond strengths to noncarious sclerotic cervical dentin are lower than bonds made to normal dentin. This is thought to be due to tubule occlusion by acid-resistant mineral salts, preventing resin tag formation following acid etching. The purpose of this review was to critically examine what is known about the structure of this type of dentin. Recent transmission electron microscopy revealed that in addition to occlusion of the tubules by mineral crystals, many parts of wedge-shaped cervical lesions contain a hypermineralized surface that resists the etching action of both self-etching primers and phosphoric acid. This layer prevents hybridization of the underlying sclerotic dentin. In addition, bacteria are often detected on top of the hypermineralized layer. Sometimes the bacteria were embedded in a partially mineralized matrix. Acidic conditioners and resins penetrate variable distances into these multilayered structures. Examination of both sides of the failed bonds revealed a wide variation in fracture patterns that involved all of these structures. Microtensile bond strengths to the occlusal, gingival, and deepest portions of these wedge-shaped lesions are significantly lower than similar areas artificially prepared in normal teeth. When resin bonds to sclerotic dentin are extended to include peripheral sound dentin, their bond strengths are probably high enough to permit retention of class V restorations by adhesion, without additional retention.

F.R. Tay (✉)
Department of Endodontics, The Dental College of Georgia, Augusta University, Augusta, GA, USA
e-mail: tayfranklin7@gmail.com

M.A. Nawareg
Department of Restorative Dentistry, Faculty of Dentistry, King Abdulaziz University, Jeddah, Saudi Arabia

Biomaterials Department, Faculty of Oral and Dental Medicine, Cairo University, Egypt

D. Abuelenain
Department of Restorative Dentistry, Faculty of Dentistry, King Abdulaziz University, Jeddah, Saudi Arabia

D.H. Pashley
The Dental College of Georgia, Augusta University, Augusta, GA, USA

M. Goldberg (ed.), *Understanding Dental Caries*, DOI 10.1007/978-3-319-30552-3_10

10.1 Introduction

The efficacy of current adhesive systems is evaluated based upon their ability to bond to normal dentin. Although many dentists bond to normal dentin, a variety of abnormal dentin substrates are encountered in the clinical practice, which include carious and sclerotic dentin. It is ironic that our current knowledge on the variability of clinical bonding substrates is so limited compared with the progress that has been achieved in adhesive bonding. This review examined the ultrastructure and bonding characteristics of one type of abnormal bonding substrate – noncarious sclerotic dentin. This paper compares the obstacles in bonding to sound versus sclerotic dentin. It will be seen that there is a huge variation in substrate morphology and in the resin-dentin interfaces created by bonding to such substrates. The recent introduction of self-etching primers and all-in-one adhesives is redefining adhesive dentistry. Because these simplified adhesives have become so widely used, we have placed extra emphasis on the interfaces created by these agents on sclerotic cervical dentin.

10.2 Noncarious Cervical Sclerotic Dentin

Noncarious cervical sclerotic lesions were described by Zsigmondy in 1894 (Zsigmondy 1894) as angular defects and by Miller in 1907 (Miller 1907) as "wasting of tooth tissue." Their development was characterized by a slow and gradual loss of tooth substances resulting in smooth, wedge-shaped defects along the cementoenamel junction. The etiology of these cervical lesions has been extensively reviewed (Braem et al. 1992; Levitch et al. 1994; Gallien et al. 1994; Spranger 1995; Tyas 1995; Aw et al. 2002; Giachetti et al. 2002). There is increasing evidence of the possible role of parafunctional occlusal stress in the pathogenesis of these hard tissue defects (Xhonga 1977; Lee and Eakle 1984, 1996; Grippo 1991; Burke et al. 1995; Rees 1998, 2000, 2002; Eramo et al. 2003). Recent studies on simulation of wedge-shaped cervical lesions using various finite element analytical models of cuspal flexure confirmed the contribution of stress in the development of these so-called abfraction lesions (Kuroe et al. 2000; Palamara et al. 2000; Lee et al. 2002; Rees et al. 2003). Unrestored, angular, wedge-shaped lesions demonstrated severe stress concentration that varied with the location of the teeth in the oral cavity, with the highest stress concentrations found within maxillary incisors and premolars. These stresses were only partially relieved after the lesions were restored.

Sclerotic dentin is a clinically relevant bonding substrate in which the dentin has been pathologically altered, partly in response to the body's natural defense mechanism to stress and partly as a consequence of colonization by the oral biofilms. Sclerotic wedge-shaped cervical lesions are glossy, hard, and have a deep yellow to dark brown color. Partial or complete obliteration of the dentinal tubules with intratubular rodlike sclerotic casts is commonly observed (Gwinnett and Jendresen 1978; Harnirattisai et al. 1993; Van Meerbeek et al. 1994; Yoshiyama et al. 1996a; Kwong et al. 2000; Sakoolnamarka et al. 2000). Depending on the degree of clinical dentin sensitivity of the lesion, various levels of tubular patency were observed, with most dentinal tubules being occluded within the insensitive dentin regions (Van Meerbeek et al. 1994; Kwong et al. 2000; Nalbandian et al. 1959; Weber 1974; Yoshiyama et al. 1990; Mixson et al. 1995; Eda et al. 1996; Kawakami et al. 1996).

In the absence of undercut retention cavity designs, cervical sclerotic dentin has been found to be more difficult to bond to than normal dentin both in vitro and in vivo, even with increased etching time (Tyas 1987; Duke and Lindemuth 1990, 1991; Duke et al. 1991; Van Meerbeek et al. 1996). Many studies have shown that the sclerotic intratubular casts that obliterated the dentinal tubules are still present after acid conditioning of the sclerotic dentin, resulting in minimal or no resin tag formation. Furthermore, the hybrid layers in sclerotic dentin were found to be thinner than those observed in normal dentin (Van Meerbeek et al. 1994; Kwong et al. 2000, 2002; Yoshiyama et al. 1996b; Prati et al. 1999; Sakoolnamarka et al. 2002).

Due to the thinness of hybrid layers in sclerotic dentin, and the complexity of the resin-bonded interface, regional tensile bond strength to cervical sclerotic root dentin with most contemporary adhesives was found to be 20–44 % lower than those bonded to artificial wedge-shaped lesions created in normal cervical root dentin (Yoshiyama et al. 1996b; Kwong et al. 2002). This was attributed to multiple factors: (a) the presence of sclerotic casts within dentinal tubules that prevented optimal resin infiltration into sclerotic dentin and/or (b) the presence of a hypermineralized surface layer that is more resistant to acid etching. It was opined that an adhesive technique which involved resin adhesion by the formation of a resin-dentin interdiffusion zone, combined with resin tag formation into the dentinal tubules, would be less effective when applied to the hypermineralized sclerotic dentin (Kwong et al. 2002; Gwinnett and Kanca 1992a). Contrary to that opinion, one study suggested that phosphoric acid etching was detrimental to resin bonding to sclerotic dentin and that sclerotic dentin which was treated with a hydrophilic primer exhibited better marginal adaptation of resin composites than similarly primed normal dentin (Kusunoki et al. 2002). Those authors recommended that the layer of sclerotic dentin be preserved for optimal bonding in cervical lesions. Such adhesive therapy conserves more dentin than techniques which recommend roughing up sclerotic dentin to try to reach more normal underlying dentin.

Scanning electron microscopy (SEM) of such surfaces does not provide sufficient detail to understand the complex subsurface structures or reveal how well these structures are demineralized during etching (Sakoolnamarka et al. 2000, 2002). This information is best obtained using transmission electron microscopy (TEM). In this review, extensive TEM examinations are used to document the biologic variations in sclerotic cervical dentin. This paper is not an exhaustive review of the literature on noncarious cervical lesions or in resin bonding to sclerotic dentin. Rather, it is an attempt to summarize a number of studies that provide a rationale for why resin bonds to noncarious, sclerotic wedge-shaped cervical lesions are lower than those made to normal dentin at the same sites. This review will be divided into two sections. In the first section, the microstructural differences that exist in noncarious, sclerotic cervical dentin will be summarized. The second section is a review of the application of adhesive resins to this altered bonding substrate.

10.3 Microstructural Changes in Sclerotic Dentin

10.3.1 Tubular Occlusion

The hallmark of sclerotic dentin is the presence of rhombohedral, whitlockite crystallites (Fig. 10.1a) within the dentinal tubules (Kwong et al. 2000; Yoshiyama et al. 1989, 1990; Kawakami et al. 1996; Daculsi et al. 1987; Schüpbach et al. 1992). A high degree of ultrastructural variation can be observed even within a single lesion. While some tubules may be completely devoid of intratubular crystallites, others may be heavily obliterated with them and/or peritubular dentin (Fig. 10.1b). Near the surface of the lesion, these crystallites are reduced in size and form mineralized casts that completely plug the tubular orifices. They are often referred to as sclerotic casts (Fig. 10.2a). At an ultrastructural level, these tiny, electron-dense crystallites (Fig. 10.2b) were surrounded by a tubelike membranous structure (Yoshiyama et al. 1996a; Kwong et al. 2000) that probably represented a mineralized lamina limitans of the dentinal tubule.

10.3.2 Hypermineralized Surface Layer in Shiny Sclerotic Lesions

Unlike tubular occlusion, the presence of a hypermineralized surface layer in natural cervical sclerotic wedge-shaped lesions can only be seen through the use of microradiography (Weber 1974) or FTIR photoacoustic spectroscopic analysis (Mixson et al. 1995). Although it has been speculated that the hypermineralized surface layer is devoid of collagen fibrils (Duke and Lindemuth 1991), the ultrastructural features of this layer

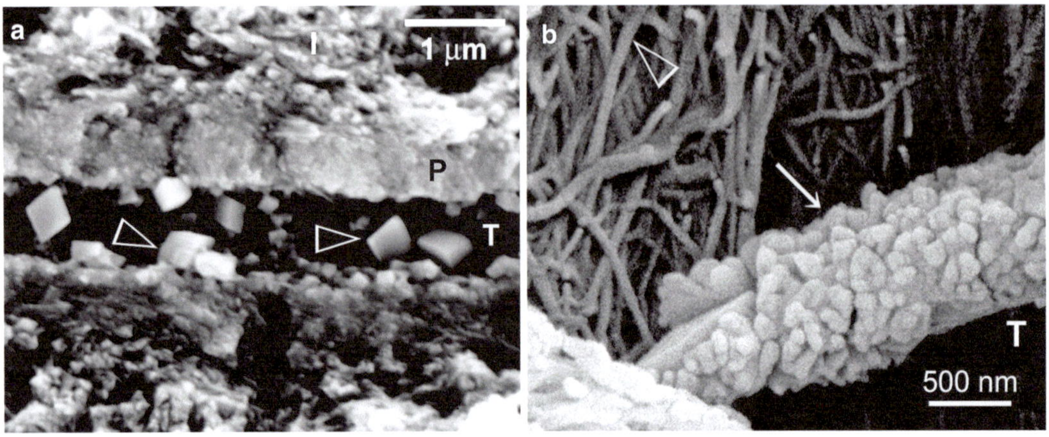

Fig. 10.1 (**a**) SEM micrograph of sclerotic dentin lesion showing a dentinal tubule that was heavily occluded with large cubic whitlockite crystallites (pointers) (Modified from Tay and Pashley (2004a)) (**b**) SEM of a fractured surface of sclerotic dentin showing how many small mineral deposits can coalesce into a solid cast within dentinal tubules in a sclerotic lesion. *T* dentinal tubule (Modified from Tay and Pashley (2004a))

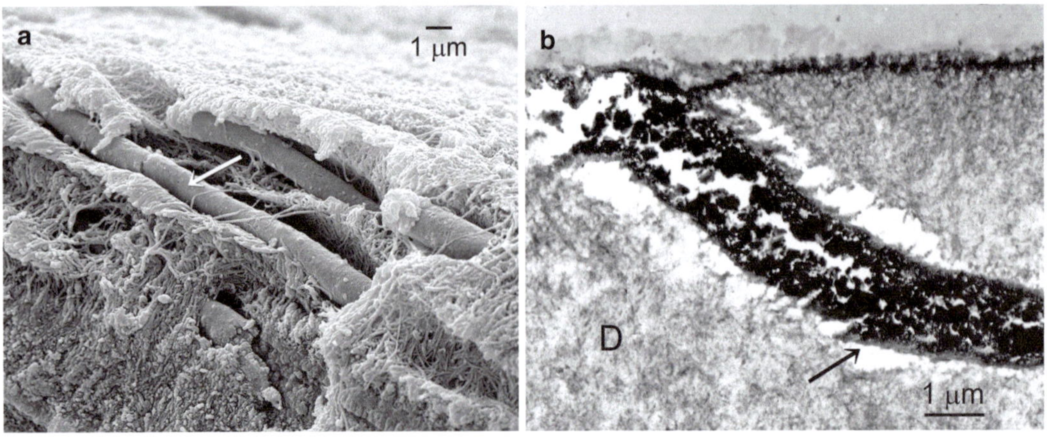

Fig. 10.2 (**a**) SEM micrograph of intratubular sclerotic casts (*white arrow*) that blocked the dentinal tubules along the surface of a sclerotic lesion (Modified from Tay and Pashley (2004a)) (**b**) TEM micrograph taken from an undemineralized section of the surface of a bonded sclerotic lesion. Tubules were obliterated with sclerotic casts that consisted of both fine electron-dense crystallites and spherical aggregates of crystals (*black arrow*). A thin, electron-dense, hypermineralized layer was also evident along the surface of the lesion (Modified from Tay and Pashley (2004a))

were only verified recently. Figure 10.3 is a toluidine blue-stained, undemineralized thin section taken from the deepest part of a wedge-shaped defect. In the preparation of the specimen, the surface of the lesion was not cleaned, but was fixed in Karnovsky's fixative prior to the preparation (Duke and Lindemuth 1991). A surface layer composed of stained, unmineralized filamentous bacteria could be seen, beneath which was an approximately 15 μm thick hypermineralized layer. Mineralized bacteria could be faintly seen within this layer. At a higher magnification (Figs. 10.4a, b), platelike minerals could be recognized within the matrix around the bacteria.

The ultrastructure of the surface hypermineralized layer was highly variable within the deepest part of the wedge-shaped lesions. The mineralized layer was retained after complete demineralization of the underlying sclerotic dentin. The hypermineralized (HM) layer in Fig. 10.5

consists of several thin, discontinuous layers that were sandwiched among different bacterial species. Each colony of bacteria was mineralized prior to the deposition of the next colony. It is pertinent to point out that the specimens that contained bacteria were brushed cleaned with a mixture of chlorhexidine and pumice prior to laboratory processing. Such lesions appeared as clean, highly shiny lesions when examined under magnification.

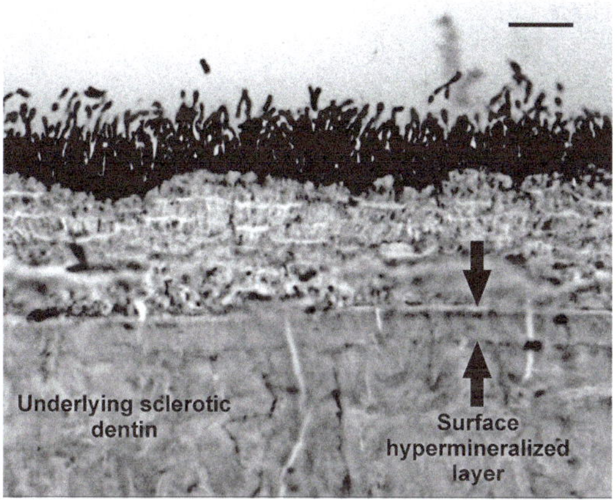

Fig. 10.3 Light microscopic image of an undemineralized section taken from the deepest part of a stained, unmineralized wedge-shaped sclerotic lesion. Bacteria cover the underlying hypermineralized layer of an untreated noncarious cervical sclerotic lesion. The hypermineralized nature of the surface layer was recognized by comparing its electron density with the underlying sclerotic dentin (Modified from Tay and Pashley (2004a))

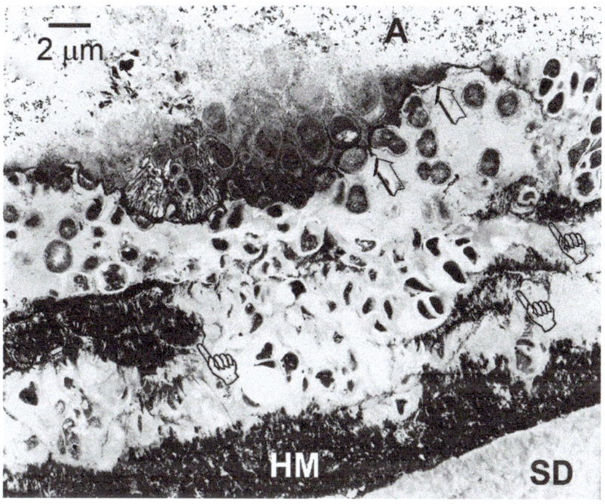

Fig. 10.5 Variation in the ultrastructure of the complex hypermineralized layer in noncarious cervical sclerotic lesions. Demineralized TEM micrograph showing a hypermineralized layer (HM) within the deepest part of a wedge-shaped lesion that was 14 µm thick. Bacteria colonies were trapped inside this thick layer (*open arrows*). Another species of bacteria (pointers) accumulated along the surface of the hypermineralized layer (Modified from Tay and Pashley (2004a))

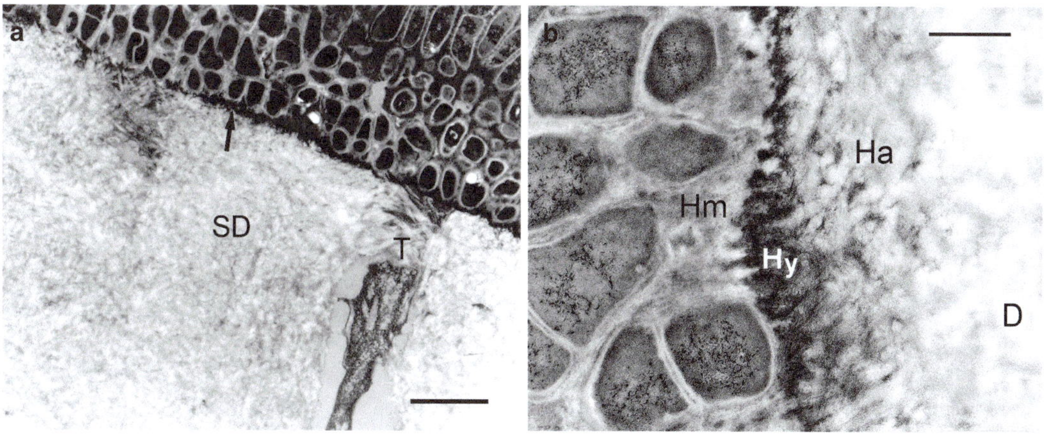

Fig. 10.4 (**a**) Undemineralized TEM micrograph of multiple layers of bacteria growing on top of a hypermineralized layer (*arrow*). The intermicrobial matrix (i.e., the material between adjacent bacteria) was partially mineralized. Note lamina limitans sheath within an open dentinal tubule (Modified from Tay and Pashley (2004a)) (**b**) Resin-hybridized sclerotic dentin. Ha designates an authentic hybrid layer created by a mild self-etching primer/adhesive. Hy designates the resin-hybridized hypermineralized layer on the dentin surface. Hm refers to resin hybridization of the bacterial organic matrix. *D* underlying sclerotic dentin; bar = 300 nm (Modified from Tay and Pashley (2004a))

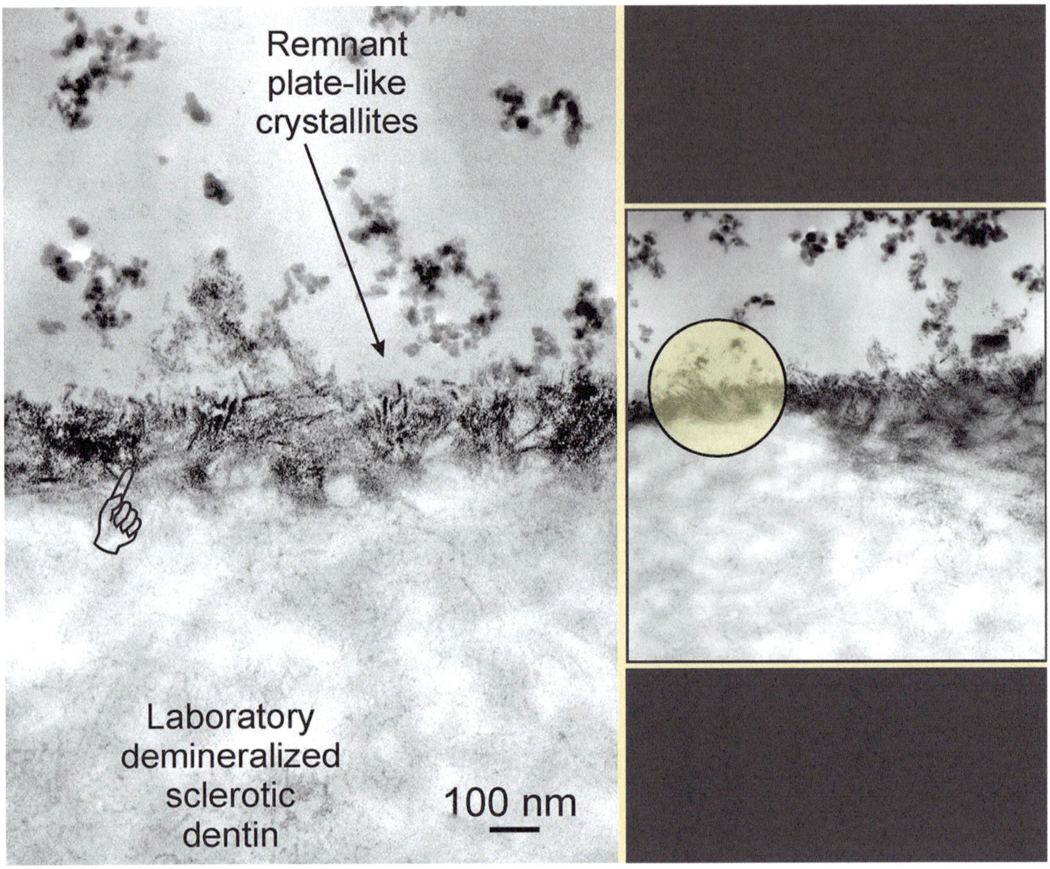

Fig. 10.6 Crystallites (*arrow*) within a surface hypermineralized layer (pointer) were platelike and were aligned along the c-axis. The lesion surface was etched by a self-etching primer, causing blunting and rounding of the partially dissolved crystallites

The presence of bacteria on the surface of sclerotic wedge-shaped lesions is consistent with the report of Spranger (Spranger 1995). The structures beneath bacterial plaque change over time depending on the metabolism of the microorganisms. This results in substantial pH fluctuations along the tooth surface (Scheie et al. 1992). Bacterial products may trigger gingival inflammation. If a plentiful supply of fermentable carbohydrates is available, the microbes would release organic acids that lower the plaque pH and tend to demineralize the underlying dental hard tissue. When the carbohydrate source is depleted, the local salivary buffering would increase the pH of the lesion, and remineralization of the dental hard tissue and mineralization of the dental plaque could occur. In the absence of carbohydrates, these bacteria may remain viable for prolonged periods (Svensäter et al. 2001), utilizing glycogen-like intracellular polysaccharide (IPS) as a metabolizable source of carbon (Spatafora et al. 1999). They may also metabolize amino acids and other nitrogenous substrates, creating ammonia and other basic chemicals that may elevate plaque pH and promote mineralization and, perhaps, hypermineralization (Sanz and Newman 1994).

Along the occlusal wall of the wedge-shaped lesions, both the surface bacterial layer and the hypermineralized layer are usually thin (1–2 μm thick). Similarly, the gingival wall of a wedge-shaped lesion, which is usually more accessible to toothbrushing, is usually devoid of bacteria. However, a very thin surface hypermineralized layer may sometimes be observed (Fig. 10.6) on the gingival wall. Such a layer, if present, is 200–300 nm thick and may be readily seen in undemineralized sections by its increased electron density, as well as the characteristic arrangement of the crystallites, which will be discussed in the next section.

10.3.3 Mineral Distribution

Mineral crystallites present within the hypermineralized layer are larger in size compared with those within the underlying sclerotic dentin (Fig. 10.6). Unlike crystallites within the underlying dentin that are randomly arranged, those found in the hypermineralized layer were longitudinally aligned along the c-axis of the crystallites. Piezoelectric potentials have been reported to be generated when teeth are subjected to parafunctional loading (Marino and Gross 1989). Some have speculated that polarization of the remineralized crystallites caused by piezoelectric potentials created during eccentric tooth flexure results in their attraction and repulsion by dipole interaction.

10.3.4 STEM/EDX Analysis

Hypermineralization implies that the density of the mineral within the surface layer of the defect is higher than that of the underlying sclerotic dentin. This is confirmed by a qualitative STEM/EDX line scan of the calcium and phosphorus distribution longitudinally across the surface layer of the defect into the underlying sclerotic dentin (Fig. 10.7). Also evident in the line scan is the presence of a region of decreased calcium and phosphorus counts along the top 500 nm of the hypermineralized layer that is attributed to partial demineralization by a self-etching primer (Fig. 10.7) that was used to bond to sclerotic lesions (Tay and Pashley 2004a).

Quantitative energy dispersive X-ray spectra of the elemental content of crystallites present within (a) the surface hypermineralized layer, (b) the underlying intertubular dentin, and (c) within the dentinal tubules of the wedge-shaped defect are illustrated in Fig. 10.8 (Tay and Pashley 2004a). As the analysis was performed using 70 nm thick undemineralized sections, this enabled estimation of the calcium/phosphate ratio of these crystallites without additional ZAF correction (Karan et al. 2009). The Ca/P ratios of the crystallites within the hypermineralized layer and the underlying dentin approach the theoretical value of 1.67 calculated for hydroxyapatite (Daculsi et al. 1979). The larger apatite crystallites observed in the surface hypermineralized layer are similar to larger apatite crystallites reported in remineralized carious dentin (Daculsi et al. 1979) and cementum (Tjäderhane et al. 2013b). Conversely, the Ca/P ratio of crystallites from the sclerotic casts within the dentinal tubules is slightly lower than the calculated value of 1.50 for tricalcium phosphate (Daculsi et al. 1979). The additional presence of about 5 % magnesium suggests that these crystallites are whitlockite (Mg-substituted β-tricalcium phosphate). All trivalent phosphate solids should be regarded as solid buffer that is difficult to solubilize. A recent microRaman study of the mineral distribution of noncarious, sclerotic cervical lesions came to similar conclusions (Karan et al. 2009).

10.3.5 Status of the Collagen Fibrils Within the Surface Hypermineralized Layer

An important question that has remained unanswered is whether the surface hypermineralized layer is devoid of collagen (Duke and Lindemuth 1990). Using special staining for collagen, it can be seen that the supporting matrix for the crystallites within the hypermineralized layer consists of a bed of denatured collagen (Fig. 10.9a). The transition from denatured collagen (gelatin) to intact collagen with crossbanding is evident at the base of the hypermineralized layer, where some of the collagen fibrils are observed to unravel into microfibrillar subunits (Tay and Pashley 2004a). This transition from banded collagen to denatured microfibrils is further illustrated beneath a layer of bacteria in Fig. 10.9b, in which unraveling of collagen fibrils created a network of microfibrillar strands that no longer showed crossbanding.

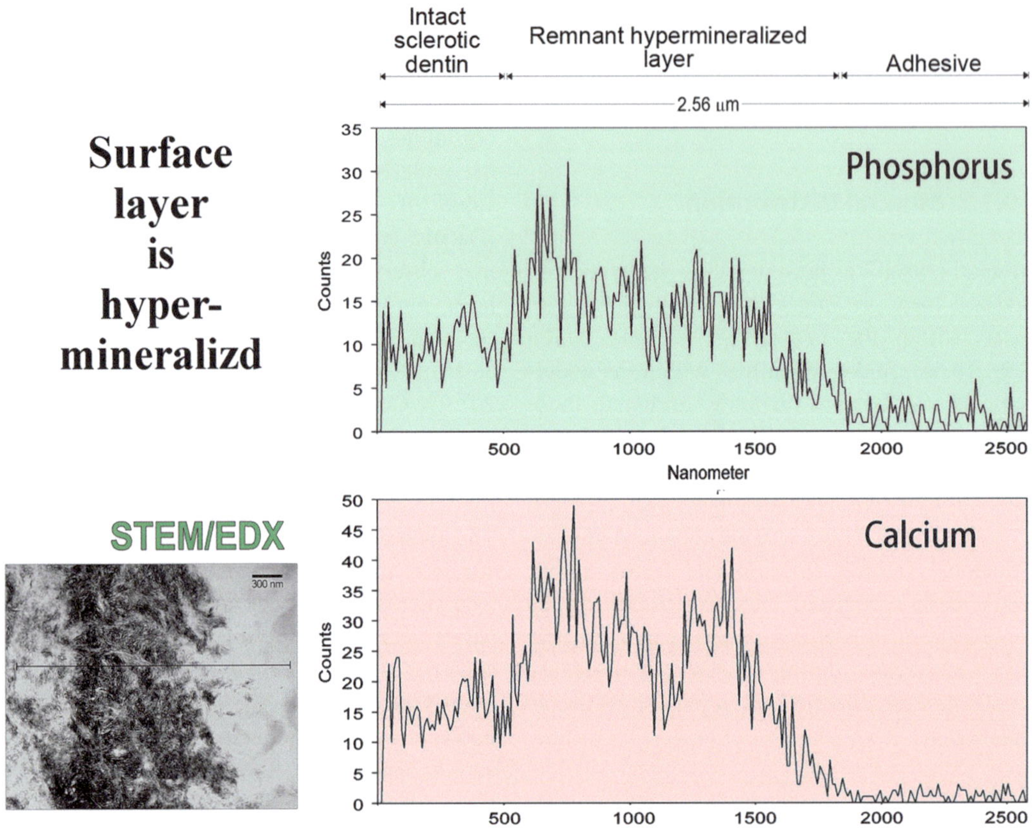

Fig. 10.7 Bright-field STEM image showing the location of a line scan that was performed across the surface hypermineralized layer of a noncarious cervical sclerotic lesion. Qualitative energy dispersive line scans showing the distribution of phosphorus (*upper scan*) and calcium (*lower scan*) along the adhesive, the surface hypermineralized layer of the lesion, and the underlying intact sclerotic dentin (Modified from Tay and Pashley (2004a))

It is possible that colonization of bacteria along the surface of the wedge-shaped defect results in the production of acidic by-products that demineralize dentin collagen fibrils (Fig. 10.9a, b). It is now thought that bacterially derived organic acids expose and activate previously inactive proforms of the endogenous matrix metalloproteinases of dentin (Pashley et al. 2004; Breschi et al. 2008; Tjäderhane et al. 2013a, b). The loss of phosphoproteins (Brackett et al. 2010) and subsequent remineralization of the surface bed of denatured collagen under the possible influence of piezoelectric charges generated from eccentric flexural deformation (Spranger 1995) may result in the characteristic orientation of the crystallites within the denatured microfibrillar matrix of the hypermineralized layer.

10.3.6 Summary of the Microstructural Changes in Noncarious Sclerotic Cervical Dentin

Sclerotic dentin is an abnormal bonding substrate that exhibits a high degree of variability both in terms of occlusion of the dentinal tubules as well as the thickness of the surface hypermineralized layer. The latter, in particular, is invariably associated with bacteria. It is

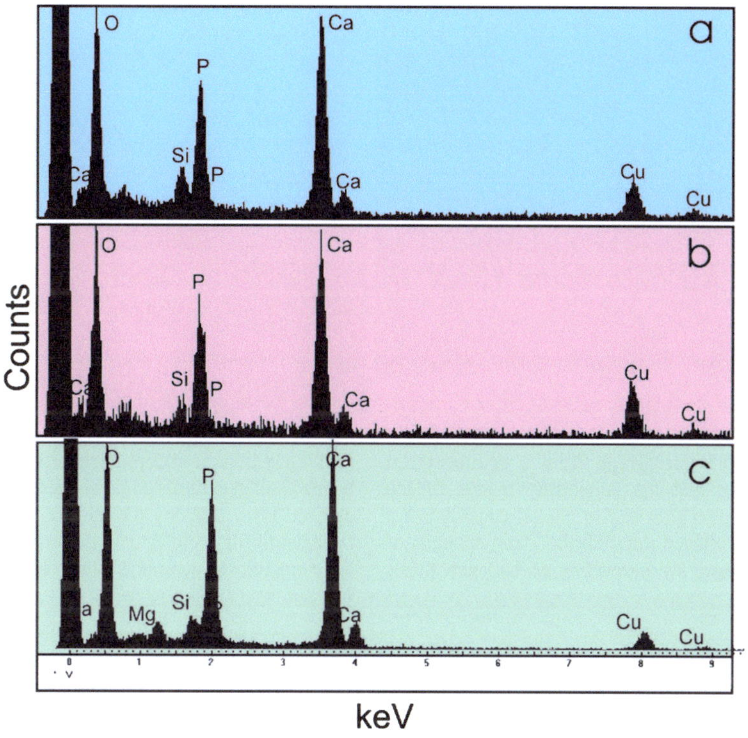

Regions from which crystallites were analyzed	Mg (wt%)	Ca (wt%)	P (wt%)	Ca/P ratio*
a Surface hypermineralized layer	0	62.5 0.9	37.5 0.9	1.7 0.1
b Underlying sclerotic dentin	0	63.1 0.5	36.9 0.5	1.7 0.1
c Sclerotic casts with dentinal tubules	4.6 1.0	55.3 1.8	40.2 1.3	1.4 0.1

Fig. 10.8 Energy spectra from different locations of a noncarious cervical sclerotic lesion. (**a**) Spectrum showing composition of crystallites within the surface hypermineralized layer. (**b**) Spectrum of crystallites within the underlying intact sclerotic dentin. (**c**) Spectrum of crystallites occupying the lumen of a dentinal tubule. Spectra were obtained using a 7 nm spot for 200 live seconds at 200 kV. The relative concentration of Ca, P, and Mg and the calculated Ca/P ratios are shown in the table beneath the spectra (Modified from Tay and Pashley (2004a))

possible that bacteria are involved in the pathogenesis of the hypermineralized layer. That is, dentin may first require demineralization before it can be hypermineralized. Also, mineral crystallites cannot accumulate without a scaffold. The presence of bacteria, apart from demineralizing the dentin, also denatures the existing collagen matrix, resulting in a bed of denatured collagen. This may act as a scaffold upon which the demineralized dentin may be

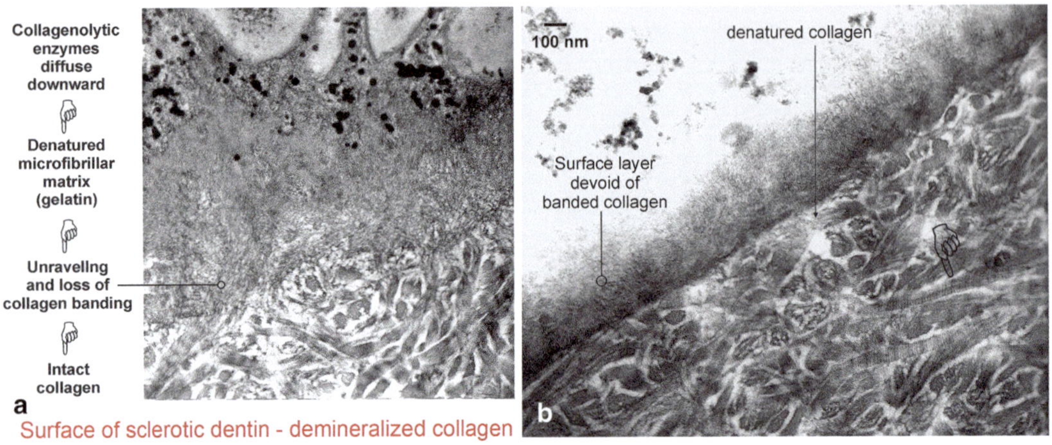

Fig. 10.9 (**a**) TEM micrograph from a demineralized specimen, showing that the supporting matrix of the hypermineralized layer (*top half of image*) consisted of a bed of denatured collagen microfibrils. These subunits of collagen were formed by unraveling of collagen fibrils (*circle*). Within the underlying sclerotic dentin, intact larger banded collagen fibrils could be seen. (**b**) A thin hypermineralized layer showing the transition from intact, banded collagen fibrils (pointer) into denatured collagen (gelatin), appearing ultrastructurally as microfibrillar strands

subsequently remineralized. The formation of the hypermineralized layer is probably also enhanced by the presence of high concentrations (10 ppm) of fluoride ions (Perdigão et al. 1994; Goncalves et al. 1999; Pashley and Carvalho 1997). As denaturing of the collagen fibrils probably removes some of the restrictions on the size of crystallite formation, this may enable larger crystallites to be formed during the process of remineralization. The unique arrangement of the crystallites further suggests the complex role of parafunctional stress on the formation of the surface hypermineralized layer in these natural wedge-shaped lesions (Rees 1998; Gwinnett and Jendresen 1978). The presence of bacteria, mineralized bacterial matrices, hypermineralized surfaces, and dentinal tubules occluded with mineralized crystals makes sclerotic cervical dentin a unique multilayered bonding substrate. This implies that bonding studies which attempt to generate hypermineralized dentin in vitro by immersing partially demineralized dentin in a remineralizing solution containing a high fluoride content (Perdigão 2002; Van Meerbeek et al. 2003) do not simulate the actual bonding conditions that clinicians are likely to encounter when bonding to noncarious cervical sclerotic dentin.

10.4 Bonding Adhesive Resins to Sclerotic Dentin

Current dentin adhesives employ two different means to achieve the goal of micromechanical retention between resin and dentin (Nakabayashi et al. 1982; Gwinnett and Kanca 1992b; Kanca 1992). The first method, the total-etch or etch-and-rinse technique, attempts to remove the smear layer completely via acid etching and rinsing. The second approach, the self-etching technique, aims at demineralizing and incorporating the smear layer as a bonding substrate.

10.4.1 Total-Etch Technique

Most self-priming, single-bottle adhesives available to date attempt to bond to dentin that is etched with 37 % phosphoric acid. Following rinsing of the conditioners with water, retention is accomplished by means of resin infiltration into the exposed, demineralized collagen matrix to form a hybrid layer of resin-impregnated dentin (Gwinnett and Kanca 1992b; Kanca 1992; Gwinnett 1994). Systems containing hydrophilic primer resins solvated in acetone or ethanol were found to produce higher bond strengths when

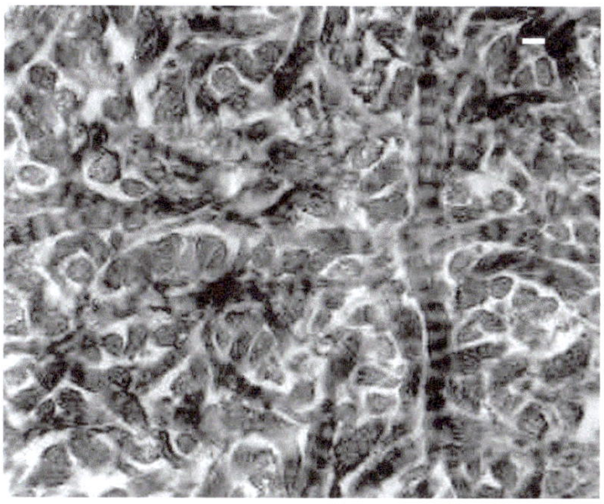

Fig. 10.10 Dentin collagen fibrils from a hybrid layer in normal dentin that was produced using a total-etch technique. Randomly oriented interfibrillar channels must be maintained open for optimal acid etching and resin infiltration. This is achieved using the wet-bonding technique. Bonded with One-Step (Bisco). Bar = 50 nm

acid-conditioned dentin was left visibly moist prior to bonding (Titley et al. 1994). This technique is often referred to as "wet bonding" (Pashley et al. 2000). The benefit of wet bonding stems from the ability of water to keep the interfibrillar channels within the collagen network from collapsing during resin infiltration (Pashley et al. 2003; Tao et al. 1988). These channels, which are about 20 nm wide when fully extended (Fig. 10.10), must be maintained open to facilitate optimal diffusion of resin monomers into the demineralized intertubular dentin (Eick et al. 1991; Watanabe et al. 1990).

10.4.2 Self-Etching Technique

Self-etching techniques in dentin bonding have reintroduced the concept of utilizing the smear layer as a bonding substrate, but with improved formulations that could etch through the smear layer and beyond, into the underlying dentin matrix. Failure to etch beyond the smear layer, exemplified by some of the early adhesives that were applied directly to the smear layer, resulted in weak bonds due to the complete absence of a hybrid layer in underlying intertubular dentin (Chigira et al. 1994; Finger and Balkenhol 1999). Contemporary self-etching adhesives have been developed by replacing the separate acid-conditioning step with increased concentrations of acidic resin monomers in a primer. Two-step self-etching primers combine etching and priming into a single step. The primed surfaces are subsequently covered with a more hydrophobic, solvent-free adhesive layer that is light cured. In the presence of water as an ionizing medium, these adhesives etch through smear layers and bond to the underlying intact dentin (Fig. 10.11) (Peschke et al. 2000; Ferrari and Tay 2003). The recent introduction of single-step, single-bottle, self-etching adhesives represents a further reduction in bonding steps that eliminates some of the technique sensitivity and practitioner variability that are associated with the use of total-etch adhesives (Watanabe et al. 1994; Nakabayashi and Saimi 1996; Sano et al. 1999; Tay and Pashley 2001).

When applied to sound dentin, the milder self-etching adhesives produce a hybridized complex that consists of a surface zone of hybridized smear layer and a thin, subsurface hybrid layer in the underlying intertubular dentin (Prati et al. 1998; Yoshiyama et al. 1998; Pereira et al. 1999). Despite the presence of a hybrid layer that was generally less than 2 μm thick, high initial bond strengths have been reported for sound dentin (Tay et al. 2000a; Ogata et al. 2002; Toida et al. 1995; Igarashi et al. 1997). The more aggressive self-etching adhesives completely dissolve smear plugs and demineralize dentin to the extent that is comparable with phosphoric acid etching (Pereira et al. 1999). There has been some concern that mild self-etching adhesives may not be able to penetrate through thick smear layers, such as those produced clinically by rough diamond burs (Prati et al. 1998; Yoshiyama et al. 1998; Pereira et al. 1999; Tay et al. 2000a; Ogata et al. 2002; Toida et al. 1995; Igarashi et al. 1997; Miyasaka and Nakabayashi 1999). The adjunctive use of phosphoric acid preconditioning has been suggested as a means to improve bonding of self-etching primers to sound dentin with thick smear layers (Tay et al. 2000b; Eick et al. 1997; Gwinnett et al. 1996). Ground dentin surfaces are often produced clinically and have been shown to improve bond strength (Coli et al. 1999).

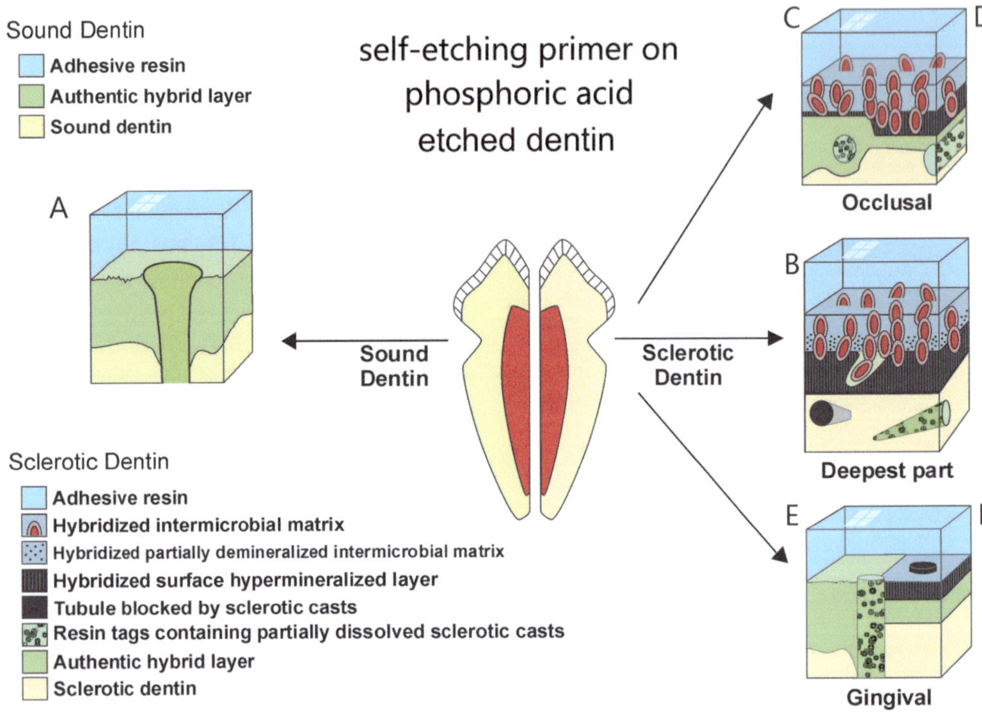

Fig. 10.11 Schematic showing the ultrastructural differences seen when bonding normal cervical dentin with 40 % phosphoric acid (**a**) versus bonding to wedge-shaped cervical sclerotic lesions preconditioned with 40 % phosphoric acid and then bonded with a mild self-etching primer/adhesive to (**c**) the occlusal wall of specimen with thin hypermineralized layer or (**d**) thicker hypermineralized layer or (**b**) to the deepest part of the wedge-shaped lesion or (**e**) to the gingival with or without a hypermineralized layer or (**f**) with a hypermineralized layer

10.4.3 Problems in Bonding to Sclerotic Dentin

Regardless of the use of a total-etch or a self-etching technique, bonding to pathologically altered substrates such as sclerotic dentin from noncarious cervical lesions generally leads to compromised bonding (Yoshiyama et al. 1996b; Prati et al. 1999; Kwong et al. 2002; Daculsi et al. 1979). Reduced bonding efficacy was attributed to a combination of factors that included the obliteration of dentinal tubules with sclerotic casts, the presence of an acid-resistant hypermineralized layer, and the presence of bacteria on the lesion surface. The presence of the hypermineralized layer, bacteria, and tubular mineral casts in sclerotic dentin is analogous to the presence of the smear layer and smear plugs in sound dentin, being potential diffusion barriers for primer and resin infiltration. The concern that a self-etching primer may not etch through the superficial layers on sound dentin may likewise be applicable to sclerotic dentin. Phosphoric acid preconditioning prior to the application of a self-etching primer may thus be a useful technique when bonding to sclerotic dentin (Fig. 10.12a) (Kwong et al. 2002).

10.4.4 Obstacles in Bonding to Acid-Etched, Sound Dentin

Adhesive strategies that rely mostly on micromechanical retention are hampered by obstacles that jeopardize infiltration of resin into dental tissues (Hashimoto et al. 2002). In abraded sound dentin, the smear layer is effectively removed in adhesive systems that utilize a separate acid-conditioning and rinsing step. In order to achieve optimal resin infiltration, acid-etched demineralized dentin

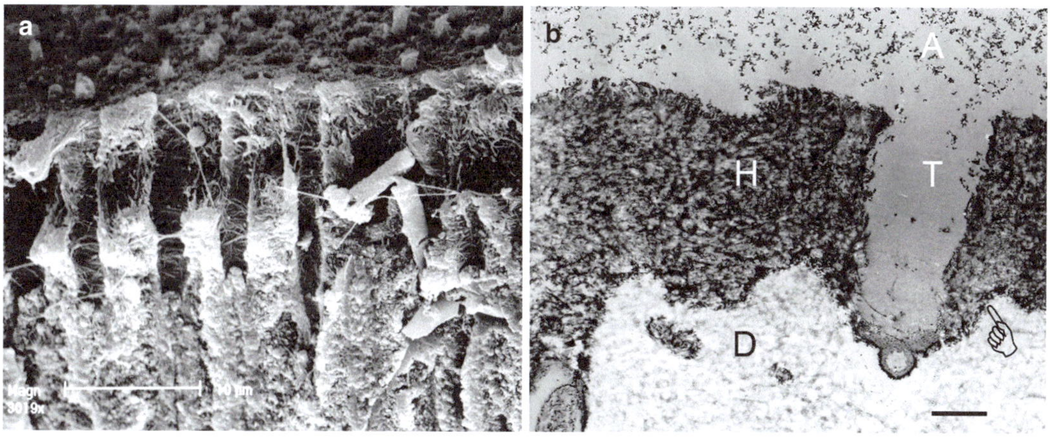

Fig. 10.12 (**a**) Sclerotic dentinal tubules that were filled with mineralized casts which block resin infiltration, after etching with 37 % phosphoric acid to solubilize those casts, opening the tubules for resin tag formation. (**b**) Combined action of 40 % phosphoric acid to demineralize hypermineralized dentin more deeply than can a self-etching adhesive, followed by a water rinse and application of a self-etching adhesive, creates well-primed thick hybrid layers in sclerotic dentin. The smear layer was completely removed. The hybrid layer (*H*) was about 4 μm thick. Pointer: base of hybrid layer. A: filled adhesive containing nanofillers (Modified from Tay and Pashley (2004a))

must be suspended in water to prevent collapsing of the interfibrillar spaces. This is effectively accomplished using the wet-bonding technique. Interfacial strength is dependent upon the ability of resins to engage the deepest extent of demineralized intertubular dentin (Wang and Spencer 2002, 2003; Vasiliadis et al. 1983; Vargas et al. 1997; Inai et al. 1998). The collagen matrix may thus be viewed as a diffusion barrier or obstacle for resin infiltration in acid-etched dentin.

10.4.5 Obstacles in Bonding to Acid-Etched Sclerotic Dentin

Unlike sound dentin, application of the same adhesive strategy to sclerotic dentin results in substantial variation in both hybrid layer and resin tag morphology. Potential obstacles of resin infiltration into uninstrumented natural lesions include the hypermineralized surface layer, an additional partially mineralized surface bacterial layer, and intratubular mineral casts which are comparatively more acid resistant (Gwinnett and Jendresen 1978; Van Meerbeek et al. 1994; Kwong et al. 2000). As these inclusions vary considerably along the occlusal, gingival, and the deepest part of a wedge-shaped lesion, variation in the ultrastructure of the resin-sclerotic dentin interfaces are possible in these different regions. While it is reasonable to assume that the extent of tubular occlusion (Fig. 10.12a) would vary according to the severity of dentin sclerosis (Tay et al. 2002), both the superficial bacterial and hypermineralized layers are found to vary from site to site, being thicker along the deepest part of the wedge-shaped lesions (Kwong et al. 2002). The surface hypermineralized layer was usually thinner in gingival and occlusal surfaces than in the apical or deepest part of the wedge-shaped defects and was often partially or completely dissolved when phosphoric acid was applied to sclerotic dentin. As a result, the thickness of the hybrid layers in the gingival and occlusal sites was similar to those seen in acid-etched sound dentin and remained fairly consistent at about 5 μm (Fig. 10.12b). Bacteria, if present, tended to be tenaciously attached to the dentin surfaces and in the dentinal tubules and were retained even after rinsing.

Thicker diffusion barriers are found within the deepest part of wedge-shaped lesions, which hamper the penetration of acids through the underlying intact sclerotic dentin. As a result, alterations in hybrid layer morphology and thickness are seen in these regions. One example is

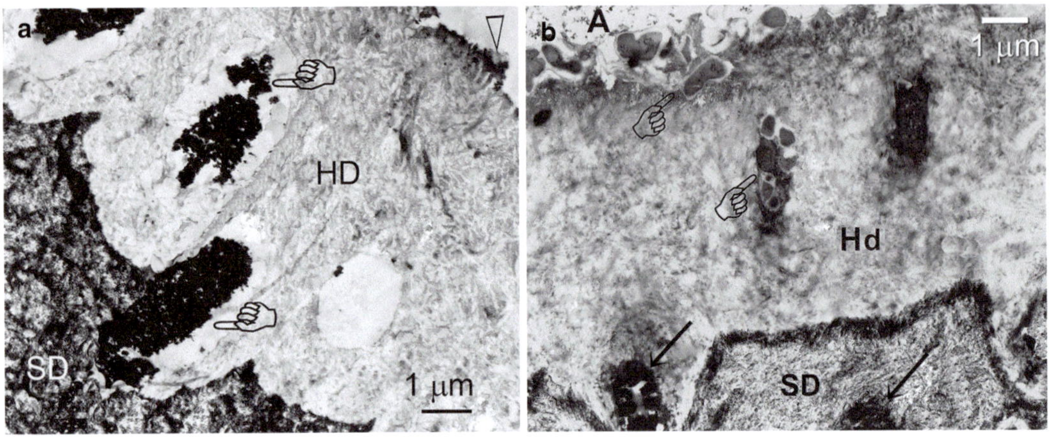

Fig. 10.13 (**a**) Application of the etch-and-rinse adhesive One-Step (Bisco) to 37% phosphoric acid-etched sclerotic dentin (SD). This stained undemineralized section was taken from the gingival surface of a wedge-shaped lesion. Remnants of a very thin, electron-dense, hypermineralized layer (*arrowhead*) could be seen on the surface of the hybrid layer. Some tubules remain occluded with sclerotic casts (pointers) that became surrounded by resin tags (pointers) (Modified from Tay and Pashley (2004a)). (**b**) Stained, undemineralized TEM section showing application of a filled adhesive to the occlusal surface of a phosphoric acid-etched, sclerotic lesion. Bacteria (pointers) were trapped in the hybrid layer (Hd) surface and in the tubules. Other tubules were filled with sclerotic casts (*arrows*) (Modified from Tay and Pashley (2004a))

shown in Fig. 10.13a. The surface hypermineralized layer from the deepest part of a wedge-shaped lesion was about 3 µm thick and was trapped within the resin-sclerotic dentin interface. The phosphoric acid apparently etched through the hypermineralized layer and created a hybrid layer of about 2 µm thick within the underlying intact sclerotic dentin. Rhombohedral whitlockite crystallites from the sclerotic casts may also be identified within dentinal tubules in the underlying sclerotic dentin. Figure 10.13b shows a specimen where the hypermineralized surface layer was destroyed. Bacteria remain on the surface and within tubules within the hybrid layer (Hd).

Figure 10.14 is a stained, demineralized TEM micrograph taken from the deepest part of another acid-etched, wedge-shaped natural sclerotic lesion. Within the 50 µm wide region of the micrograph, the thickness of the hybrid layer in sclerotic dentin changed abruptly from 2 µm to 5 µm. This aspect of uneven etching may also be seen in areas in which the acid etched laterally within the subsurface sclerotic dentin, producing lateral hybrid layer extensions which are separated from areas above that are not infiltrated with resin. This feature is distinct from incompletely resin-infiltrated hybrid layers that are observed in air-dried, acid-etched sound dentin.

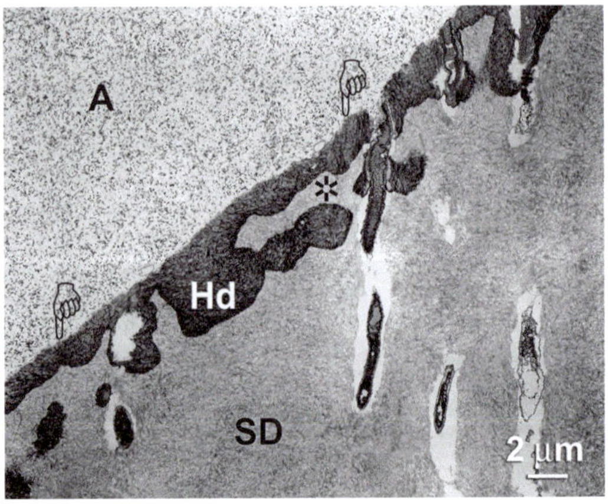

Fig. 10.14 Undemineralized section taken from the deepest part of a wedge-shaped natural sclerotic lesion that was etched with 40% phosphoric acid and bonded using self-etching primer/adhesive. Hd: hybridized hypermineralized layer that varied in thickness from 2 µm (pointers) to 5 µm (Hd). *A* adhesive containing nanofillers. A lateral extension of the hybrid layer could be seen below an area that was not infiltrated with adhesive resin (*asterisk*). *A* adhesive, *SD* sclerotic dentin (Reprinted from Tay and Pashley 2004b, with permission from Elsevier)

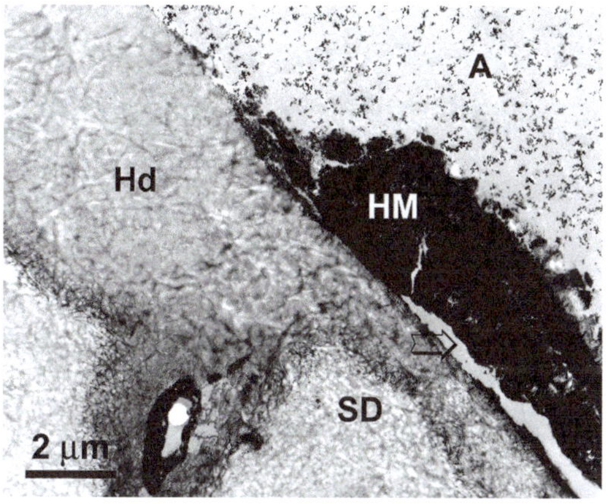

Fig. 10.15 Undemineralized TEM micrograph from the deepest part of a phosphoric acid-etched, natural sclerotic lesion. The hybrid layer (Hd) in intact sclerotic dentin (SD) was 5 µm thick when there was no overlying hypermineralized layer. This thickness was reduced to 2 µm thick beneath the hypermineralized layer (HM). The separation of the hypermineralized layer (*arrow*) was an artifact produced during specimen processing. *A* filled adhesive, *SD* sclerotic dentin (Reprinted from Tay and Pashley 2004b, with permission from Elsevier)

These "eccentric" hybrid layers in abnormal dentin substrates have never been observed in bonded sound dentin.

Unlike sound dentin in which the morphology of the hybrid layer remains fairly consistent as long as a wet-bonding technique is used, extensive variations are found in different specimens or locations within cervical sclerotic lesions. Figure 10.15 is a demineralized, stained TEM micrograph taken from the deepest part of a natural lesion. Whereas a thin hypermineralized layer and the presence of bacteria did not prevent the penetration of acid or resin into the underlying sclerotic dentin, the thickness of the hybrid layer was greatly reduced in the presence of a thick hypermineralized layer. These thick hypermineralized layers probably serve as diffuse barriers and prevent the penetration of both phosphoric acid and adhesive monomers. Reduced hybrid layer thickness may have no correlation with reduced regional microtensile bond strength in natural sclerotic dentin (Yoshiyama et al. 1996b; Kwong et al. 2002; Daculsi et al. 1979). However, the presence of thin hybrid layers should clearly be differentiated from the total absence of hybrid layer formation in the bonding substrate. Under such circumstances, the adhesive will be bonding directly to the diffusion barriers that impede acid etching. The resultant bond strength will depend on the strength of the attachment of such obstacles to the underlying sclerotic dentin. It is remarkable that these morphological fluctuations are continuous and vary within a very small region of a lesion that is covered by these micrographs. Such extreme variations in hybrid layer morphology are probably responsible for the large standard deviations in microtensile bond strength measurements of bonding to sclerotic dentin. It is likely that these segregated areas of deficient hybrid layer formation act as weak links, or stress raisers, that contribute to the initiation of adhesive failures in bonded sclerotic dentin.

10.4.6 Obstacles to Bonding in Sound Dentin Treated with a Self-Etching Primer Alone

The use of two-step and single-step self-etching adhesives represents an alternative means to acquire micromechanical retention in dentin. They are attractive in that they may be used on dry dentin and, after mixing, require only one primer application, which is subsequently air-dried rather than rinsed. The latest single-step self-etching adhesives further incorporate all the resin monomers, photoinitiator, and tertiary amine accelerator into a single bottle and eliminate an additional mixing step. Despite the physical appearance of thin hybrid layers and short, hybridized smear plugs in a two-step self-etching adhesive (Fig. 10.16), high initial bond strength have been reported. This suggests that there is no correlation between hybrid layer thickness and bond strength as long as a uniform demineralization front is created in sound intertubular dentin (Ogata et al. 2002; Wang and Spencer 2002; Pashley et al. 1988, 1992).

There was concern, in normal dentin, that thick and rough smear layers may interfere with

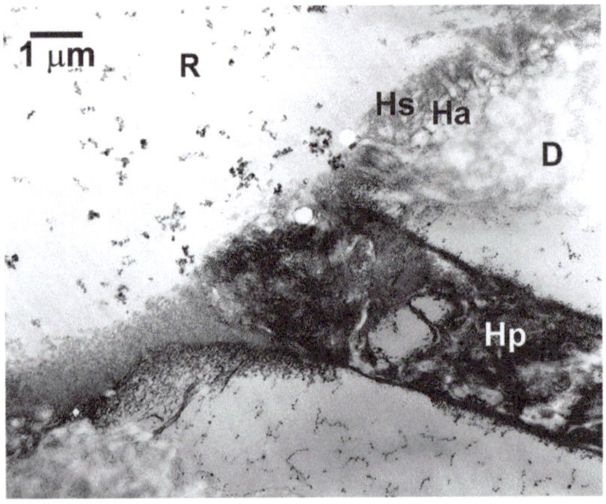

Fig. 10.16 Demineralized TEM micrograph of the application of a self-etching primer/adhesive to sound normal dentin (artificial wedge-shaped lesion). To achieve effective bonding, a self-etching primer must not only create a hybridized smear layer (Hs) but also an authentic hybrid layer in the underlying intact sound dentin (Ha). The dentinal tubule was sealed by a hybridized smear plug (Hp). *R* adhesive resin, *D* sound dentin

diffusion of self-etching primers into the underlying intact dentin. This may be due to the physical presence of thick smear layers as a diffusion barrier, or their ability to buffer the acidic monomers, making the pH too high to demineralize the underlying intertubular dentin. Recent studies showed that mildly aggressive self-etching adhesives penetrated through smear layers up to 3–4 μm thick and still retained sufficient acidity to demineralize the underlying intertubular dentin to a depth of 0.4–0.5 μm (Yu et al. 1990). This suggests that either the buffering capacity of the smear layer is weak or the smear layer does not impose much of a physical barrier to the primer compared with the underlying mineralized dentin matrix. The looseness of the surface portion of the smear layer and/or the presence of diffusion channels between its constituents may facilitate diffusion of the self-etching primer through the smear layer (Ferrari et al. 1996). Disaggregation of the smear layer into globular subunits (Gwinnett 1993) further provides micro-channels for diffusion of the self-etching adhesives. These micro-channels, in theory, should be more permeable to resin monomers than the interfibrillar spaces (ca. 20 nm) of demineralized intertubular dentin.

10.4.7 Obstacles in Bonding to Self-Etching Primer Treated Sclerotic Dentin

The smear layers in sound, cut dentin do not impose much of a restriction to the bonding of contemporary self-etching adhesives because of their loose organization. Unless they are instrumented, shiny sclerotic cervical lesions are free of smear layers. In lieu of smear layers, other diffusion barriers in shiny cervical sclerotic lesions include the much denser surface hypermineralized layer, as well as the more loosely arranged, partially mineralized bacterial biofilms. Some of the hypermineralized layers in sclerotic dentin are so thick that they restrict the penetration of strong inorganic acids such as phosphoric acid that usually etches 5 μm or beyond into sound dentin. Being less acidic in nature, mild self-etching primers only etch 0.5 μm into sound dentin that is covered with smear layers. As sclerotic dentin is highly variable in its ultrastructure, different morphologic expressions of the resin-dentin interfaces can be anticipated when a mild self-etching primer is applied to this abnormal bonding substrate. This may be classified into three categories, depending on the thickness and continuity of the surface hypermineralized layer at different locations of the wedge-shaped lesion.

10.4.7.1 Sclerotic Dentin with a Thin Hypermineralized Layer (<0.5 μm Thick)

Thin hypermineralized layers are usually located along the gingival and occlusal aspects of wedge-shaped lesions. Figure 10.17a represents a straightforward situation in which a very thin hypermineralized layer is present, without bacteria, along the occlusal aspect of a natural wedge-shaped lesion. This layer may be recognized by the characteristic arrangement of the partially dissolved crystallite remnants. The difference in hybrid layer morphology that results from uneven etching is readily apparent. On the right side of Fig. 10.17a, the effect of the self-etching primer is restricted to the surface layer alone, producing a 0.1 μm thick, hybridized hypermineralized

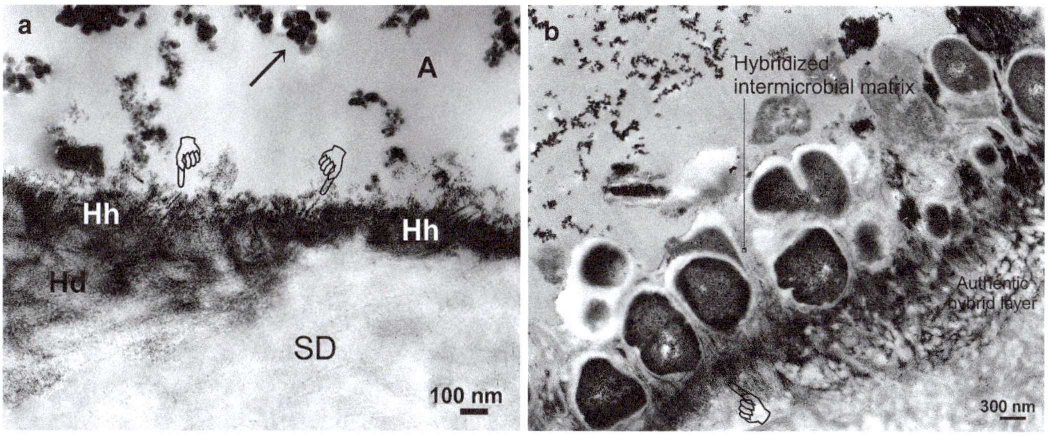

Fig. 10.17 (**a**) Demineralized TEM micrograph of the gingival aspect of a wedge-shaped sclerotic lesion that was treated with a self-etching primer (*A*). Uneven etching was evident. *On the left* a 300 non-thick thin hybridized layer was formed in the hypermineralized layer (Hh) within which were platelike crystallite remnants (pointers). *On the right*, a 100 nm thick layer of hybrid layer in sclerotic dentin (Hb) was formed. *SD* sclerotic dentin. *Arrow*: nanofillers (Modified from Tay and Pashley (2004a)). (**b**) The bonded interface from the occlusal aspect of a sclerotic lesion that contained a thin hypermineralized layer (pointer) covered with surface bacterial deposits. The hybridized complex consisted of (1) a hybridized intermicrobial matrix, (2) a hybridized hypermineralized layer (pointer), and (3) an authentic hybridized layer. The latter was absent on the *left side* of the micrograph (pointer)

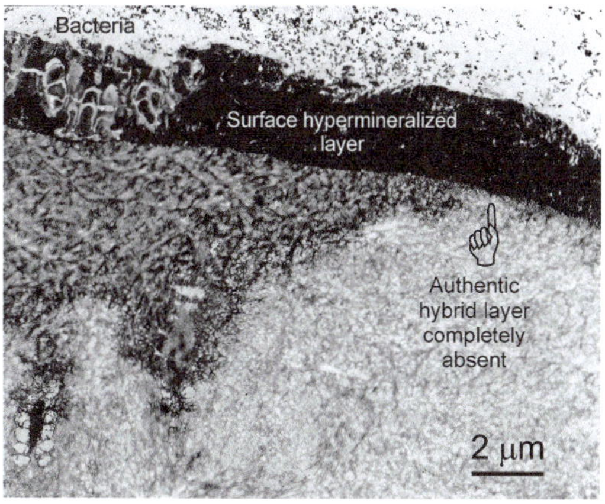

Fig. 10.18 (**a**) The hybridized complex in sclerotic dentin created by 40% phosphoric acid followed by self-etching primer/adhesive, showing bacteria invading a hypermineralized surface. An authentic 2–3 µm hybrid layer formed under the hypermineralized layer than was being eroded by bacteria on the left, but not under the intact hypermineralized layer (Modified from Fig. 18, Tay and Pashley (2004a))

layer. On the left, the primer etched beyond the surface layer to form an additional layer of hybridized dentin that was about 0.5 µm thick.

A similar uneven etching effect may be seen in thin hypermineralized layers that contain additional surface bacterial attachments (Fig. 10.17b). This complicates etching by the fact that the self-etching primer must first infiltrate through the matrix between the bacteria and then through the hypermineralized layer in order to demineralize the underlying intact sclerotic dentin. Unlike the hypermineralized layer that consists of densely arranged crystallites, the intermicrobial matrix is more easily penetrable by the self-etching primer. The hybridized complex, thus, consisted of three components: the hybridized intermicrobial matrix, the hybridized hypermineralized layer, and the layer of hybridized dentin. In this micrograph, the layer of hybridized dentin (Hd) was about 0.5–0.8 µm on the right, but was completely absent on the left. This illustrates the kind of biological variation that may be expected along the entire lesion surface. The features are not the rare, one-of-a-kind phenomenon that is observed only in one single lesion. Figure 10.18 is a high magnification of similar features observed in another specimen. These were taken from the same 1 mm x 1 mm section of the gingival aspect of a bonded sclerotic lesion. Where the hypermineralized layer was dissolved by bacteria, the phosphoric acid etch demineralized the dentin matrix to a depth of 5 μm. However, where the hypermineralized layer was not eroded by bacteria, the hypermineralized layer resisted the etching action of 40 % phosphoric acid, thereby preventing the formation of an authentic hybrid layer.

10.4.7.2 Sclerotic Dentin with a Thick, Continuous Hypermineralized Layer (>0.5 μm)

Thicker hypermineralized layers are found along the occlusal aspects and sometimes within the deepest part of wedge-shaped, sclerotic lesions. As the etching effect of a self-etching primer is limited, it cannot etch beyond the hypermineralized layer into the underlying sclerotic dentin (Fig. 10.17a). At a higher magnification, the crystallites within the bonded hypermineralized layer are shorter and more sparsely arranged, when compared with the underlying unaffected hypermineralized layer. This partially demineralized zone was about 0.5 μm in depth. Porosities created for resin infiltration within this zone are reminiscent of acid-etched, aprismatic enamel. It has been shown that bonding to the surface hypermineralized layer alone resulted in relatively high bond strength (Kwong et al. 2002). The ultimate strength of the entire bonded assembly, however, depends on the strength of the attachment of the hypermineralized layer to the underlying sclerotic dentin.

10.4.8 Summary of Obstacles in Bonding to Sound Versus Sclerotic Dentin

Potential barriers to resin infiltration following total etching or self-etching in sound and sclerotic dentin are summarized schematically in Fig. 10.19 (Kwong et al. 2000). The left side of the figure illustrates the response of ground dentin to acid etching and bonding with a self-etching primer adhesive system alone, while the right side illustrates the response of sclerotic dentin to bonding with the same self-etching primer. The thickness of the hybrid layer is fairly consistent both for self-etching and wet-bonded, acid-etched sound dentin, but is much thicker in the latter group. Conversely, application of the same adhesive strategy to sclerotic dentin results in substantial variation in the hybrid layer morphology in both treatment techniques. Absence of a hybrid layer in some parts of a lesion suggests that both treatment protocols are ineffective in completely overcoming the diffusion barriers in sclerotic dentin. This situation is comparable to the early-generation dentin adhesives that were directly applied to the smear layers in sound dentin (Chigira et al. 1994). Similar to the junction between the partially infiltrated smear layer and the underlying intact sound dentin, areas devoid of hybrid layer formation are potential weak links that may be responsible for the lower bond strengths observed when bonding to sclerotic dentin.

Fig. 10.19 Schematic of wide variation in ultrastructure of resin bonds made to normal vs. sclerotic dentin. Normal dentin (*left*) etched with 40 % phosphoric and bonded with etch-and-rinse adhesive. On the *right* is shown normal dentin etched with a mild self-etching primer. The self-etching primer does not remove the smear layer or smear plug that infiltrates into them. The lower panels are of sclerotic, wedge-shaped lesions that have an occlusal wall, a deep apex, and a gingival wall. The specimens on the right side were bonded with a mild self-etching primer, while the specimens on the left were pre-etched with 40 % phosphoric acid in an attempt to partially or totally remove the hypermineralized layer, followed by bonding with a two-bottle mild self-etching primer followed by an adhesive. The figure legends define the symbols used within the schematics (Modified from Tay and Pashley (2004a))

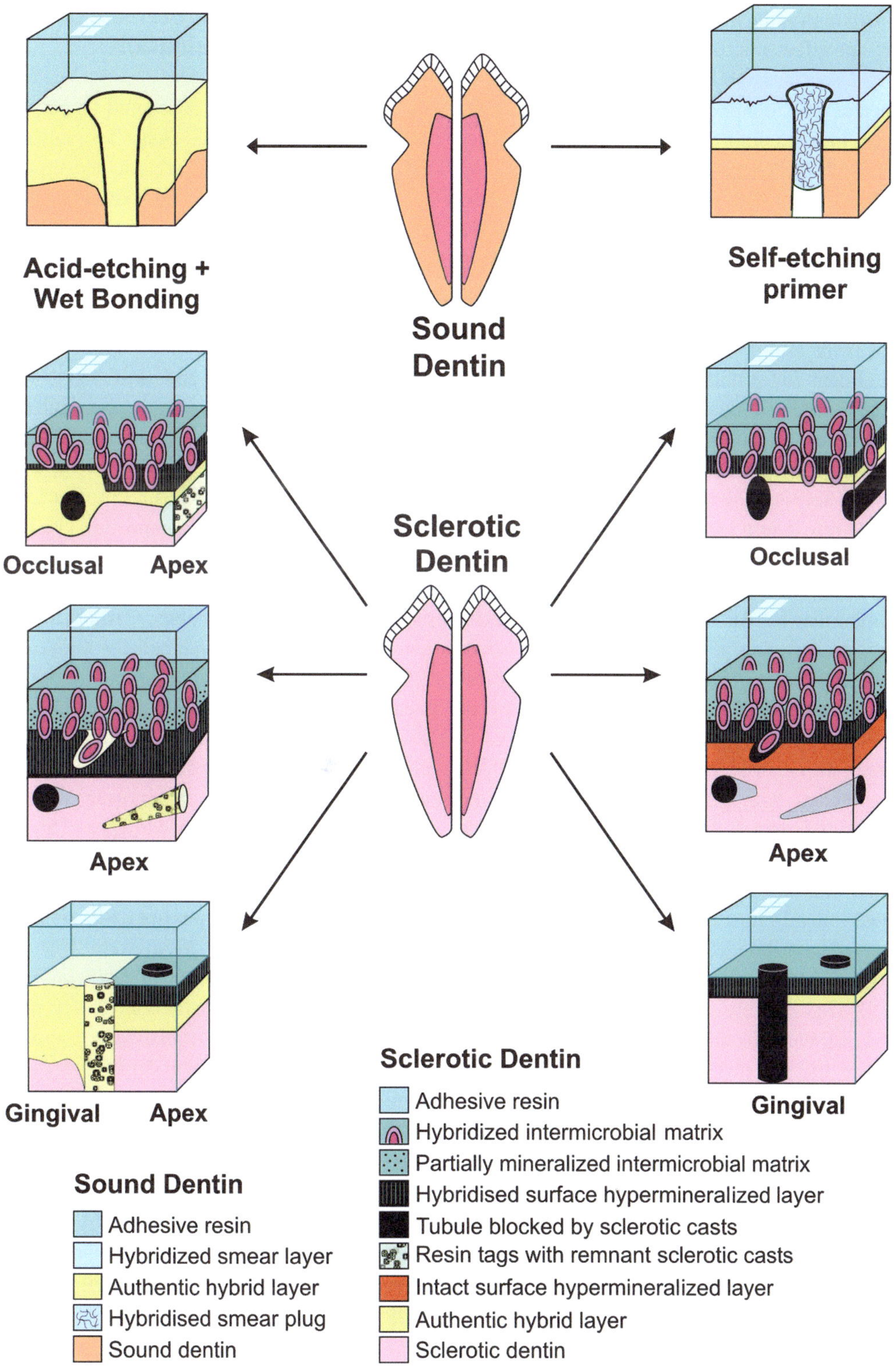
Acid-etching +
Wet Bonding
Sound
Dentin
Self-etching
primer
Occlusal
Apex
Sclerotic
Dentin
Occlusal
Apex
Apex
Gingival
Apex
Gingival
Sclerotic Dentin
Adhesive resin
Hybridized intermicrobial matrix
Partially mineralized intermicrobial matrix
Hybridised surface hypermineralized layer
Tubule blocked by sclerotic casts
Resin tags with remnant sclerotic casts
Intact surface hypermineralized layer
Authentic hybrid layer
Sclerotic dentin
Sound Dentin
Adhesive resin
Hybridized smear layer
Authentic hybrid layer
Hybridised smear plug
Sound dentin

Although reduction in hybrid layer thickness may not affect micromechanical retention, sporadic absence of the hybrid layer and resin tags indicates that both treatment techniques are inadequate in overcoming diffusion barriers in sclerotic dentin. Physical removal of the superficial obstacle layers with a bur may improve intertubular retention. In highly sclerotic lesions however, this may be offset by moving the bonding interface pulpward into an area where bonding requires increasing contribution from intratubular resin infiltration. Moreover, the formation of a smear layer that consists of acid-resistant hypermineralized dentin chips and whitlockite crystals derived from the sclerotic casts also creates additional diffusion barriers for both total-etch and self-etching adhesives.

Sclerotic dentin located at the apex of wedge-shaped natural lesions is derived from deep dentin. Consequently, resin tag formation should play an important role in achieving strong immediate bond strength in the sclerotic cervical lesion. However, resin tag formation is sporadic regardless of the conditioning methods. Absence of intratubular infiltration may even be observed in some of the occlusal parts of natural lesions which were etched with phosphoric acid, where the thickness of intertubular infiltration is comparable to that present in sound dentin. Similar to the results of Ferrari et al. (1996) and Prati et al. (1999), lateral branches of resin tags were rarely observed when bonded sclerotic dentin was examined by TEM (Kwong et al. 2002; Daculsi et al. 1979). This is likely caused by the acid-resistant nature of the mineral-dense sclerotic casts that occlude the dentinal tubules. It has been suggested that 20 % of the strength of an interfacial bond was contributed by resin infiltration derived from resin tag formation (Pashley et al. 1995) and another 20 % from hybridization of the intertubular dentin (Shono et al. 1999; Phrukkanon et al. 1999). Regional tensile bond strength from cervical sclerotic root dentin was found to be 20–45 % lower than those obtained from artificial lesions prepared in sound root dentin (Yoshiyama et al. 1996b; Kwong et al. 2002). This reduction may be due to the absence of resin tags and incomplete hybridization in sclerotic dentin.

10.5 Regional Microtensile Bond Strength Evaluation

Because of the unique location and shape of non-carious, sclerotic wedged-shape lesions, it was important to prepare similarly shaped lesions in normal dentin as microtensile bond strength controls so that both types of dentin had similar C-factors.

Microtensile bond strength measurements (Pashley et al. 1999) comparing resin bonds to the occlusal, gingival, and the apex or deepest part of natural lesions and artificially wedge-shaped defects created in sound cervical dentin were reported by Tay and Pashley (2004) using the microtensile bond test. Lesions were restored with a flowable resin composite, Protect Liner F (Kuraray) and Z100 resin composite (3 M ESPE) following treatment with a self-etching primer adhesive, with or without phosphoric acid preconditioning of the lesions. Using the non-trimming technique developed by Shono et al. (1999), beams with a mean area of 0.46 ± 0.03 mm^2 were prepared and stressed to failure. The use of a non-trimming technique (Fig. 10.20) facilitated preparation of a series of slabs, thus allowing more than one beam to be harvested from each lesion (Phrukkanon et al. 1999; Uno et al. 2001; Ogata et al. 2001).

The mean tensile bond strengths of bonds produced by the self-etching primer adhesives alone to natural lesions (48.7 MPa) were 26 % lower (Fig. 10.21) than those from artificial lesions (65.8 MPa) when all of the bonds were pooled, and the result was statistically significant ($p < 0.001$). Similarly pooled data on bonds made using the self-etching primer adhesives with adjunctive phosphoric acid preconditioning (Torii et al. 2002) to natural lesions (53.1 MPa) were also 24 % lower ($p < 0.005$) than those produced from artificial lesions (69.8 MPa). Pooled data, however, showed no significant difference among the bonds made by self-etching or total-etching adhesives to either sound dentin ($p = 0.415$) or sclerotic dentin ($p = 0.314$). Of the three factors (substrate, conditioning method, and location) tested, only the difference in the type of substrate (i.e., sound dentin vs. sclerotic

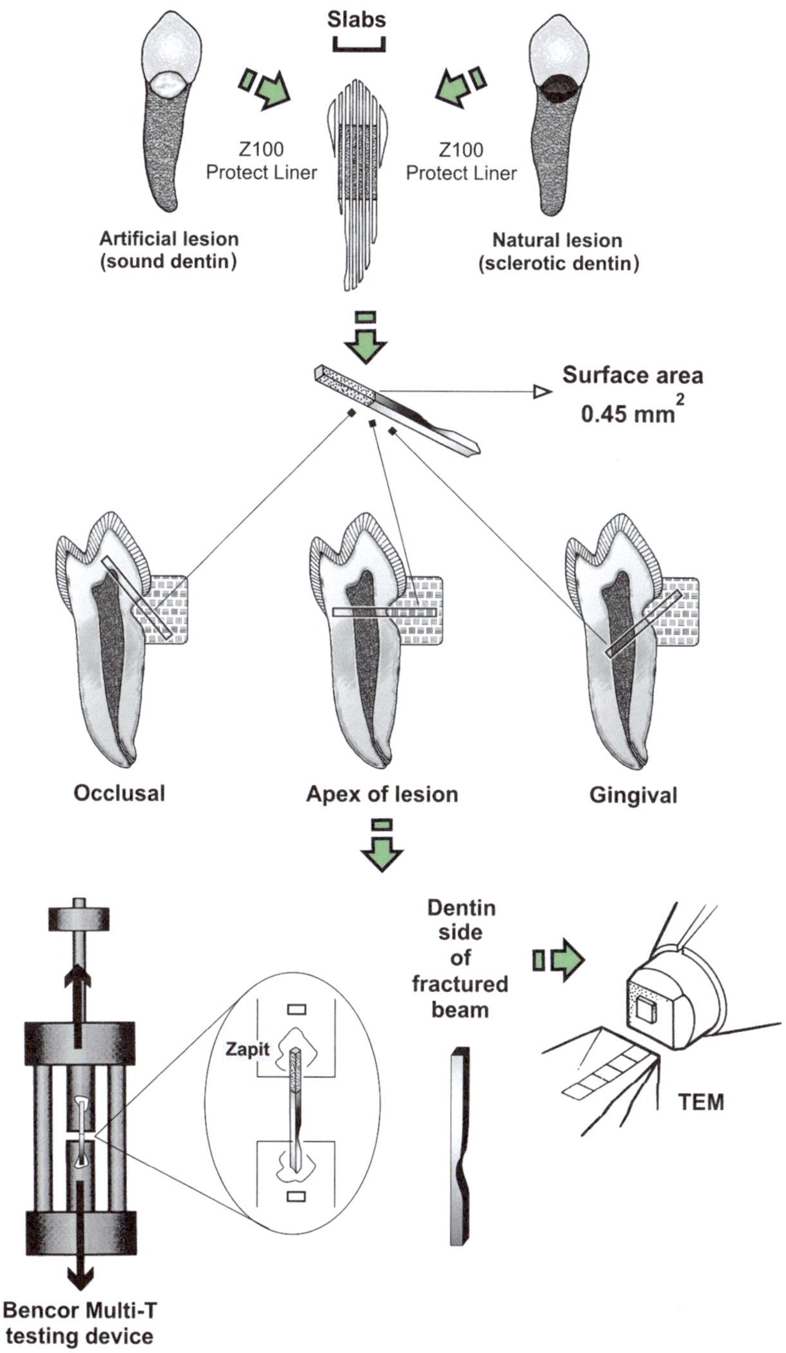

Fig. 10.20 Schematic showing how normal sound mandibular cuspids and bicuspids had artificial wedge-shaped "lesions" prepared (*left side* of schematic) to simulate the configuration of natural sclerotic wedge-shaped lesions (*right side*). After applying the adhesive to the dentin, it was covered with a low-filled, flowable resin composite (Clearfil Protect F to permit ultramicrotomy) that, in turn, was covered with 3 M ESPE Z-100 to provide a resin composite "handle" for bond testing. After immersion in 37 °C water for 24 h, the teeth were sectioned longitudinally into 0.6–0.7 mm thick slabs. Each slab was, in turn, sectioning into 0.7 mm thick "sticks" at various angles to permit bond testing of the "occlusal," "apical," and "gingival" portions of the wedge-shaped restorations. Each "stick" was then pulled to failure in tension in a testing jig (Danville Engineering, Danville, CA, USA) mounted in a universal testing machine. The sticks were fixed to the jig using viscous cyanoacrylate (Zapit brand, Dental Ventures of America, Ventura, CA, USA) (Modified from Tay and Pashley (2004a))

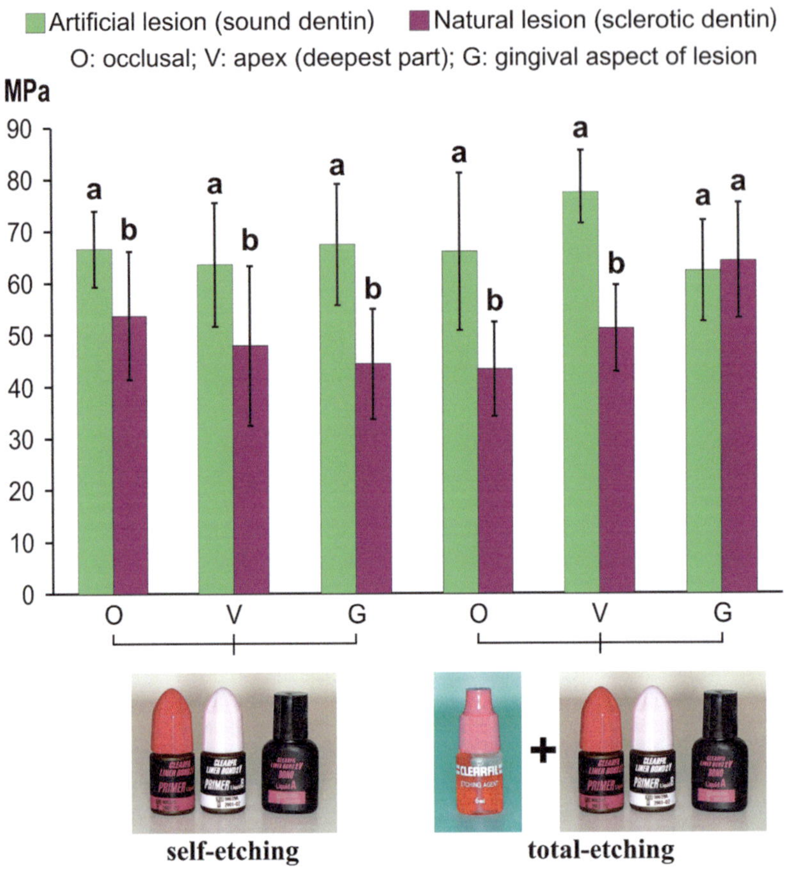

Fig. 10.21 Microtensile bond strengths of self-etching primer/adhesive to sound dentin (*green bars*) or sclerotic (*purple bars*) dentin. Height of bars are the means; brackets indicate ± 1 S.D.; bars identified with different lowercase letters are significantly different ($p<0.05$). Note that all bonds made to sclerotic dentin were significantly ($p<0.05$) lower than those made to normal dentin, except for those made to the gingival floor of specimens that were pre-etched with 40 % phosphoric acid prior to being bonded with the self-etching primer/adhesive. Number of teeth from which slabs were made in each group = 10 (Modified from Fig. 23, Tay and Pashley (2004a))

dentin) was found to have a significant influence on bond strength ($p<0.05$). Multiple comparison tests showed that there was no difference in self-etching or total-etching sclerotic dentin except for the gingival aspect of the lesions, in which higher bond strengths were obtained for total etching (Fig. 10.21) (Tay and Pashley 2004a).

These results are comparable to those of Yoshiyama et al. (1996b) in that lower bond strengths were found in natural sclerotic lesions and to the work of Phrukkanon et al. (1999) showing that bonding of a self-etching primer adhesive to sound dentin is independent of the tubular orientation. The orientation of dentinal tubules in the occlusal or upper wall of wedge-shaped lesions is approximately parallel to the surface, while their orientation in the gingival wall is perpendicular to the prepared surface (Walker et al. 2000; Ogata et al. 1999). Many believed that resin tag formation would be more prominent in surfaces where the tubules are oriented perpendicular to the surface rather than parallel. However, measurement of microtensile bond strengths of self-etching primers and total-etch adhesives to these walls in wedge-shaped cavities prepared in normal dentin revealed significantly higher bond strengths to dentin in which the bonded surfaces were oriented parallel to the tubules (i.e., occlusal walls) (Walker et al. 2000; Ogata et al. 1999).

Double etching of dentin by phosphoric acid followed by a self-etching primer adhesive has been shown to increase bond strengths to enamel, but to lower bond strengths in dentin (Gwinnett and García-Godoy 1992). That result may have been caused by incomplete infiltration of the adhesive into the phosphoric acid-etched dentin (Gwinnett and Kanca 1992a). Using Clearfil Liner Bond 2, Ogata et al. (2001) found that multiple applications of the primer to wedge-shaped lesions increased bond strength due to the weak acidity of the primer. Although this has not been tested in sclerotic dentin, the same result would be expected. That is, multiple applications of weakly acidic agents using constant agitation should improve bonding.

TEM examination of the failed bonds exhibited by bonds made to sclerotic dentin revealed a wide variation in the modes of failure, which included all of the different structural components that are present within the resin-sclerotic dentin interfaces (Kwong et al. 2002). The complexity of failure modes indicates that reduced bond strength in sclerotic dentin is not related to any single factor. Similar to other biological variations, it is possible that each factor contributes to a variable degree in different lesions. The summation of all these factors, however, leads to an overall reduction in bond strength.

The presence of a partially mineralized bacterial zone in sclerotic lesions is analogous to the presence of a smear layer on sound, abraded dentin. This zone is porous, allowing easy penetration of acids and primers to form a zone of hybridized intermicrobial matrix. The presence of a hybridized intermicrobial matrix may not affect bonding, at least in the short term, providing that the self-etching primer can effectively etch through this layer into the underlying bonding substrate. This is analogous to the hybridized smear layers in sound dentin. It remains to be seen whether the eventual degradation of the bacteria in this layer would lead to decrease in bond strength with time. The large standard deviation in bond strength results in natural sclerotic lesions may simply reflect the large biological variation in the thickness of such a layer. Based on the results of a 2-year clinical trial, it has been suggested that micromechanical retention produced by acid etching with 40 % phosphoric acid, is still indispensable for the clinical success of cervical class V composite restorations (Van Meerbeek et al. 1993).

The presence of a hybridized hypermineralized layer together with an underlying zone of hybridized dentin does not necessarily result in low bond strength. This is comparable to the infiltration of a self-etching primer through smear layer-covered sound dentin. Provided that the acids can penetrate the overlying diffusion barriers to engage the underlying substrate with even a very thin hybrid layer, strong initial bonds may still be achieved. However, erratic bonds may be expected when the hypermineralized layer in sclerotic dentin is too thick for acids to etch through. Resin attachment to the partially demineralized surface of this layer is still strong and may be comparable with bonding to unground, aprismatic enamel (Tani et al. 2001). However, since a layer of hybridized dentin is not produced, the strength of the bond will be highly dependent upon the strength of the union between the hypermineralized layer to the intact sclerotic dentin.

The fact that higher bond strength was observed along the gingival site of total-etched natural lesions (Fig. 10.21) merits further discussion. This suggests that the inability of the adhesive to form resin tags in tubule lumina which are blocked by mineral deposits is an important parameter that leads to the reduction in bond strength. If the above hypothesis is correct, then grinding of the surface hypermineralized layer of these cervical wedge-shaped defects prior to bonding (Handelman and Shey 1996) should not result in an increase in bond strength, since the underlying sclerotic dentin still contains dentinal tubules which are blocked by whitlockite crystallites. Application of stronger phosphoric acid to these defects could have resulted in partial dissolution of the sclerotic casts and/or complete removal of the surrounding peritubular dentin, allowing resin infiltration into the dentinal tubules. This may result in higher bond strength along the gingival site of phosphoric acid-etched, sclerotic dentin.

10.6 Restoring the Class V Sclerotic Lesion

Maintaining the marginal integrity and retention of class V resin composite restorations without the use of additional retention has always been a challenge for clinicians. One major factor already analyzed is the difficulty in bonding to sclerotic dentin. Removing the hypermineralized surface layers by grinding or by using stronger acids (Fig. 10.21) are possible strategies to improve micromechanical retention in sclerotic dentin. While it is possible to produce hybrid layers in sclerotic dentin with thin diffusion barriers, these hybrid layers become erratic or even nonexistent in the presence of thick barriers. As clinicians have no way of discerning these differences at a clinical level, removal of the surface layer of sclerotic dentin prior to bonding should be adopted (Kwong et al. 2002; Handelman and Shey 1996). Although such a recommendation may not result in an increase in bond strength to sclerotic dentin, it does remove one potential source of inconsistency that leads to bond failure. The notion that wedge-shaped cervical sclerotic lesions must be preconditioned with 40 % phosphoric acid has been challenged. Several authors maintained that sclerotic dentin, being a part of the body's natural defense mechanism, should be preserved as much as possible and that acid etching should be avoided to promote the marginal integrity of resin composites that are bonded to these lesions (Kusunoki et al. 2002; Yoshiyama et al. 2002).

While one may remove bacteria overgrowths from the surface hypermineralized layer, it is not possible to remove bacteria entirely from dentinal tubules. This is analogous to the application of fissure sealants to stained enamel fissures (Handelman and Shey 1996; Simonsen 2002) or the bonding of resins to the inner layer of carious dentin (Yoshiyama et al. 2002, 2003). The use of bactericidal solutions (i.e., chlorhexidine) or adhesive resins with antibacterial activity (Imazato et al. 1998, 2003) would be helpful. However, the longevity of bonds that contain dead, degradable bacteria should be further investigated. This is particularly applicable to adhesives that contain an increasing amount of hydrophilic resin monomers that absorb water such as all-in-one adhesives. Other studies showed that both hydrophilic resins (Ichim et al. 2007a, b) and collagen fibrils within the hybrid layer (Hashimoto et al. 2000, 2001, 2003; Armstrong et al. 2004; Ichim et al. 2007a) degrade upon long-term water storage.

Swain's group (Brunton et al. 1999) believes that restoration of noncarious sclerotic cervical lesions should not be done with stiff (18 GPa), heavily filled resin composites, but with much more elastic (1 GPa) materials. This recommendation was based upon the use of nonlinear FEA studies of stress-strain relationships in wedge-shaped lesion simulations.[143,144] They made a plea for the development of such a low modulus material. Currently, the closest material would be a low-filled resin-modified glass ionomer with an elastic modulus of 2 GPa.

Conclusions

The structural complexity of noncarious sclerotic cervical dentin is remarkable. The common presence of adherent bacteria on such surfaces, and their incorporation into the bonded restorations is disconcerting. This raises issues such as whether these bacteria are dormant and whether their confinement by adhesives will create any long-term liability. These questions have also been raised in reports that residual bacteria are present in resin-bonded caries-affected dentin (Yoshiyama et al. 2002, 2003). The presence of bacteria on these surfaces justifies the use of 2 % chlorhexidine disinfectant treatment or the use of antibacterial adhesives to disinfect the substrate prior to bonding.

Microtensile bond strengths of self-etching primers to sclerotic dentin were comparable with those made to phosphoric acid-etched sclerotic dentin, although they were lower than those attained with sound dentin. These bond strengths are probably high enough to retain class V restorations even under heavy loads, if bonding is performed with etching of the enamel to create additional micromechanical retention. Although there are clinical studies that showed encouraging results with the use of dentin adhesives on noncarious cervical lesions (Brunton et al. 1999; van Dijken 2000; Tyas and Burrow 2002), the failure rates of some specific adhesives have been reported to be high in other studies. For example, the retention rate for One-Step, a total-etch single-bottle adhesive, in noncarious cervical lesions involving sclerotic dentin was only half of that of non-sclerotic dentin (Kwong et al. 2002). The retention rate of the same adhesive in noncarious cervical lesions was reduced from the original 100 % at 6 months to 75 % after 3 years.

If viable bacteria are entombed by adhesive resin during bonding, do they die or remain dormant? It is likely that bacterial products from colonies on hypermineralized layers would never reach the pulp because most of the tubules are occluded with mineralized structures.

When many of the papers cited in this review were written (2000–2004), the role of the endogenous proteases of dentin on the durability of resin-dentin bonds had not yet been clarified (Pashley et al. 2004; Breschi et al. 2008). However, the durability of resin composite used to restore wedge-shaped lesions has been reported to be retained well for 24 months (Brackett et al. 2002) or 36 months (Matis et al. 1996) or 8 years (Neo and Chew 1996). There are also other clinical studies that reported more favorable retention rates when glass ionomer-based restorative materials were compared with dentin adhesives/resin composites in restoring these lesions. Unfortunately, there are no TEM studies that examine the bonding of glass ionomer cements and resin-modified glass ionomer cements to sclerotic dentin. Admittedly, TEM work on these types of restorative materials that are susceptible to dehydration is difficult to perform. However, this should be done to complete our understanding of this alternative type of chemical/micromechanical interaction with sclerotic dentin.

Acknowledgments This work was supported by grant DE015306 from the NIDCR. The authors are grateful to Michelle Barnes for secretarial support. DHP was also supported as a Highly Cited Scholar by the Faculty of Dentistry of King Abdulaziz University, Jeddah, Saudi Arabia.

References

Armstrong SR, Vargas MA, Chung J, Pashley DH, Campbell JA, Laffoon JE, Qian F. Resin-dentin interfacial and micromechanical dentin bond strength after 5-year water storage. Oper Dent. 2004;29(6):705–12.

Aw TC, Lepe X, Johnson GH, Mancl L. Characteristics of noncarious cervical lesions: a clinical investigation. J Am Dent Assoc. 2002;133:725–33.

Brackett MG, Dib A, Brackett WW, Estrada BE, Reyes AA. One-year clinical performance of a resin-modified glass ionomer and a resin composite restorative material in unprepared class V restorations. Oper Dent. 2002;27:112–6.

Brackett MG, Dib A, Franco G, Estrada BE, Brackett WW. Two-year clinical performance of Clearfil SE and Clearfil S3 in restoration of unabraded non-carious class V lesions. Oper Dent. 2010;35(3):273–8.

Braem M, Lambrechts P, Vanherle G. Stress-induced cervical lesions. J Prosthet Dent. 1992;67:718–22.

Breschi L, Mazzoni A, Ruggeri A, Cadenaro M, Di Lenarda R, DeStefano DE. Dental adhesion: aging and stability of the bonded interface. Dent Mater. 2008;24:90–101.

Brunton PA, Cowan AJ, Wilson MA, Wilson NH. A three-year evaluation of restorations placed with a smear-layer-mediated dentin bonding agent in non-carious cervical lesions. J Adhes Dent. 1999;1:333–41.

Burke FJT, Whitehead SA, McCaughey AD. Contemporary concepts in the pathogenesis of the class V non-carious lesion. Dent Update. 1995;22:28–32.

Chigira H, Manabe A, Hasegawa T, Yukitani W, Fujimitsu T, Itoh K, Hisamitsu H, Wakumoto S. Efficacy of various commercial dentin bonding systems. Dent Mater. 1994;10:363–8.

Coli P, Alaeddin S, Wennerberg A, Karlsson S. *In vitro* dentin pretreatment: surface roughness and adhesive shear bond strength. Eur J Oral Sci. 1999;107:400–13.

Daculsi G, Kerebel B, Le Cabellec MT, Kerebel LM. Qualitative and quantitative data on arrested caries in dentin. Caries Res. 1979;13:190–202.

Daculsi G, LeGeros RZ, Jean A, Kerebel B. Possible physico-chemical processes in human dentin caries. J Dent Res. 1987;66:1356–9.

Duke ES, Lindemuth J. Polymeric adhesion to dentin: contrasting substrates. Am J Dent. 1990;3:264–270.

Duke ES, Lindemuth J. Variability of clinical dentin substrates. Am J Dent. 1991;4:241–6.

Duke ES, Robbins JW, Snyder DS. Clinical evaluation of a dentinal adhesive system: three-year results. Quintessence Int. 1991;22:889–95.

Eda S, Hasegawa H, Kawakami T. Crystals closing tubules in sclerosed root dentin of the aged. In: Shimono M, Maeda T, Suda H, Takahashi K, editors. Proceedings of the international conference on dentin/pulp complex 1995 and the international meeting on clinical topics of dentin/pulp complex. Osaka: Quintessence Publishing Co, Inc.; 1996. p. 283–4.

Eick JD, Cobb CM, Chappell RP, Spencer P, Robinson SJ. The dentinal surface: its influence on dentinal adhesion. Part I. Quintessence Int. 1991;22:967–77.

Eick JD, Gwinnett AJ, Pashley DH, Robinson SJ. Current concepts on adhesion to dentin. Crit Rev Oral Biol Med. 1997;8:306–35.

Eramo S, Baldi M, Marci MC, Monaco A. Histopathological and therapeutical aspects of cervical lesions. Minerva Stomatol. 2003;52:69–74.

Ferrari M, Tay FR. Technique sensitivity in bonding to vital acid-etched dentin. Oper Dent. 2003;28:3–8.

Ferrari M, Cagidiaco MC, Kugel G, Davidson CL. Dentin infiltration by three adhesive systems in clinical and laboratory conditions. Am J Dent. 1996;9:240–04.

Finger WJ, Balkenhol M. Practitioner variability effects on dentin bonding with an acetone-based one-bottle adhesive. J Adhes Dent. 1999;1:311–4.

Gallien GS, Kaplan I, Owens BM. A review of noncarious dental cervical lesions. Compendium. 1994;15: 1366–74.

Giachetti L, Ercolani E, Bambi C, Landi D. Sclerotic dentin: aetio-pathogenetic hypotheses. Minerva Stomatol. 2002;51:285–92.

Goncalves SE, de Araujo MA, Damiao AJ. Dentin bond strength: influence of laser irradiation, acid etching, and hypermineralization. J Clin Laser Med Surg. 1999;17:77–85.

Grippo JO. Abfractions: a new classification of hard tissue lesions of teeth. J Esthet Dent. 1991;3:14–9.

Gwinnett AJ. Quantitative contribution of resin infiltration/hybridization to dentin bonding. Am J Dent. 1993;6:7–9.

Gwinnett AJ. Chemically conditioned dentin: a comparison of conventional and environmental scanning electron microscopy findings. Dent Mater. 1994;10:150–5.

Gwinnett AJ, García-Godoy F. Effect of etching times and acid concentration on resin shear bond strength to primary tooth enamel. Am J Dent. 1992;5:237–0.

Gwinnett AJ, Jendresen M. Micromorphological features of cervical erosion after acid conditioning and its relation with composite resin. J Dent Res. 1978;7:543–9.

Gwinnett AJ, Kanca JA. Interfacial morphology of resin composite and shiny erosion lesions. Am J Dent. 1992a;5:315–7.

Gwinnett AJ, Kanca JA. Micromorphology of the bonded dentin interface and its relationship to bond strength. Am J Dent. 1992b;5:73–7.

Gwinnett AJ, Tay FR, Pang KM, Wei SH. Quantitative contribution of the collagen network in dentin hybridization. Am J Dent. 1996;9:140–4.

Handelman SL, Shey Z. Michael Buonocore and the Eastman Dental Center: a historic perspective on sealants. J Dent Res. 1996;75:529–34.

Harnirattisai C, Inokoshi S, Shimada Y, Hosoda H. Adhesive interface between resin and etched dentin of cervical erosion/abrasion lesions. Oper Dent. 1993;18:138–43.

Hashimoto M, Ohno H, Kaga M, Endo K, Sano H, Oguchi H. *In vivo* degradation of resin-dentin bonds in humans over 1 to 3 years. J Dent Res. 2000;79:1385–91.

Hashimoto M, Ohno H, Kaga M, Endo K, Sano H, Oguchi H. Resin-tooth adhesive interfaces after long-term function. Am J Dent. 2001;14:211–5.

Hashimoto M, Ohno H, Kaga M, Sano H, Tay FR, Oguchi H, Araki Y, Kubota M. Over-etching effects on micro-tensile bond strength and failure patterns for two dentin bonding systems. J Dent. 2002;30:99–105.

Hashimoto M, Ohno H, Sano H, Kaga M, Oguchi H. Degradation patterns of different adhesives and bonding procedures. J Biomed Mater Res. 2003; 66B:324–30.

Ichim IP, Loughran QL, Swain MV, Kieser JA. Restoration of non-carious cervical lesions. Part I: modelling of restorative fracture. Dent Mater. 2007a;23:1553–61.

Ichim IP, Schmidlin PR, Li Q, Kieser JA, Swain MV. Restoration of non-carious cervical lesions. Part II: restorative material selection to minimize fracture. Dent Mater. 2007b;23:1562–9.

Igarashi K, Toida T, Nakabayashi N. Effect of Phenyl P/HEMA primer on bonding to demineralized dentin by phosphoric acid. Jpn J Dent Mater. 1997;16:55–60.

Imazato S, Ehara A, Torii M, Ebisu S. Antibacterial activity of dentin primer containing MPDB after curing. J Dent. 1998;26:267–71.

Imazato S, Kinomoto Y, Tarumi H, Ebisu S, Tay FR. Antibacterial activity and bonding characteristics of an adhesive resin containing antibacterial monomer MDPB. Dent Mater. 2003;19:313–9.

Inai N, Kanemura N, Tagami J, Watanabe LG, Marshall SJ, Marshall GW. Adhesion between collagen depleted dentin and dentin adhesives. Am J Dent. 1998;11:123–7.

Kanca JA. Resin bonding to wet substrate. 1. Bonding to dentin. Quintessence Int. 1992;23:39–41.

Karan K, Yao X, Xu C, Wang Y. Chemical profile of the dentin substrate in non-carious cervical lesions. Dent Mater. 2009;25:1205–12.

Kawakami T, Takei N, Eda S. Crystals closing tubules in sclerosed coronal dentin of the aged. In: Shimono M, Maeda T, Suda H, Takahashi K, editors. Proceedings of the international conference on dentin/pulp complex 1995 and the international meeting on clinical topics of dentin/pulp complex. Osaka: Quintessence Publishing Co, Inc.; 1996. p. 285–6.

Kuroe T, Itoh H, Caputo AA, Konuma M. Biomechanics of cervical tooth structure lesions and their restoration. Quintessence Int. 2000;1:267–74.

Kusunoki M, Itoh K, Hisamitsu H, Wakumoto S. The efficacy of dentin adhesive to sclerotic dentin. J Dent. 2002;30:91–7.

Kwong SM, Tay FR, Yip HK, Kei LH, Pashley DH. An ultrastructural study of the application of dentin adhesives to acid-conditioned sclerotic dentin. J Dent. 2000;7:515–28.

Kwong SM, Cheung GS, Kei LH, Itthagarun A, Smales RJ, Tay FR, Pashley DH. Micro-tensile bond strengths to sclerotic dentin using a self-etching and a total-etching technique. Dent Mater. 2002;18: 359–69.

Lee WC, Eakle WS. Possible role of tensile stress in the etiology of cervical erosive lesions of teeth. J Prosthet Dent. 1984;2:374–80.

Lee WC, Eakle WS. Stress-induced cervical lesions: review of advances in the past 10 years. J Prosthet Dent. 1996;75:487–94.

Lee HE, Lin CL, Wang CH, Cheng CH, Chang CH. Stresses at the cervical lesion of maxillary premolar – a finite element investigation. J Dent. 2002;30:283–90.

Levitch LC, Bader JD, Shugars DA, Heymann HO. Non-carious cervical lesions. J Dent. 1994;22:195–207.

Marino AA, Gross BD. Piezoelectricity in cementum, dentin and bone. Arch Oral Biol. 1989;34:507–9.

Matis BA, Cochran M, Carlson T. Longevity of glass-ionomer restorative materials: results of a 10-year evaluation. Quintessence Int. 1996;27:373–82.

Miller WD. Experiments and observations on the wasting of tooth tissue variously designated as erosion, abrasion, chemical abrasion, denudation, etc. Dent Cosmos. 1907;49:1–23, 109–124, 225–247, 677–689.

Mixson JM, Spencer P, Moore DL, Chappell RP, Adams S. Surface morphology and chemical characterization of abrasion/erosion lesions. Am J Dent. 1995;8:5–9.

Miyasaka K, Nakabayashi N. Combination of EDTA conditioner and Phenyl-P/HEMA self-etching primer for bonding to dentin. Dent Mater. 1999;15:153–7.

Nakabayashi N, Saimi Y. Bonding to intact dentin. J Dent Res. 1996;75:1706–15.

Nakabayashi N, Kojima K, Masuhara E. The promotion of adhesion by the infiltration of monomers into tooth substrates. J Biomed Mater Res. 1982;16:265–73.

Nalbandian J, Federico G, Sognnaes RF. Sclerotic age changes in root dentin of human teeth as observed by optical, electron, and x-ray microscopy. J Dent Res. 1959;39:598–607.

Neo J, Chew CL. Direct tooth-colored materials for non-carious lesions: a 3-year clinical report. Quintessence Int. 1996;27:183–8.

Ogata M, Nakajima M, Sano H, Tagami J. Effect of dentin primer application on regional bond strength to cervical wedge-shaped cavity walls. Oper Dent. 1999;24:81–8.

Ogata M, Okuda M, Nakajima M, Pereira PN, Sano H, Tagami J. Influence of the direction of tubules on bond strength to dentin. Oper Dent. 2001;26:27–35.

Ogata M, Harada N, Yamaguchi S, Nakajima M, Tagami J. Effect of self-etching primer vs phosphoric acid etchant on bonding to bur-prepared dentin. Oper Dent. 2002;27:447–54.

Palamara D, Palamara JE, Tyas MJ, Messer HH. Strain patterns in cervical enamel of teeth subjected to occlusal loading. Dent Mater. 2000;16:412–9.

Pashley DH, Carvalho RM. Dentin permeability and dentin adhesion. J Dent. 1997;25:355–72.

Pashley DH, Tao L, Boyd L, King GE, Horner JA. Scanning electron microscopy of the substructure of smear layers in human dentin. Arch Oral Biol. 1988;33:265–70.

Pashley DH, Horner JA, Brewer PD. Interactions of conditioners on the dentin surface. Oper Dent. 1992;(Suppl) 5:137-50.

Pashley DH, Sano H, Ciucchi B, Carvalho RM, Russell CM. Bond strength versus dentin structures: a modeling approach. Arch Oral Biol. 1995;40:1109–18.

Pashley DH, Carvalho RM, Sano H, Nakajima M, Yoshiyama M, Shono Y, Fernandes CA, Tay F. The micro-tensile bond test: a review. J Adhes Dent. 1999;1:299–309.

Pashley DH, Zhang Y, Agee K, Rouse CJ, Carvalho RM, Russell CM. Permeability of demineralized dentin to HEMA. Dent Mater. 2000;1:7–14.

Pashley DH, Agee KA, Carvalho RM, Lee KW, Tay FR, Callison TE. Effects of water and water-free polar solvents on the tensile properties of demineralized dentin. Dent Mater. 2003;19:347–52.

Pashley DH, Tay FR, Yiu C, Hashimoto M, Breschi L, Carvalho RM, Ito S. Collagen degradation by host-derived enzymes during aging. J Dent Res. 2004;83:216–21.

Perdigão J. Dentin bonding as a function of dentin structure. Dent Clin North Am. 2002;46:277–301.

Perdigão J, Swift Jr EJ, Denehy GE, Wefel JS, Donly KJ. *In vitro* bond strengths and SEM evaluation of dentin bonding systems to different dentin substrates. J Dent Res. 1994;73:44–55.

Pereira PNR, Okuda M, Sano H, Yoshikawa T, Burrow MF, Tagami J. Effect of intrinsic wetness and regional difference on dentin bond strength. Dent Mater. 1999;15:46–53.

Peschke A, Blunck U, Roulet JF. Influence of incorrect application of a water-based adhesive system on the marginal adaptation of Class V restorations. Am J Dent. 2000;13:239–44.

Phrukkanon S, Burrow MF, Tyas MJ. The effect of dentin location and tubule orientation on the bond strengths between resin and dentin. J Dent. 1999;27:265–274.

Prati C, Chersoni S, Mongiorgi R, Pashley DH. Resin-infiltrated dentin layer formation of new bonding systems. Oper Dent. 1998;23:185–94.

Prati C, Chersoni S, Mongiorgi R, Montanari G, Pashley DH. Thickness and morphology of resin-infiltrated dentin layer in young, old, and sclerotic dentin. Oper Dent. 1999;24:66–72.

Rees JS. The role of cuspal flexure in the development of abfraction lesions: a finite element study. Eur J Oral Sci. 1998;106:1028–32.

Rees JS. A review of the biomechanics of abfraction. Eur J Prosthodont Restor Dent. 2000;8:139–44.

Rees JS. The effect of variation in occlusal loading on the development of abfraction lesions: a finite element study. J Oral Rehabil. 2002;29:188–93.

Rees JS, Hammadeh M, Jagger DC. Abfraction lesion formation in maxillary incisors, canines and premolars: a finite element study. Eur J Oral Sci. 2003;111:149–54.

Sakoolnamarka R, Burrow MF, Prawer S, Tyas MJ. Micromorphological investigation of noncarious cervical lesions treated with demineralizing agents. J Adhes Dent. 2000;2:279–87.

Sakoolnamarka R, Burrow MF, Tyas MJ. Micromorphological study of resin-dentin interface of non-carious cervical lesions. Oper Dent. 2002;27:493–9.

Sano H, Yoshikawa T, Peireira PNR, Kanemura N, Morigami M, Tagami J, Pashley DH. Long-term durability of dentin bonds made with a self-etching primer, *in vivo*. J Dent Res. 1999;78:906–11.

Sanz M, Newman MG. Dental plaque and calculus. In: Nisengard RJ, Newman MG, editors. Oral microbiology and immunology. Philadelphia: WB Saunders; 1994. p. 320–40.

Scheie AA, Fejerskov O, Lingström P, Birkhed D, Manji F. Use of palladium touch microelectrodes under field conditions for *in vivo* assessment of dental plaque pH in children. Caries Res. 1992;26:44–52.

Schüpbach P, Lutz F, Guggenheim B. Human root caries: histopathology of arrested lesions. Caries Res. 1992;26:153–64.

Shono Y, Ogawa T, Terashita M, Carvalho RM, Pashley EL, Pashley DH. Regional measurement of resin-dentin bonding as an array. J Dent Res. 1999;78: 699–705.

Simonsen RJ. Pit and fissure sealant: review of the literature. Pediatr Dent. 2002;24:393–414.

Spatafora GA, Sheets M, June R, Luyimbazi D, Howard K, Hulbert R, Barnard D, el Janne M, Hudson MC. Regulated expression of the *Streptococcus mutans* dlt genes correlates with intracellular polysaccharide accumulation. J Bacteriol. 1999;181:2363–72.

Spranger H. Investigation into the genesis of angular lesions at the cervical region of teeth. Quintessence Int. 1995;26:149–54.

Svensäter G, Björnsson O, Hamilton IR. Effect of carbon starvation and proteolytic activity on stationary-phase acid tolerance of *Streptococcus mutans*. Microbiology. 2001;147:2971–9.

Tani C, Itoh K, Hisamitsu H, Wakumoto S. Efficacy of dentin bonding to cervical defects. Dent Mater J. 2001;20:359–68.

Tao L, Pashley DH, Boyd L. The effect of different types of smear layers on dentin and enamel bond strengths. Dent Mater. 1988;4:208–16.

Tay FR, Pashley DH. Aggressiveness of contemporary self-etching adhesives. Part I: depth of penetration beyond dentin smear layers. Dent Mater. 2001;17: 296–308.

Tay FR, Pashley DH. Bonding of a self-etching primer to noncarious cervical sclerotic dentin: a review. J Dent. 2004a;32:173–96.

Tay FR, Pashley DH. Resin bonding to cervical sclerotic dentin: a review. J Dent. 2004b;32(3):173–96.

Tay FR, Sano H, Carvalho R, Pashley EL, Pashley DH. An ultrastructural study of the influence of acidity of self-etching primers and smear layers thickness on bonding to intact dentin. J Adhes Dent. 2000a;2:83–98.

Tay FR, Carvalho R, Sano H, Pashley DH. Effect of smear layers on the bonding of a self-etching primer to dentin. J Adhes Dent. 2000b;2:99–116.

Tay FR, King NM, Chan KM, Pashley DH. How can nanoleakage occur in self-etching adhesive systems that demineralize and infiltrate simultaneously? J Adhes Dent. 2002;4:255–69.

Titley K, Chernecky R, Maric B, Valiquette N, Smith D. The morphology of the demineralized layer in primed dentin. Am J Dent. 1994;7:22–6.

Tjäderhane L, Nascimento FD, Breschi L, Mazzoni A, Tersariol ILS, Geraldeli S, Tezvergil-Mutluay A, Carrilho MR, Carvalho RM, Tay FR, Pashley DH. Optimizing dentin bond durability: control of collagen degradation by matrix metalloproteinases and cysteine cathepsins. Dent Mater. 2013a;29:116–35.

Tjäderhane L, Nascimento FD, Breschi L, Mazzoni A, Tersariol ILS, Geraldeli S, Tezvergil-Mutluay A, Carrilho M, Carvalho RM, Tay FR, Pashley DH. Strategies to prevent hydrolytic degradation of the hybrid layer – a review. Dent Mater. 2013b;29:999–1011.

Toida T, Watanabe A, Nakabayashi N. Effect of smear layer on bonding to dentin prepared with bur. Jpn J Soc Dent Mater Devices. 1995;14:109–16.

Torii Y, Itou K, Nishitani Y, Ishikawa K, Suzuki K. Effect of phosphoric acid etching prior to self-etching primer application on adhesion of resin composite to enamel and dentin. Am J Dent. 2002;15:305–8.

Tyas MJ. Clinical performance of three dentin bonding agents in class V abrasion lesions without enamel etching. Aust Dent J. 1987;33:177–80.

Tyas MJ. The class V lesion – aetiology and restoration. Aust Dent J. 1995;40:167–70.

Tyas MJ, Burrow MF. Three-year clinical evaluation of one-step in non-carious cervical lesions. Am J Dent. 2002;15:309–11.

Uno S, Inoue H, Finger WJ, Inoue S, Sano H. Microtensile bond strength evaluation of three adhesive systems in cervical dentin cavities. J Adhes Dent. 2001;3: 333–41.

van Dijken JW. Clinical evaluation of three adhesive systems in class V non-carious lesions. Dent Mater. 2000;16:285–91.

Van Meerbeek B, Braem M, Lambrechts P, Vanherle G. Two-year clinical evaluation of two dentin-adhesive systems in cervical lesions. J Dent. 1993;21: 195–202.

Van Meerbeek B, Braem M, Lambrechts P, Vanherle G. Morphological characterization of the interface between resin and sclerotic dentin. J Dent. 1994;22: 141–6.

Van Meerbeek B, Peumans M, Gladys S, Braem M, Lambrechts P, Vanherle G. Three-year clinical effectiveness of four total-etch dentinal adhesive systems in cervical lesions. Quintessence Int. 1996;27:775–84.

Van Meerbeek B, De Munck J, Yoshida Y, Inoue S, Vargas M, Vijay P, Van Landuyt K, Lambrechts P, Vanherle G. Buonocore memorial lecture. Adhesion to enamel and dentin: current status and future challenges. Oper Dent. 2003;28:215–35.

Vargas MA, Cobb DS, Armstrong SR. Resin-dentin shear bond strength and interfacial ultrastructure with and without a hybrid layer. Oper Dent. 1997;22:159–66.

Vasiliadis L, Darling AI, Levers BG. The histology of sclerotic human root dentin. Arch Oral Biol. 1983;28:693–700.

Walker MP, Wang Y, Swafford J, Evans A, Spencer P. Influence of additional acid etch treatment on resin cement dentin infiltration. J Prosthodont. 2000;9:77–81.

Wang Y, Spencer P. Quantifying adhesive penetration in adhesive/dentin interface using confocal Raman microspectroscopy. J Biomed Mater Res. 2002;59:46–55.

Wang Y, Spencer P. Hybridization efficiency of the adhesive/dentin interface with wet bonding. J Dent Res. 2003;82:141–5.

Watanabe I, Nikaido T, Nakabayashi N. Effect of adhesion promoting monomers on adhesion to ground dentin. Jpn J Soc Dent Mater Devices. 1990;9:888–93.

Watanabe I, Nakabayashi N, Pashley DH. Bonding to ground dentin by a phenyl-P self-etching primer. J Dent Res. 1994;73:1212–20.

Weber DF. Human dentin sclerosis: a microradiographic survey. Arch Oral Biol. 1974;19:163–9.

Xhonga FA. Bruxism and its effect on the teeth. J Oral Rehabil. 1977;4:65–76.

Yoshiyama M, Masada J, Uchida A, Ishida H. Scanning electron microscopic characterization of sensitive versus insensitive human radicular dentin. J Dent Res. 1989;68:1498–502.

Yoshiyama M, Noiri Y, Ozaki K, Uchida A, Ishikawa Y, Ishida H. Transmission electron microscopic characterization of hypersensitive human radicular dentin. J Dent Res. 1990;9:1293–7.

Yoshiyama M, Suge T, Kawasaki A, Ebisu S. Morphological characterization of tube-like structures in hypersensitive human radicular dentin. J Dent. 1996a;24:57–63.

Yoshiyama M, Sano H, Ebisu S, Tagami J, Ciucchi B, Carvalho RM, Johnson MH, Pashley DH. Regional strengths of bonding agents to cervical sclerotic root dentin. J Dent Res. 1996b;75:1404–13.

Yoshiyama M, Matsuo T, Ebisu S, Pashley DH. Regional bond strengths of self-etching/self-priming adhesive systems. J Dent. 1998;26:609–16.

Yoshiyama M, Tay FR, Doi J, Nishitani Y, Yamada T, Itou K, Carvalho RM, Nakajima M, Pashley DH. Bonding of self-etch and total-etch adhesives to carious dentin. J Dent Res. 2002;81:556–60.

Yoshiyama M, Tay FR, Torii Y, Nishitani Y, Doi J, Itou K, Ciucchi B, Pashley DH. Resin adhesion to carious dentin. Am J Dent. 2003;16:47–52.

Yu XY, Wieczkowski G, Davis EL, Joynt RB. Scanning electron microscopic study of dentinal surfaces treated with various dentinal bonding agents. Quintessence Int. 1990;21:989–99.

Zsigmondy U. Über die keilförmigen Defekte an den Facialflächen der Zajnhälse. Österr Ungar Vjhrschr Zahnärzte. 1894;1:439–42.

The Pulp Reaction Beneath the Carious Lesion

11

Michel Goldberg

Abstract

The carious lesion may develop at a slow rate. In such case, they are involved in the formation of reactionary (or tertiary) dentin. Rapidly progressing carious lesions lead to the formation of an atubular dentin of the osteodentin type or to the complete absence of tertiary dentin. This rapidly progressing lesion management often leads to pulp necrosis, followed by the formation of a periapical lesion. Type I, III, V, and VI collagens are associated with phosphorylated and non-phosphorylated proteins form a loosely network. Combined with proteins, CS-4 and CS-6 and KS appear as proteoglycans. MMPs, TIMPs, and other proteases are involved in matrix components degradation. Reactionary dentin results from the synthetic and secretory activities of altered odontoblasts. The dentinal layer is mostly tubular and deposited beneath a calciotraumatic line. Reparative dentin is under the control of pulp cells. It appears as an osteodentin, with osteoblast-like cells being residing in osteocyte lacunae, with tiny interconnections between cells. The dentin matrix proteins contains collagen type I, phosphophoryn (PP), and dentin sialoprotein (DSP), all of which play crucial roles in the dentin mineralization process. Apical cells formed a niche of stem/progenitor cells sliding from the apex toward the coronal pulp where they differentiate. Arrested caries contribute to the formation of reactionary dentin. Rapidly progressing carious lesions lead to the formation of an atubular dentin. Pulp capping induces the formation of reparative dentin. After a mild caustic effect, the pulp surface undergoes necrosis due to the alkaline of calcium hydroxide (pH 12), followed by new matrix formation and the mineralization of a dentinal bridge. The cells proliferate and form a dense extracellular matrix. The cells display

M. Goldberg
University Paris Descartes, Sorbonne, Paris Cité
and INSERM UMR-S1124, 45 rue des Saints Pères,
Cedex 06, 75270 Paris, France
e-mail: mgoldod@gmail.com

M. Goldberg (ed.), *Understanding Dental Caries*, DOI 10.1007/978-3-319-30552-3_11

odontoblast-like morphology by day 14. The mineralization of the reparative bridge is uncompleted. The bridge showing many interruptions is due to the presence of tunnels and pulp remnants. However, the reparative dentin contributes to occlude the pulp exposure. Pulp stones are either adherent to the pulp walls, or isolated within the pulp, forming calcospherites around blood vessels.

11.1 Extracellular Matrix of Sound Pulp: Composition

Primary dentin characterizes the dentin formed during odontogenesis. Secondary dentin starts to be formed while the tooth is still embedded in the jaws and is continuous after the tooth is erupted. The tubules in primary and secondary dentins form a continuum. Secretory odontoblasts and the so-called Hoehl's cell layer form primary and secondary dentins. Tertiary dentin generated in response to nonphysiological stimuli, such as caries or cavity preparation, is formed only by mesenchymal tissue and is formed by "secondary" odontoblasts, which are actually pulp cells. They are activated after primary odontoblasts have been destroyed (Mjör 2009). Dentin matrix results from the secretion of specific cells (odontoblasts and Hoehl's cells exclusively) (Figs. 11.1, 11.2, 11.3, and 11.4). In addition, dentin is composed of a mineral phase (70 %), an extracellular matrix (20 %), and water (10–12 %), formed by partially free water and bound water.

Type I collagen is the major fibrous component of the dentin matrix, but pulp matrix also contains significant amounts of type III collagen (Figs. 11.4, 11.5, and 11.6). Fibronectin and proteoglycans are also present in the dental pulp (osteoadherin/osteomodulin) (Linde 1985). *Type III collagen* constitutes 28 % of the pulp (Shuttleworth et al. 1978). It may form up to 42.6 % type III of the total collagen (see table 11.1, 41 %). *Type V collagen* comprised two different molecular species of $[a1(V)]_2$ a2(V)a2(V)a3(V), the ratio of which represented, respectively, 56,41 and 2 % of the total collagen (Tsuzaki et al. 1990). Type VI (0.5 %) is associated with microfibrillin.

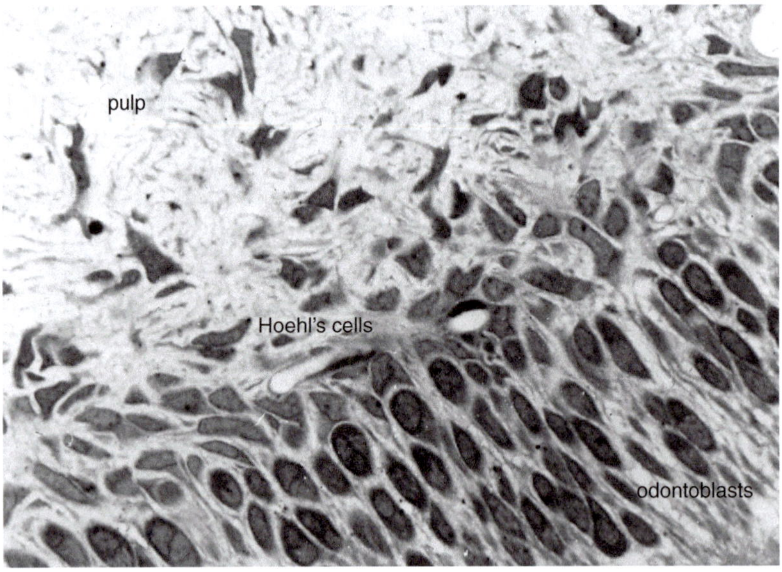

Fig. 11.1 Odontoblasts and Hoehl's cells are located at the periphery of the pulp

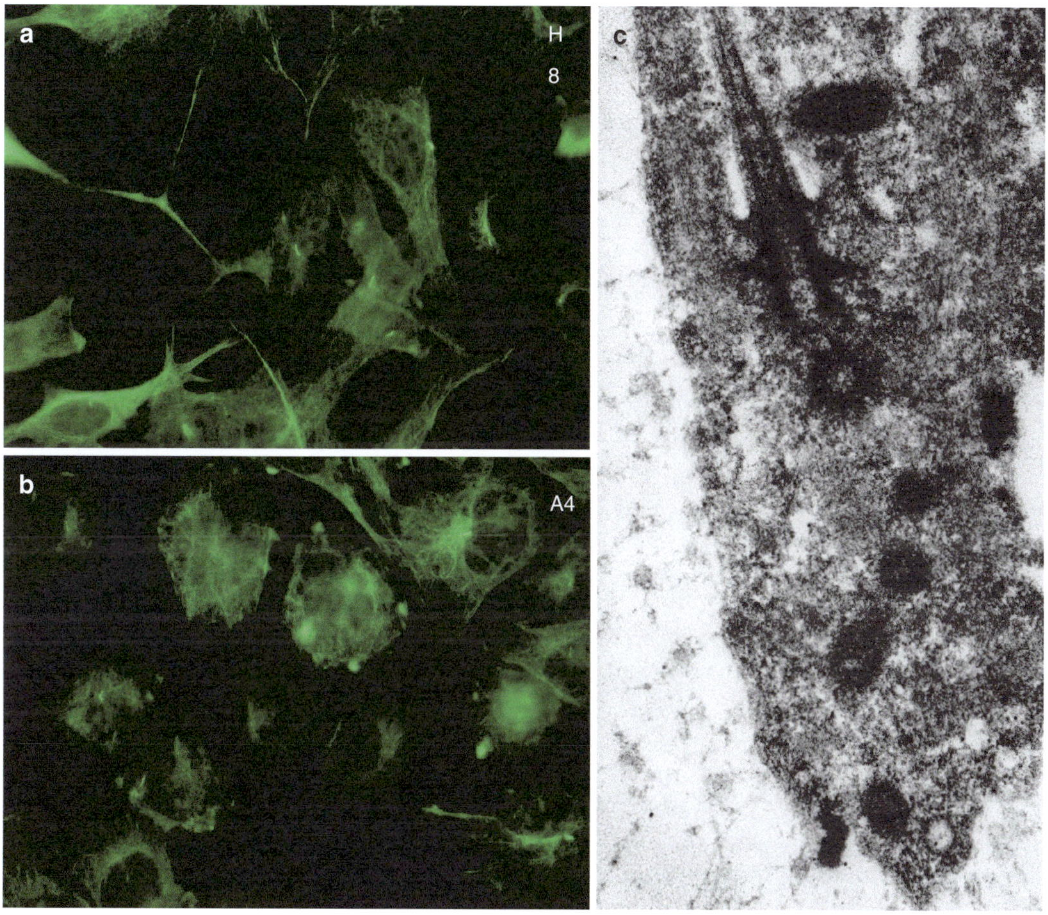

Fig. 11.2 Immunohistochemical visualization of alpha acetyl tubulin, a component of microtubules, in H8 (**a**) and A4 (**b**) cell lines. In c = a pulpoblast displays a cilium and basal body

Collagen degradation is regulated by matrix metalloproteinases (MMPs). TNF-α, IΛ – 1β, and IΛ – 6 ανδ ΤΓΦ – β1 πλαψ ρολε ιν χολλαγεν δεγραδατιον are mediated by pulp fibroblasts (Wisithphrom and Windsor 2006) (Fig. 11.6).

Phosphorylated and non-phosphorylated proteins: Osteocalcin, dentin sialophosphoprotein (DSPP), and matrix extracellular phosphoglycoprotein (MEPE) have been detected in pulp cell cultures. DSPP and MEPE expressions are regulatory pattern of DPCC with stem cell characteristics. DSPP is processed by protease (BMP-1) into three major domains: dentin sialoprotein (DSP), dentin glycoprotein (DGP), and dentin phosphoprotein (DPP). Expression of full-length *Dspp mRNA* by quantitative real-time polymerase chain reaction analysis was significantly higher in odontoblasts than in pulp (Yamamoto et al 2015). DSPP-derived proteins in porcine pulp are expressed at both the protein and mRNA levels.

Tenascin and fibronectin were found by immunohistochemistry at the periphery of the pulp, next to the odontoblasts of normal human dental pulp.

Glycosaminoglycans (GAGs) and proteoglycans (PGs) are present in the dental pulp. GAGs are formed by chondroitin sulfate, dermatan sulfate, heparan sulfate, keratan sulfate, and hyaluronic acid. CS-4 and CS-6 are the major glycosaminoglycans, hyaluronic acid and keratan sulfate being presented in minor amount (Rahamtulla 1992).

Decorin, biglycan, and fibromodulin are CS PGs (Goldberg et al. 2005, 2006) (Fig. 11.4).

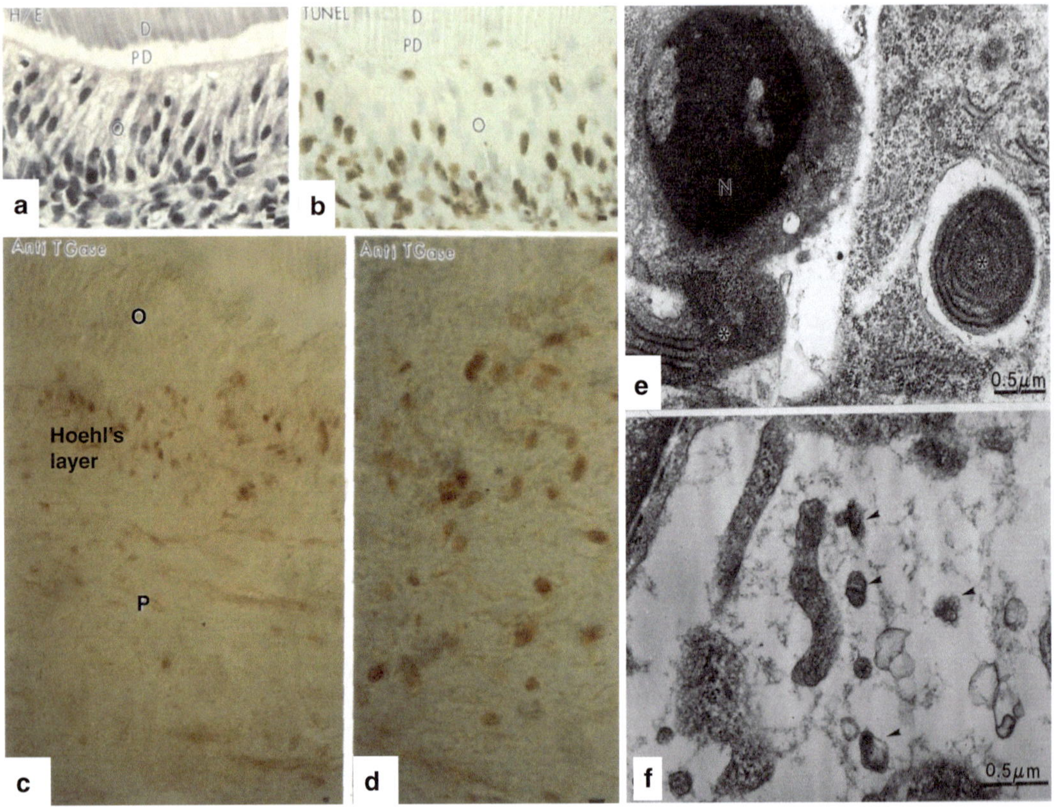

Fig. 11.3 (**a**, **b**) (**a**) Hematoxylin-eosin staining of a control semi-thin epon section. b: after TUNEL staining apoptotic cells (colored in *dark brown*) are located in the odontoblast (*o*) layer. *PD* predentin, *D* dentin. (**c**, **d**) An antibody raised against the apoptotic marker the anti-transglutaminase (anti-TGases) stains cells located in the Hoehl's layer, but not odontoblasts (*O*) or pulp (*P*) cells. (**e**) Chromatin condensation in the nucleus (*left* part of the figure) and isolated rough endoplasmic reticulum (*asterisk*) inside another pulp cell (*right* part of the figure). (**f**) Apoptotic bodies (*arrowheads*) after the apoptotic destruction of the cell

Versican, a proteoglycan aggregate, has also been extracted from the dental pulp. Versican, hyaluronan, and link protein form ternary aggregate structures in the rat dental pulp (Shibata et al. 2000).

Metalloproteinases (MMPs) and tissue-specific inhibitors (TIMPs) are implicated in the extracellular matrix degradation (Sulkala et al. 2004). cDNA microarray demonstrated the high level for MMP-13 (collagenase-3) and a lesser expression of MMP-16 (MT3-MMP) and TIMP-1, especially during caries progression. During rat tooth eruption, a disintegrin and metalloprotease with thrombospondin type 1 motifs (ADAMTS) is implicated in cleaving proteoglycans such as aggrecan, versican, and brevican. ADAMTS1, ADAMTS4, ADAMTS5, and versican were expressed in dental pulp cells (Fig. 11.5). Dental pulp cells are involved in both production and degradation of versican with secreting ADAMTS1, ADAMTS4, and ADAMTS5 (Sone et al. 2005).

11.2 Cells

The pulp periphery: At the outer border of the pulp, odontoblasts and the so-called Hoehl's cells form continuous layers. These postmitotic cells have the capacity to undergo terminal differentiation.

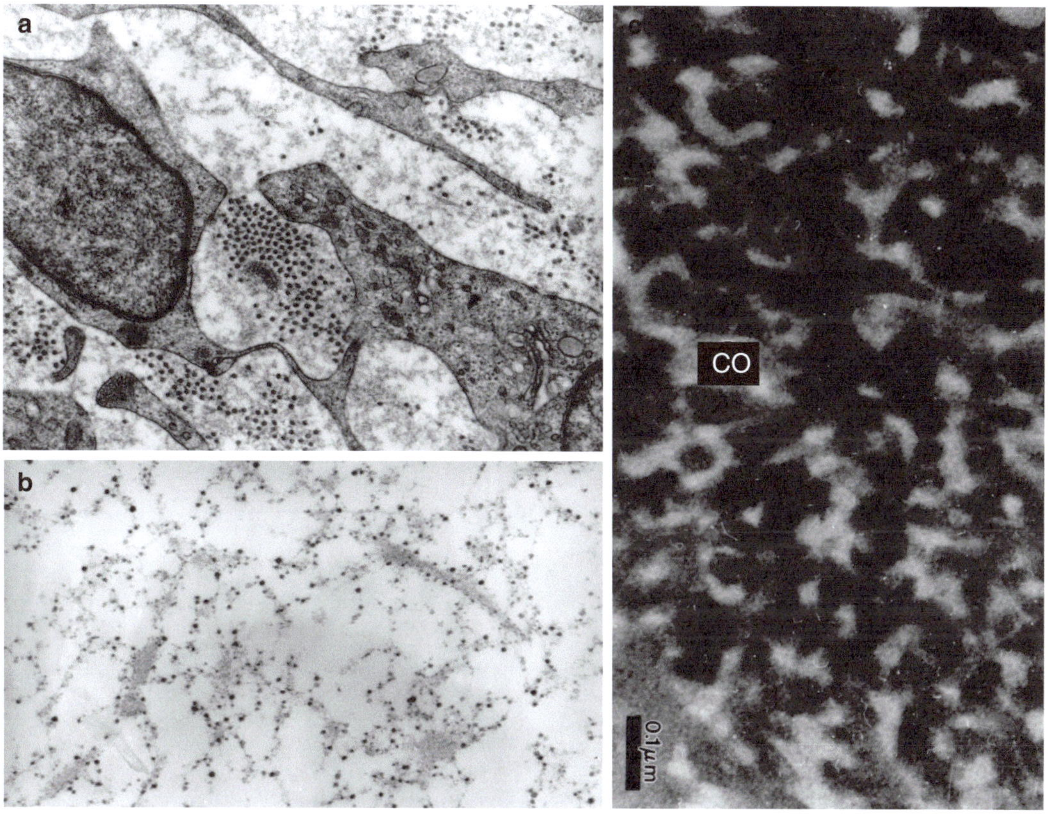

Fig. 11.4 (**a**) Pulpoblasts and collagen fibrils displaying different diameters. (**b**) Histochemical staining of glycosaminoglycans appearing as electron-dense granules aligned along collagen fibrils and pulpoblast processes. (**c**) Alcian blue stained predentin after rapid freezing freeze substitution. The collagen fibrils appear electron lucent; intercollagenic spaces are electron dense and stained by the cationic dye

Odontoblasts are implicated in the synthesis of collagen and noncollagenous extracellular matrix components. Some ECM proteins are phosphorylated (SIBLINGs), whereas others are non-phosphorylated. ECM components are implicated in predentin and dentin formation, followed by dentin mineralization. Due to a fixation artifact, the formation of a cell-free layer results in from fixation and dehydration. A cell-free area underlines odontoblasts and Hoehl's cells, which do not appear on sections after adequate fixative perfusion. Fenestrated capillary loops infiltrate the layer formed by odontoblasts and Hoehl's cells but do not cross the terminal junctions located between the distal odontoblast cell bodies nor penetrate within the predentin. In contrast, axons infiltrate the odontoblastic layer and penetrate into the predentin. A few axons penetrate into dentin tubules and occupy the inner dentin but are found only in the inner 150 micrometers (Fig. 11.1).

Pulp cells are present in the dental pulp. Fibroblasts (pulpoblasts) and fibrocytes are the prominent cells, with variable cell density. They are elongated, with thin spinous processes. A few macrophages, plasmocytes, mast cells, and leukocytes have been also identified. Pulpoblasts contain dense cytoskeletal proteins, including microfilaments, intermediary filaments, and microtubules. Immunostaining of alpha acetyl tubulin revealed the presence of microtubules (Fig. 11.2a, b) associated in cilium and basal corpuscle (Fig. 11.2c).

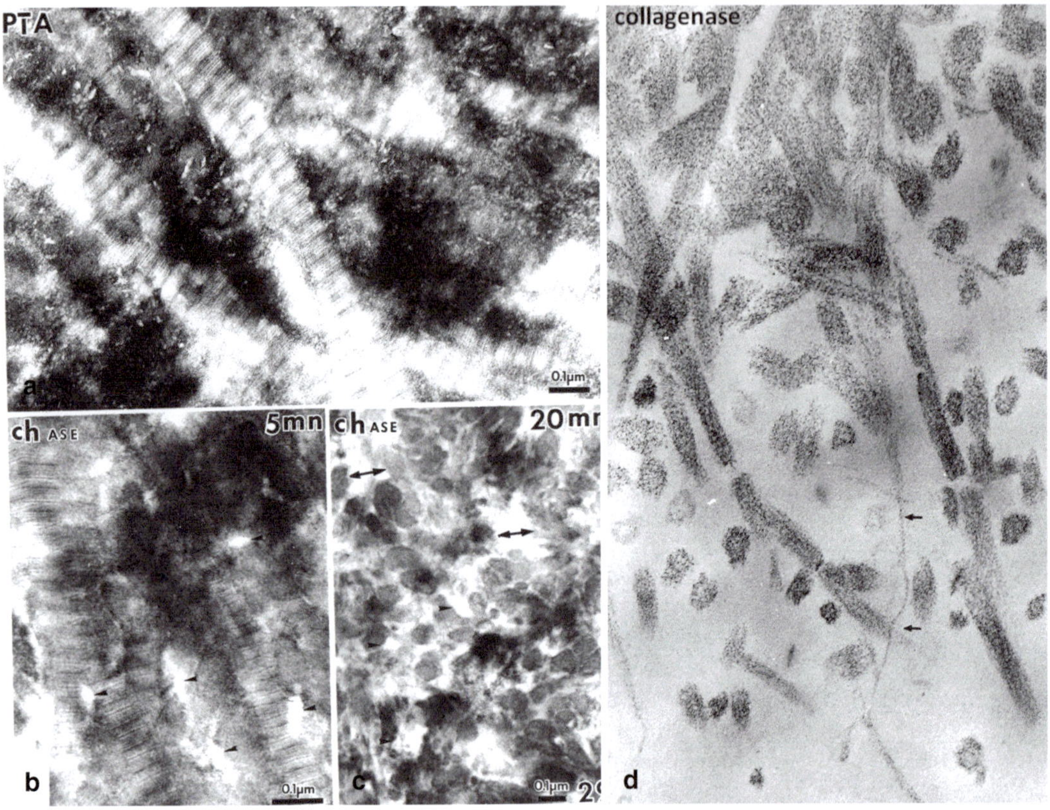

Fig. 11.5 (**a**) Dentin stained by phosphotungstic acid (PTA). The periodic banding of the collagen fibrils is clearly seen. Along the surface of collagen fibrils, and in the intercollagenic spaces, PTA positive intercollagenic spaces are densely stained. (**b**) Treatment of the section with a chondroitinase for 5 min reduce partially the PTA staining, whereas in (**c**): enzyme digestion with chase for 20 min largely suppresses the proteinaceous material located in intercollagenic spaces. Treatment of the sections with a bacterial collagenase disrupt the fibril in ¾ and ¼, (*small arrows*), and in thickness

Capillaries connect arterioles and venules. Capillaries display continuous thick or thin endothelial lining. Fenestrated endothelial cells contribute to the control and balance between the intravascular compartment and the interstitial tissue. Lymphatic capillaries have been recognized at the pulp periphery. Beneath the odontoblast compartment, the so-called Hoehl subodontoblastic compartment constitutes a second layer of cells, which may differentiate and become a second generation of odontoblasts. The renewal of odontoblasts requires newly differentiated cells, and because odontoblasts are postmitotic cells, there is a need for mesenchymal cells taking origin in the stromal pulp.

11.3 Neuropeptides in Dental Pulp

Nerve fibrils penetrate into the pulp within the apical region. They are surrounded by a myelin sheath that surrounds the axon. The role of neuropeptides, including substance P, calcitonin gene-related peptide, neurokinin A, neuropeptide Y, and vasoactive intestinal polypeptide has been discovered. Neurotransmitters or neuromodulators presumably play a variety of functions, participating in paracrine, endocrine, and neurocrine forms of communication (Caviedes-Bucheli et al. 2008).

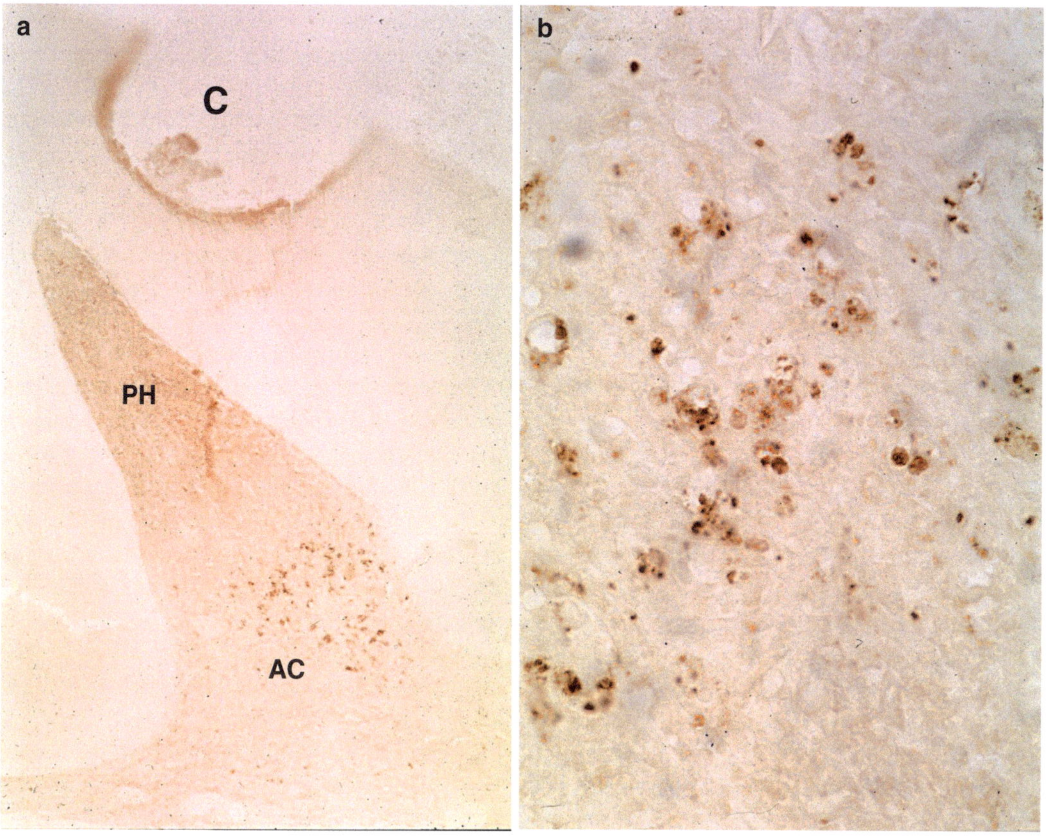

Fig. 11.6 (**a**) After the preparation of a cavity (*C*) and accumulation of cells in the pulp horn (*PH*), apoptotic cells (*AC*) are grouped in the lower part of the mesial pulp horn. (**b**) Larger magnification shows pulp cell fragmentation of apoptotic cells

Table 11.1 Composition of the pulp ECM

Component	Protein family	Specific protein
Collagen	Collagens	Type I 56 % Type III 41 % Type V 2 % Type VI 0.5 % associated with microfibrillin
Noncollagenous proteins	Phosphorylated ECM proteins	DSPP, DPP, DSP, bone sialoprotein, osteopontin, MEPE
	Non-phosphorylated proteins	Fibronectin, osteonectin
	Proteoglycans–glycosaminoglycans	Chondroitin sulfate-4 (CS-4) and CS-6 (60 %), dermatan sulfate (DS) 34 %, keratan sulfate (KS) 2 %, hyaluronic acid
	Growth factors	BMPs, type 1A and II receptors for TGFβ, activin
	Proteins taking origin from the plasma	Fibronectin
	Enzymes	Metalloproteinases (collagenases, gelatinases, stromelysine-1; tissue inhibitors of MMPs (TIMPs), alkaline and acid phosphatases, catalytic lysosomal and extracellular enzymes
	Phospholipids	Membrane and ECM phospholipids (proteolipids)

In: Goldberg (2014)

11.4 Human T-Lymphocyte Subpopulation

Pulp inflammatory cells include polymorphonuclear neutrophilic leukocytes and mast cells implicated in the defense mechanisms. Interleukin-8 expression is elevated in the irreversibly inflamed dental pulp, but lacking in the normal caries-free pulp (Huang et al. 1999).

CD45+ represented 0.94 % ± 0.65 % of cells obtained from the enzymatic digestion of the whole dental pulp cells. CD16 + CD14+ granulocyte/neutrophils (50.0 % ± 9.08 % represent the major subpopulation in CD 45+ cells, followed by CD3 T lymphocytes (32.58 ± 11 %), CD14+ monocytes (8.93 % ± 5.8 %), and HLA-DR high-Lin1+ dendritic cells (4.51 % ± 1.12 %). Minor subpopulations included CD3-CD56+ natural killer cells (2.63 % ± 1.15 %) and CD19 B lymphocytes (1.65 % ±0.89 %). In addition cells presenting a phenotype compatible with Foxp3/CD25 are seen in regulatory T lymphocytes (Gaudin et al. 2015).

Pulp cells are present for a limited period of time. Odontoblasts (Fig. 11.3a, b) are postmitotic cells that survive the initial period. Later, the so-called Hoehl's cell layer becomes apoptotic and displays a turn over more rapidly than the odontoblasts (Fig. 11.3c, d). Within the dental pulp, some pulpoblasts underwent apoptosis; their nuclei display condensed chromatin (Fig. 11.3e). Cytoplasmic inclusions contribute to the restricted aging of pulpoblasts. After the complete degradation of pulp cells, apoptotic bodies are present in the pulp extracellular matrix. They are destroyed by phagocyte or by macrophages (Fig. 11.3f). Apoptosis contributes actively to the pulp defense mechanisms.

11.5 The Carious Pulp

Carious pulps can be classified as being at the transitional stage, or displaying partial pulpitis, or total pulpitis and/or total necrosis (Di Nicolo et al. 2000).

If caries progresses slowly, there is time to form reactionary dentin or tertiary dentin (Bjorndal 2008). Pulp can be affected or infected. Bacteria are rarely seen in the unexposed pulp, whereas they are often sees in infected and necrotic pulps (Massler and Pawlak 1977). Microorganisms can reach the pulp via the dentin tubules. Often apoptotic pulpal cells at some distance from cavity preparations may display fragmentation of nuclei (Fig. 11.6a, b).

Such rapidly progressing carious lesions lead to the formation of an atubular dentin or to the complete absence of tertiary dentin. This rapidly progressing lesion leads to pulp necrosis and furthermore to periapical lesion formation. The formation of reactionary or reparative dentin is representative of the pulp response to the carious lesion. Dentin sclerosis, dead tracts, or reparative dentin are correlated with sex, age, and the type of surface location of the lesion (Stanley et al. 1983). Dentin sclerosis results from aging. The formation of translucent zone is observed in response to caries of the slow type and other mild irritations. The production of reparative dentin is directly related to the carious decay. Slowly progressing caries may become arrested caries lesions, with occlusion of the tubules by mineral deposits contributing to the formation of a "transparent zone" subjacent to the mineralized carious dentin. In this zone needle and rhombohedral crystals have been identified, together with hydroxyapatite and whitlockite crystals. They occlude the lumen of the tubules (Fig. 11.8a, b).

A gradual degradation of the dental pulp is seen. The density of the odontoblast layer slowly decreases (Fig. 11.7a), and finally, between the mineralized dentin and the pulp, an empty border is gradually inhabited.

11.6 Reactionary and Reparative Dentin Formation

Odontoblasts are postmitotic cells. After development of carious lesions, under pro-inflammatory stimuli, dental pulp cells can differentiate and produce reactionary or reparative dentin. The pro-inflammatory cytokine tumor necrosis factor α (TNFα) may be a mediator involved in dental pulp cell differentiation toward an odontoblastic phenotype. TNF-α-

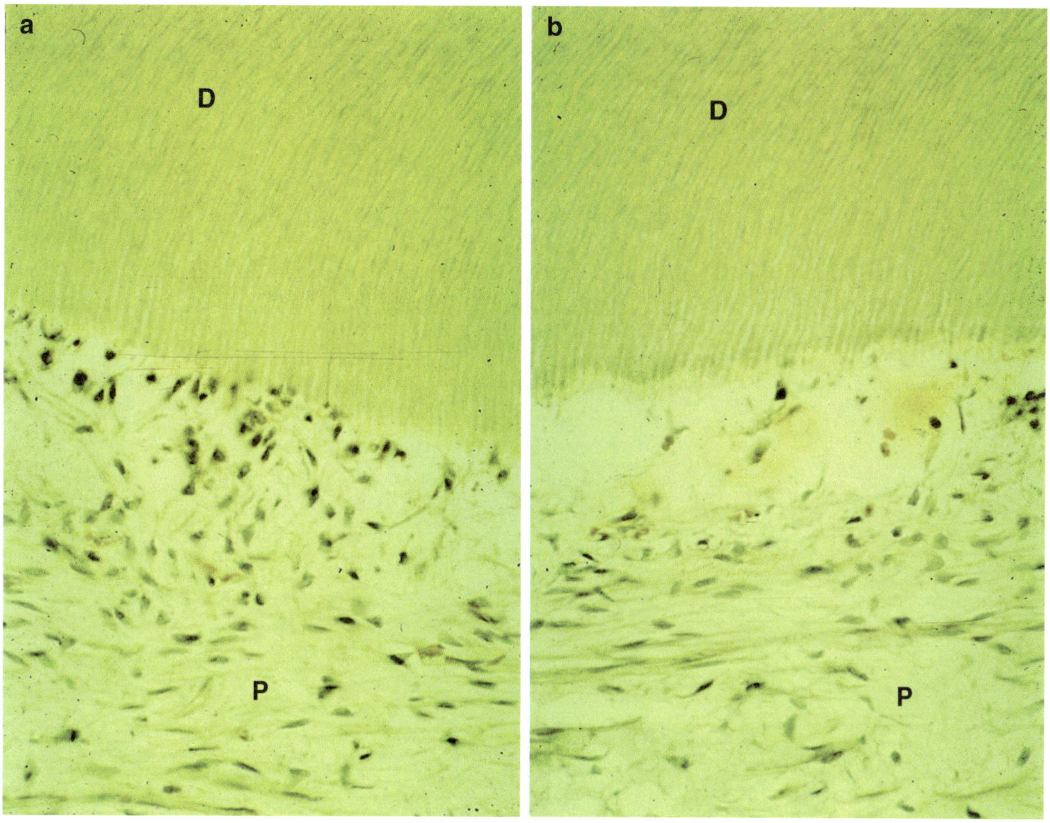

Fig. 11.7 (**a**) The preparation of a cavity induces disturbances of the odontoblast layer. *P* pulp, *D* dentin. In (**b**): the layer of odontoblast is empty. *D* dentin, *P* pulp

stimulated pulp cells display increased expression of DPP, DSP, DMP-1, and osteocalcin. The TNF-α differentiation of dental pulp cells toward an odontoblastic phenotype occurs via p38 and is negatively regulated by MMP-1 expression (Paula-Silva et al. 2009). Although there are no specific odontoblastic markers, osteocalcin, osteonectin, alkaline phosphatase, bone sialoprotein, and DSPP have been used as indicators of odontoblastic differentiation. Studies have shown that MMP-2 and MMP-9 inhibition is necessary for dentin matrices to mineralize alters dentin remodeling (Fanchon et al. 2004).

Bacterial invasion occurs in dentin that is stained bright red by 0.5 % basic fuchsine – propylene glycol solution, whereas caries-affected dentin that is bacteria-free stains pink. Collagen fibrils in infected dentin have lost their cross-banded appearance in transmission electron micrographs, indicating they are irreversibly denatured (Kuboki et al. 1977).

Reactionary dentin and reparative dentin are both strongly immunopositive for osteopontin (OPN), a phosphorylated protein of the SIBLING family, also implicated in intracellular cell signaling and inflammatory process (Aguiar and Arana-Chavez 2007). DMP-1 and collagen were associated and seem to be essential for reactionary and reparative dentin formation (Aguiar and Arana-Chavez 2010) (Figs. 11.6, 11.7, 11.8, 11.9 and 11.10).

11.6.1 Reactionary Dentin Formation

Dentin sialoprotein (DSP) may be cleaved into NH2-terminal and a COOH-terminal fragments. Using immunohistochemistry, the two DSP

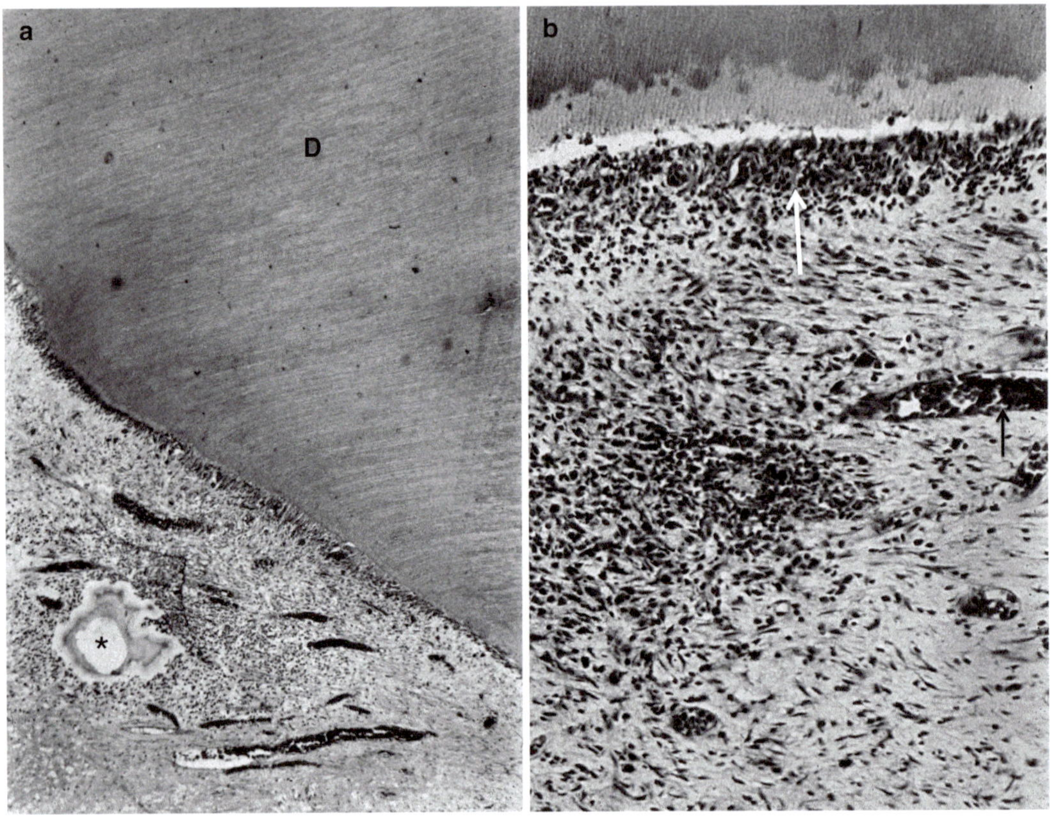

Fig. 11.8 (**a**) Accumulation of inflammatory cells and necrotic area (*asterisk*). The odontoblast layer shows continuity. *D* dentin. (**b**) Pulp cell inflammation in the subodontoblastic layer. *Red* blood accumulation is seen in vascular blood vessels (*black arrow*). Inflammation is also seen in the odontoblast layer (*white arrow*)

antibodies showed weak staining in reactionary dentin. Hence, DSP is probably less positive in reactionary dentin formation, in contrast with osteopontin, which seems to be crucial in the construction of this dentin (Yuan et al. 2012) (Figs. 11.9, 11.10, 11.11, 11.12, 11.13, 11.14, and 11.15).

11.6.2 Reparative Dentin Formation

After pulp exposure and capping with calcium hydroxide, apatite crystals were detected within *matrix vesicles* (Sela et al. 1981). Taking advantage of the A4 cell line, a multipotent stem cell derived from the molar pulp of mouse embryo, the capacity of these pulp-derived precursors to induce in vivo formation of a reparative dentin-like structure upon implantation was investigated within the pulp of a rodent incisor or a first maxillary molar after surgical exposure. One month after the pulp injury alone, a non-mineralized fibrous matrix filled the mesial part of the coronal pulp chamber. Upon A4 cell implantation, a mineralized osteodentin was formed in the implantation site without affecting the structure and vitality of the residual pulp in the central and distal parts of the pulp chamber. These results show that dental pulp stem cells can induce the formation of reparative dentin and therefore constitute a useful tool for pulp therapies (Dimitrova-Nakov et al. 2014). Differentiation of stem/progenitor cell populations of dental pulp is followed by reparative dentin formation. β-catenin was significantly upregulated during odontoblast differentiation, accompanied with reduction of Runx2 (Han et al. 2014).

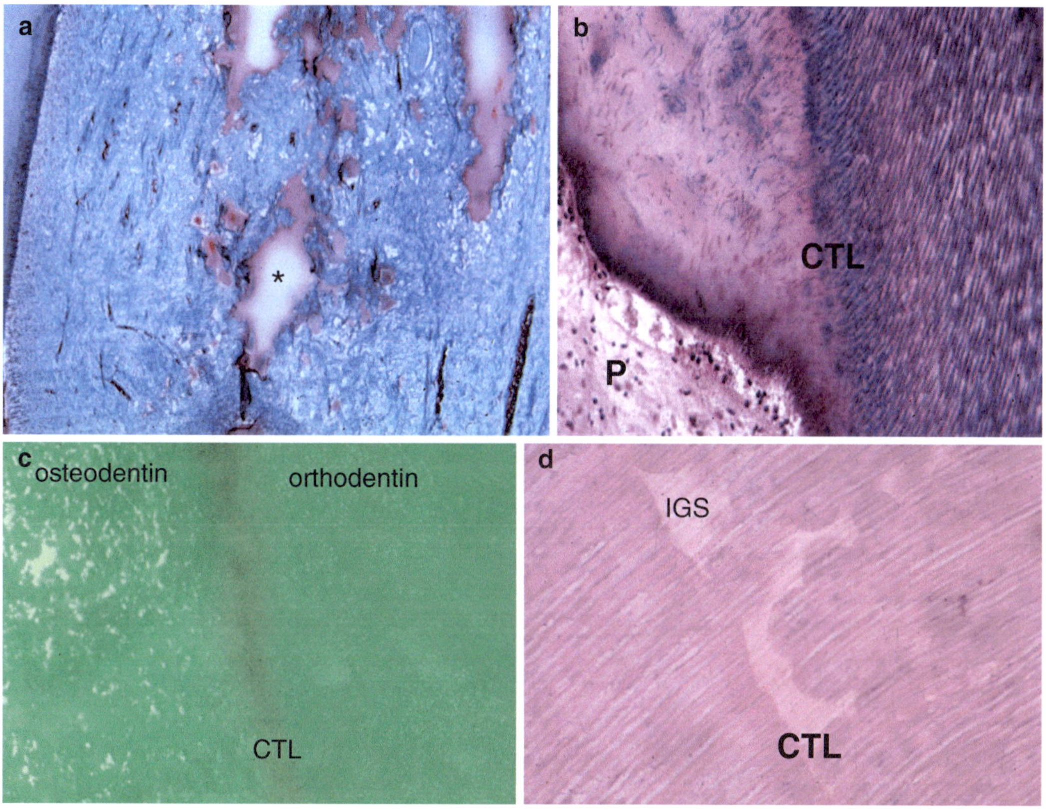

Fig. 11.9 (**a**) Necrotic empty areas (*asterisk*) where apoptotic cells melt. (**b**) Border between orthodentin (*right* part of the figure) and osteodentin (*left* part of the figure). A calciotraumatic line (*CTL*) separates the two dentin. (**c**) Stains all treated section. Near the pulp (*P*) the formation of osteodentin (*left* part of the figure) is separated from orthodentin (*right* part of the figure) by a calciotraumatic line. (**d**) Orthodentin is formed on the left. A calciotraumatic line (*CTL*) shows an interruption of dentinogenesis, revealing the presence of interglobular spaces (*IGS*)

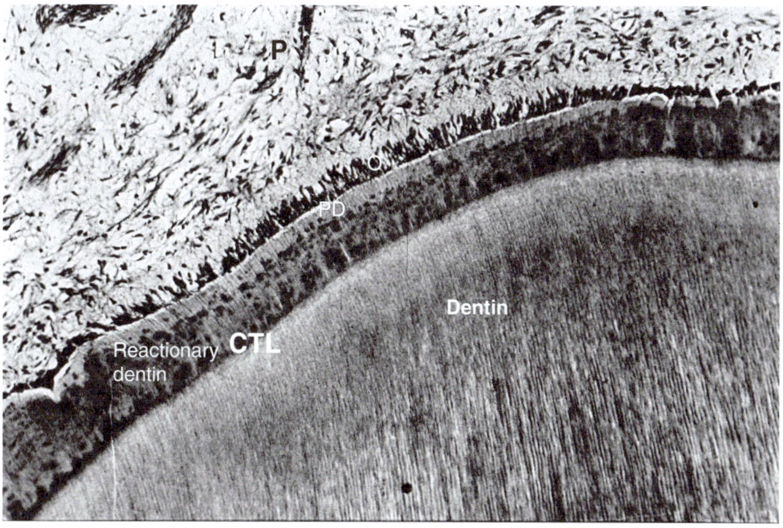

Fig. 11.10 A calciotraumatic line (*CTL*) separates the dentin from reactionary dentin. *PD* predentin, *O* odontoblasts, *P* pulp

When A4 cells were implanted in peripheral sites in dog dental pulp, elongated and polarized odontoblast-like cells were observed, whereas implanted in the center of the pulp, they produced an atubular hard tissue with lining fibroblast-like cells (Tziafas et al. 1996).

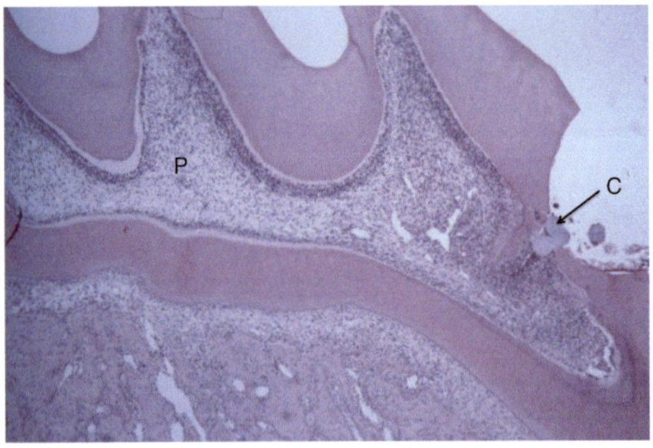

Fig. 11.11 The preparation of a cavity (*C*) provokes an inflammatory reaction in the mesial part of the pulp (*P*)

Dentin phosphophoryn (DPP) has a RGD motif and repeat sequences of aspartic acid and phosphoserine. DPP promotes cell migration in a concentration-dependent manner but has no effect on cell proliferation. Cell migration is suppressed by the addition of alpha v beta 3 integrin antibody to the culture medium (Yasuda et al. 2008).

The connective tissue growth factor/CCN family 2 (CTGF/CCN2) seems to play role in reparative dentin formation. In healthy teeth, minimal expression was evident in odontoblast subjacent to the dentin-pulp junction, whereas a strong expression was detected in the odontoblast-like cells lining the reparative dentin subjacent to dental caries. CTGH/CCN2 promoted mineralization but not proliferation (Muromachi et al. 2012).

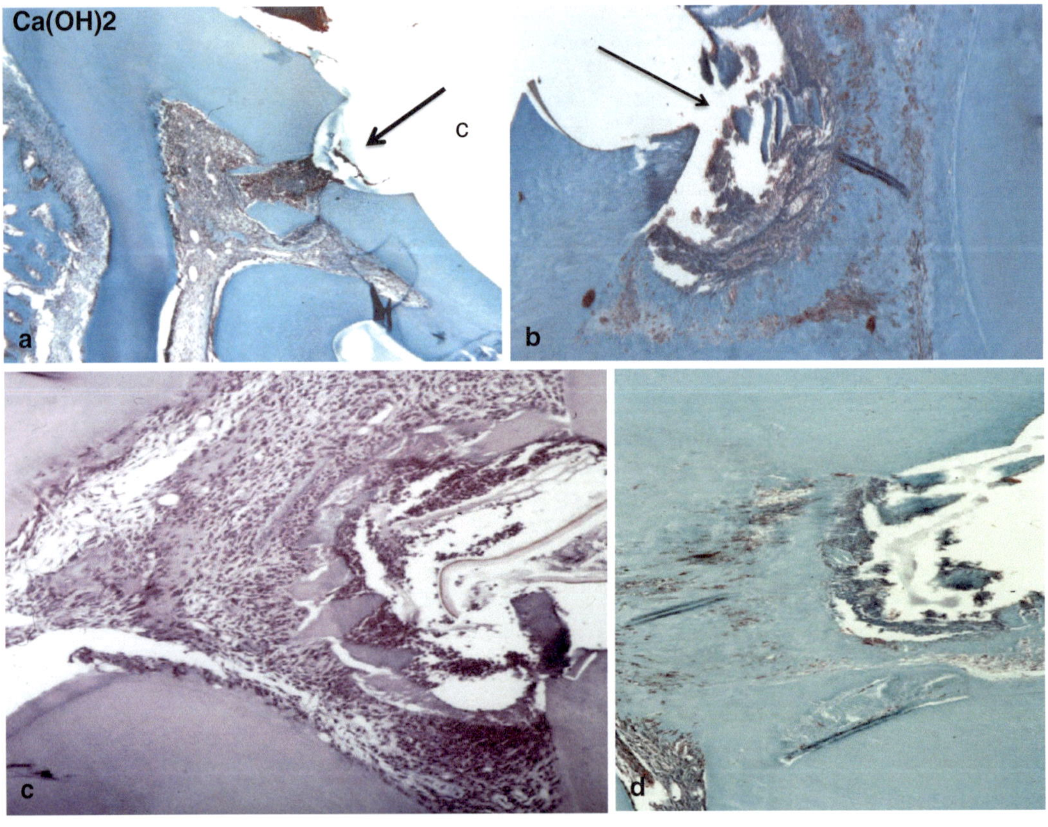

Fig. 11.12 (**a**) One week after calcium hydroxide capping (*arrow*), *c*: cavity; (**b**): a dentinal bridge starts to be formed (*arrow*). (**c**) Its thickness increases and (**d**) finally osteodentin occludes the pulp exposure

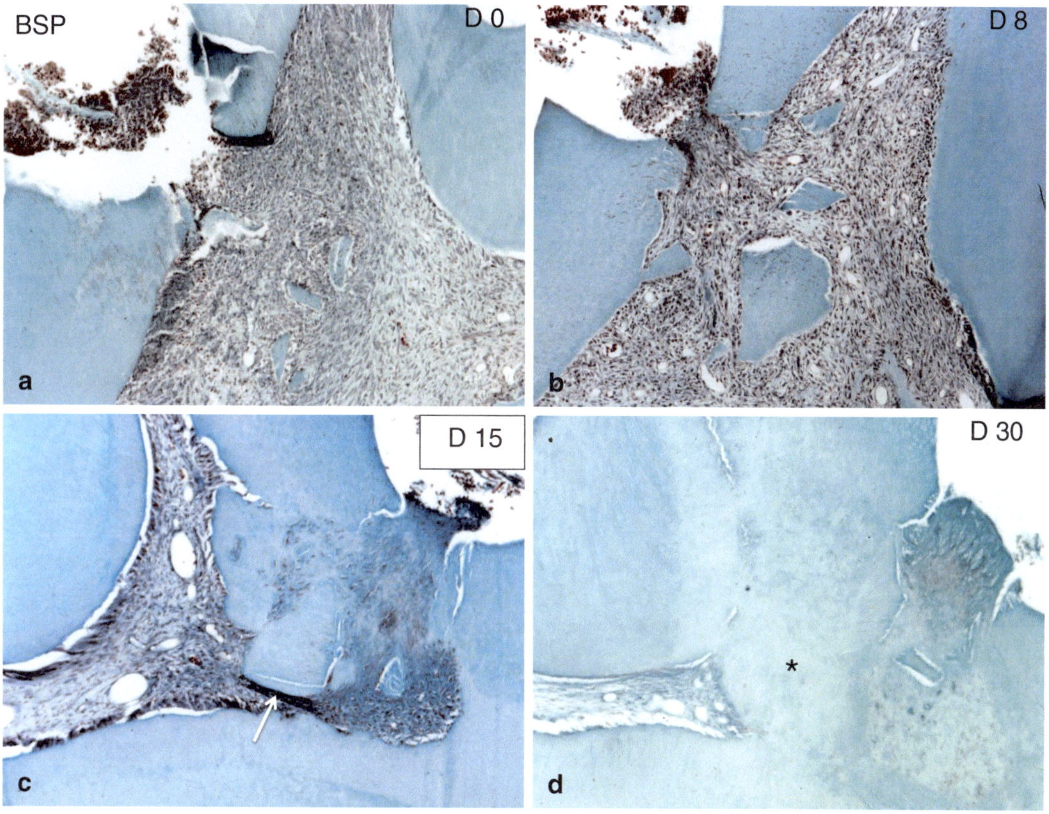

Fig. 11.13 Pulp capping with bone sialoprotein (BSP). (**a**) At day O, the pulp exposure is accompanied by the projection of dentin debris within the pulp (**b**): after 8 days, an inflammatory reaction is seen in the pulp horn. (**c**) After 15 days, dentin debris pushed in the pulp are thicker (*white arrow*) and covered with a layer of reactionary dentin. (**d**) At day 30, the pulp exposure is totally filled by reparative dentin (*asterisk*)

11.7 Pulp Capping

Using calcium hydroxide, pulp capping was introduced clinically in the year 1930 by Hermann (Schroder 1985). The chemical mechanisms of pulp capping leading to the formation of a hard tissue barrier are now better understood. The initial reaction on the dental pulp of calcium hydroxide was vascular, associated with a mild inflammation, cell migration, and proliferation (Fig. 11.11). These events were followed by cell destruction and liquefaction necrosis. The alkaline pH of calcium hydroxide demineralizes dentin matrix that solubilizes TGF-β1 and noncollagenous phosphoproteins from the matrix that recruits odontoblast-like cells to form at the site (Graham et al. 2006). Mineral trioxide aggregate (MTA) appears to have similar properties since it slowly release calcium hydroxide from the set material (Tomson et al. 2007).

Migration and proliferation of pulp cells were observed adjacent to the necrotic zone. An increased formation of the extracellular matrix, namely, *collagen*(s), concerned DNA synthesis by pulp cells. The formation of a scar involves collagen construction, with a dentin appearance. The mineralization of the barrier and cellular differentiation occurs. *Matrix vesicles* play an initial role in pulp mineralization. *Calcium carbonate* granulations initiate the mineralization of the newly formed collagen and in the differentiation of secondary odontoblasts (e.g., differentiation of the so-called Hoehl's cells and mesenchymal stem cells/pulp progenitors). One day after capping, precipitations of crystalline structures are

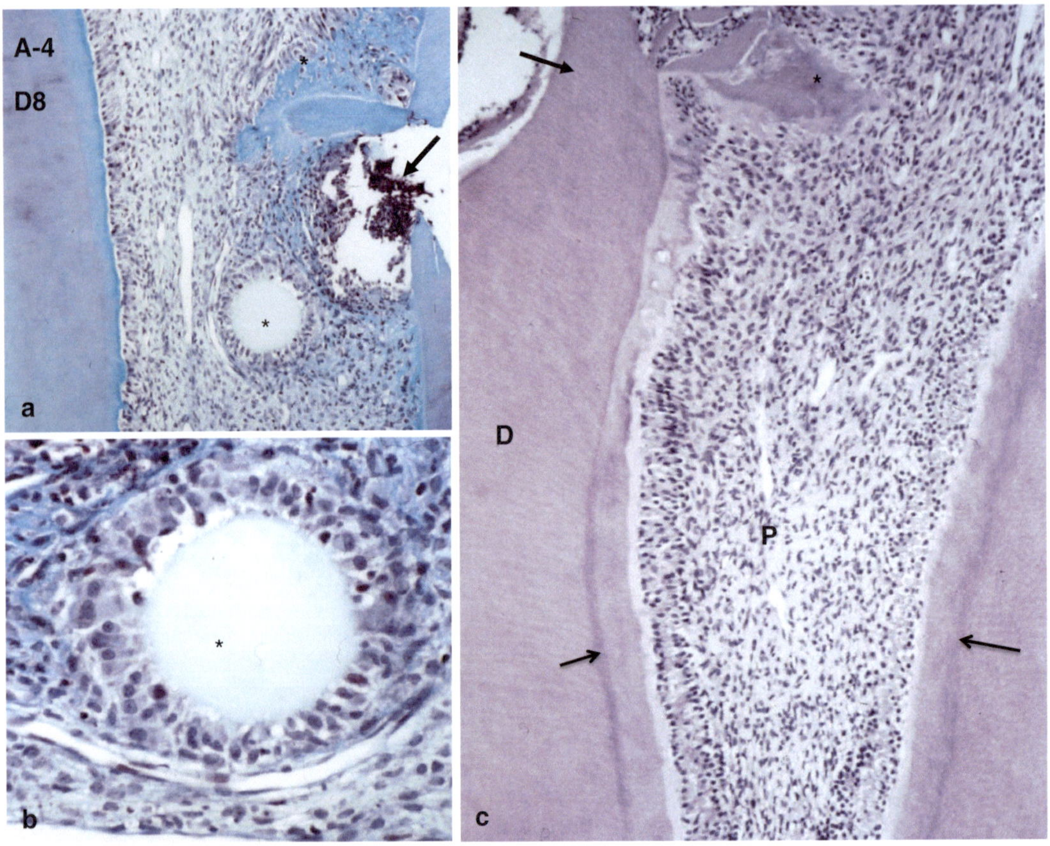

Fig. 11.14 Implantation of an amelogenin peptide (A-4) in the dental pulp. (**a**) At 8 days, implanted in the cavity (*arrow*), an inflammatory reaction is detected in the superficial area, near the agarose bead (*asterisk*). (**b**) Larger magnification of the agarose bead (see here as carrier for A-4) (*asterisk*). A ring of cells occupies the outer surface of the bead. (**c**) Pulp exposure is seen in the upper part of the root together with dentin debris (*asterisk*). No pulp inflammation (*P*) appears in the root. *Arrows* indicate the division between orthodentin (*D*) and reactionary osteodentin

observed at the interface between the superficial necrotic zone and the underlying pulp tissue. This layer is immunopositive to *fibronectin*. Odontoblast-like cells are positive at 7 to 10 days after capping. Corkscrew fiber-like fluorescent structures are visible between the cells (Yoshiba et al. 1996). Observation of adult rhesus monkeys' molars capped with Dycal or Life, $Ca(OH)_2$ calcium hydroxide implanted for 14 days, 5 weeks, and 1 and 2 years, revealed that 89 % of the dentin bridges contain tunnel defects. The tunnels fail to provide a hermetic seal (Cox et al. 1996) (Figs. 11.11, 11.12, 11.13, 11.14, 11.15, 11.16, 11.17, 11.18, and 11.19).

Capping with mineral trioxide aggregate (MTA) follows the same cascade of events reported with Ca(OH)2. After inducing a mild surface necrosis, bridging new matrix is formed and the collagenous matrix is mineralized. The cells proliferate for 3 days, appearing as *nestin*-expressing cells. They form a matrix on the fifth day. Cells displaying odontoblast-like morphology were seen by day 14. *Osteopontin* (OPN) was immunopositive just beneath the necrotic area after 1 day. OPN appears to trigger the initiation of the pulp reparative process (Kuratate et al. 2008).

MTA and Portland cements were immunostained for *dentin matrix protein-1* (DMP-1), in contrast with calcium hydroxide, which display a negative immunostaining (Neto et al. 2016). Dentin matrix protein 1 is one of the dentin noncollagenous extracellular matrix proteins implicated in regulation of mineralization. We have examined

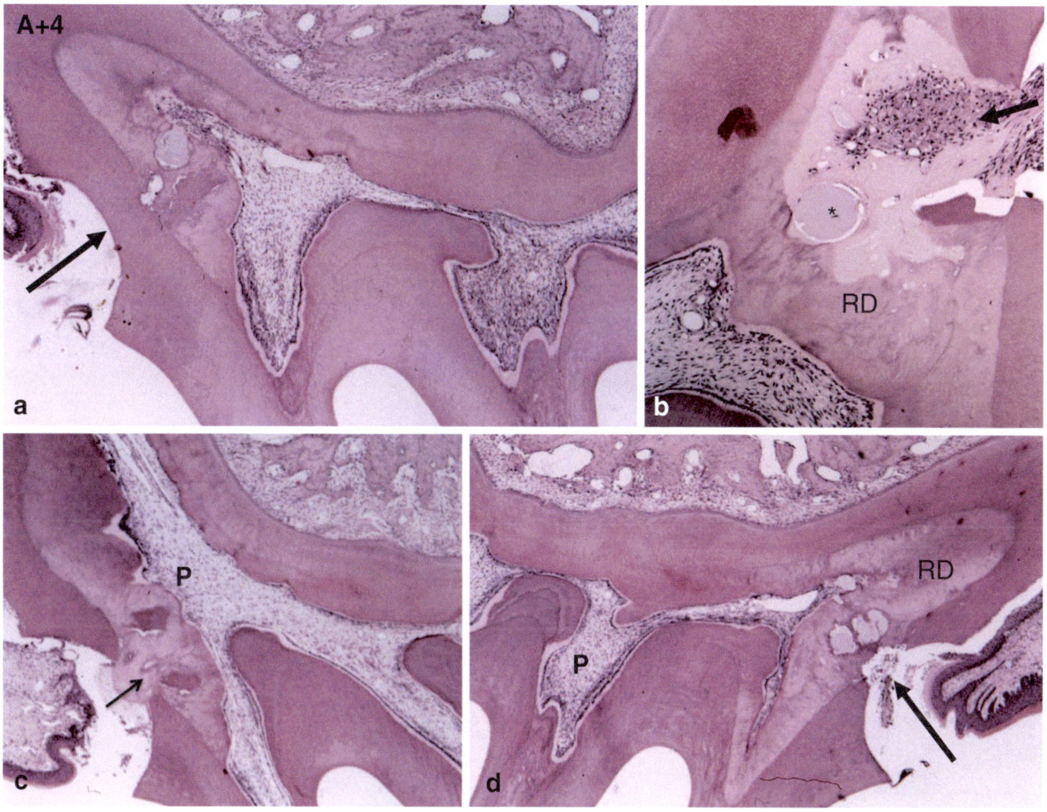

Fig. 11.15 (**a**) Reactionary dentin formation in the root, beneath a cavity (*arrow*) after implantation of A+4 amelogenin molecule. (**b**) Pulp exposure with debris pushed inside the dental pulp and an agarose bead (*asterisk*). Reparative dentin (*RD*) fills the pulp exposure. (**c**) Reparative dentin (*arrow*) fills the pulp exposure (*P*). (**d**) Connected with the mesial cavity (*arrow*), in the mesial root reparative dentin (*RD*) occludes the upper part of the root

the potential role of DMP1 in inducing cytodifferentiation of dental pulp stem cells into odontoblast-like cells and formation of reparative dentin in a rat model. Cavities were drilled and pulps exposed in maxillary first molars. Collagen matrix impregnated with recombinant DMP1 was implanted directly in group 1, while calcium hydroxide was implanted in group 2; collagen matrix that was not impregnated with rDMP1 was implanted directly in group 3, which served as control (Almushayt et al. 2006) (Figs. 11.20, 11.21, and 11.22).

When pulp exposures are capped with calcium hydroxide, positive immunostaining for *tenascin* (TN) and *fibronectin* (FN) was seen around the dentin barrier, delimitating the reparative dentin.

Bone sialoprotein (BSP) implanted in the pulp of the first maxillary molar formed a reparative dentinal bridge after 30 days. BSP stimulates the differentiation of pulp cells and contributes to the formation of a thick reparative dentinal tissue, occluding the perforation (Decup et al. 2000). After experimental pulp capping with MTA, the pulps were either capped with MTA alone or with BMP-7 followed by restoration with MTA. More complete bridge immunostaining was seen for *dentin sialoprotein* (DSP) in MTA-capped pulps, compared with BMP-7 alone, appearing as bone-like and devoid of DSP staining (Andelin et al. 2003) (Figs. 11.22, 11.23, and 11.24).

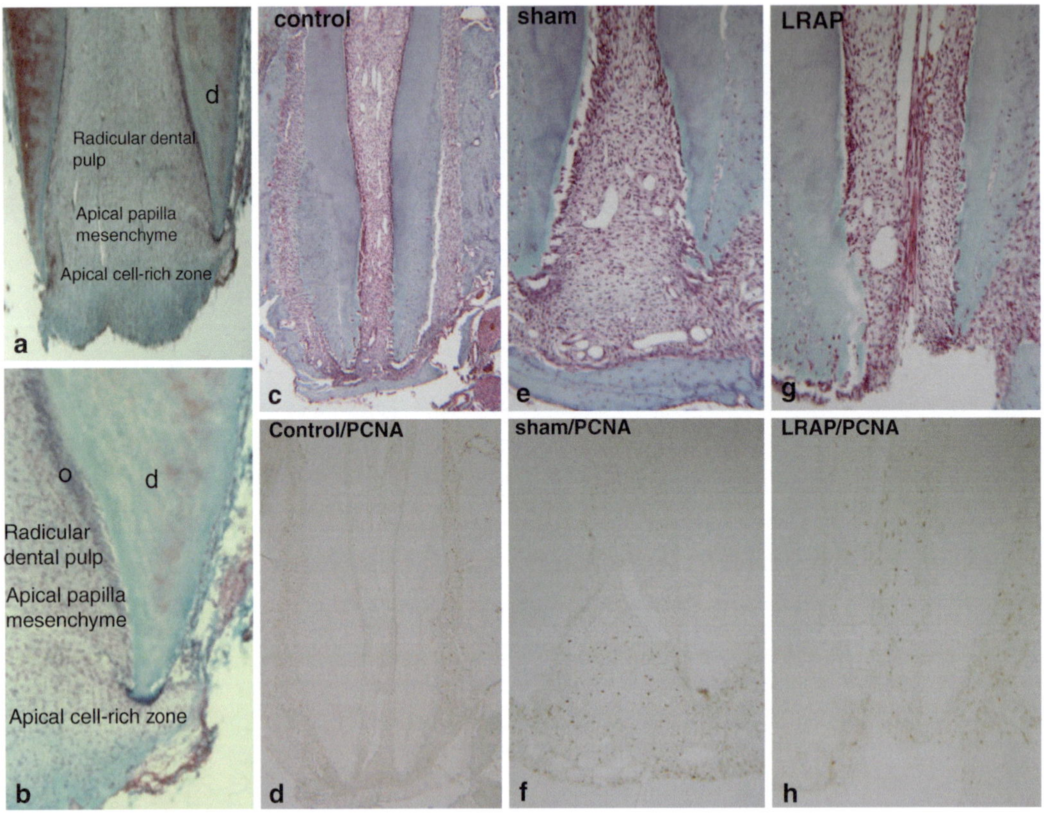

Fig. 11.16 (**a**, **b**) In the apical part of the root, three distinct zones are seen: the apical cell-rich zone, the apical papilla mesenchyme, and the radicular dental pulp. In the control teeth, (**c**, **d**) PCNA labeling is only seen in the periodontal ligament. After sham treatment, PCNA-labeled cells are detectable in the apical papilla and in the apical cell-rich zone (**e**, **f**). After amelogenin implantation in the pulp (LRAP/PCNA), proliferating labeled cells are visible in the radicular dental pulp alone (**g**, **h**)

Zone III	Apical cell-rich zone (1x1 cm^2)	Root pulp
sham	3.4	0.43
Beads implantation	2	1.33
LRAP Implantation	1	4.23

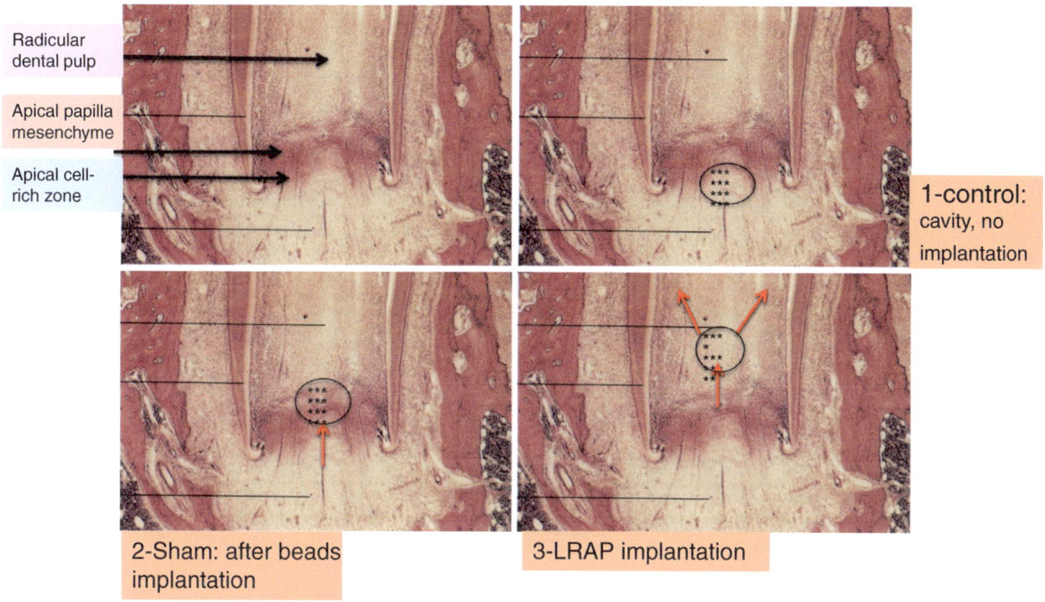

Fig. 11.17 Crude calculation of the cell density in the apical cell-rich zone and in the root pulp differs depending on the treatment (sham, bead implantation, or LRAP implantation). Labeling differs in (1) control, (2) sham, or (3) after LRAP implantation

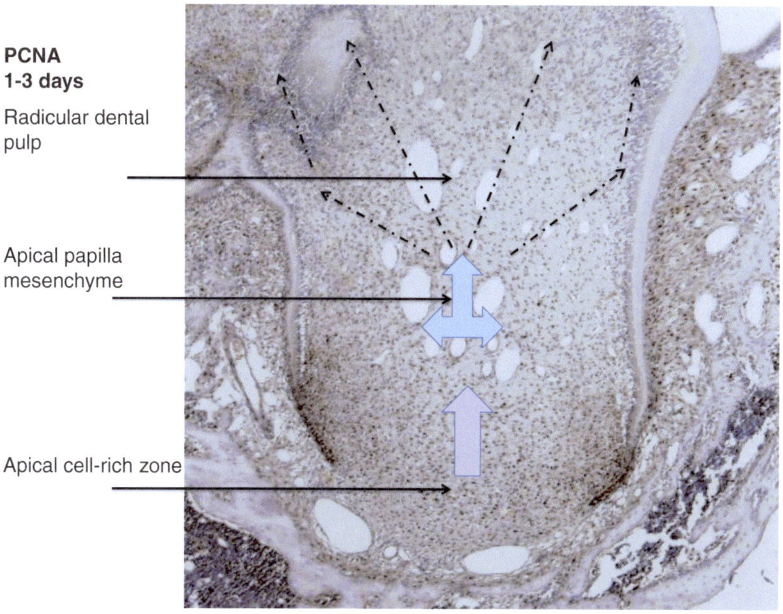

Fig. 11.18 Cells labeled in the apical cell-rich zone migrate. They move laterally in the apical papilla mesenchyme and slide in the coronal direction in the radicular dental pulp, where they become subodontoblastic and migrate in the coronal direction

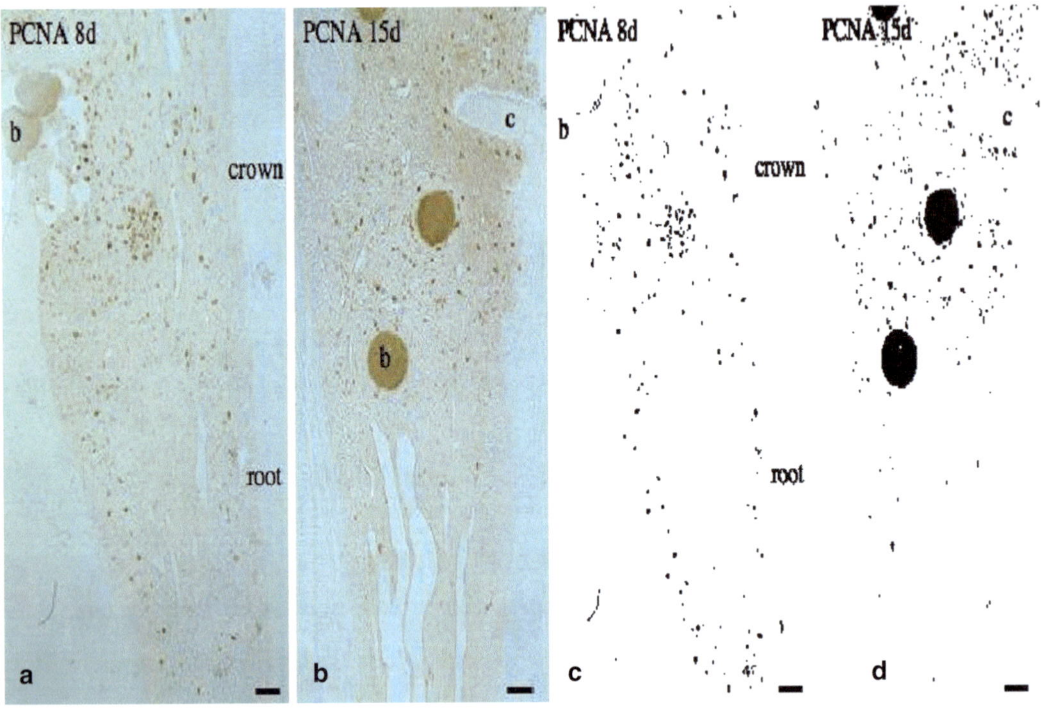

Fig. 11.19 PCNA-labeled cells are located after 8 days in the root in a subodontoblastic layer (**a**, **c**) and in the crown inside and around agarose beads. After 15 days, there is no more labeling in the root, and all the labeled cells are groups in the crown part (**b**, **d**)

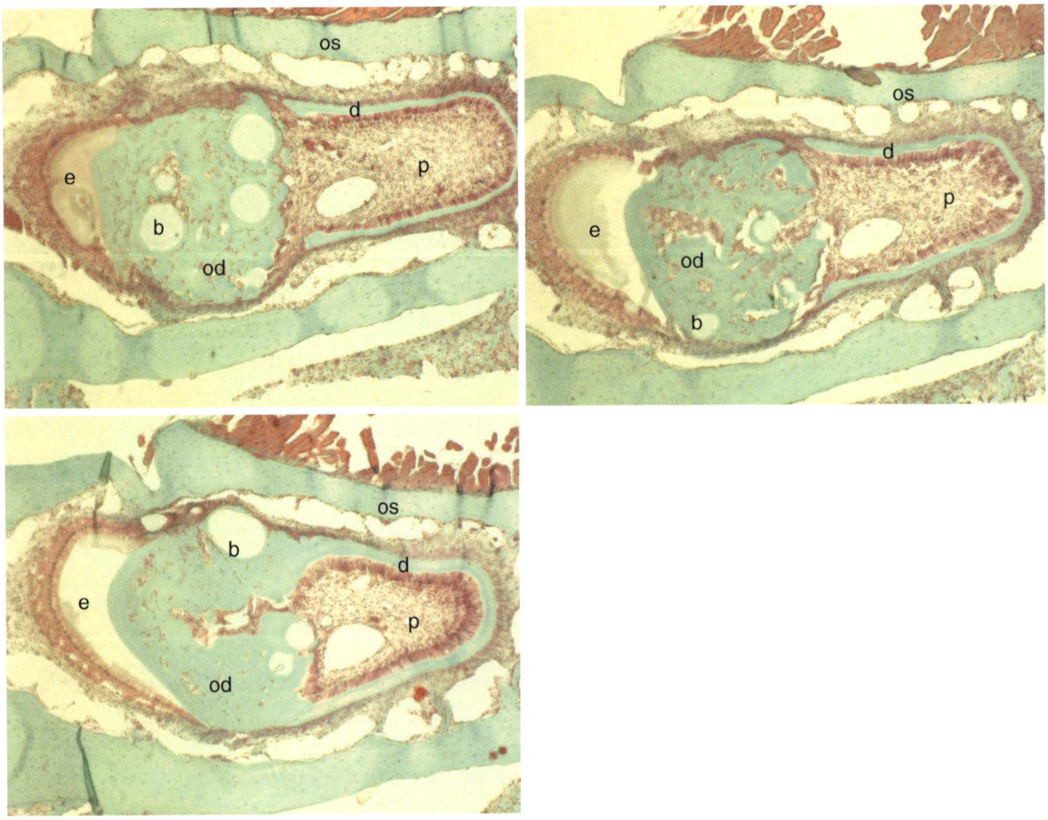

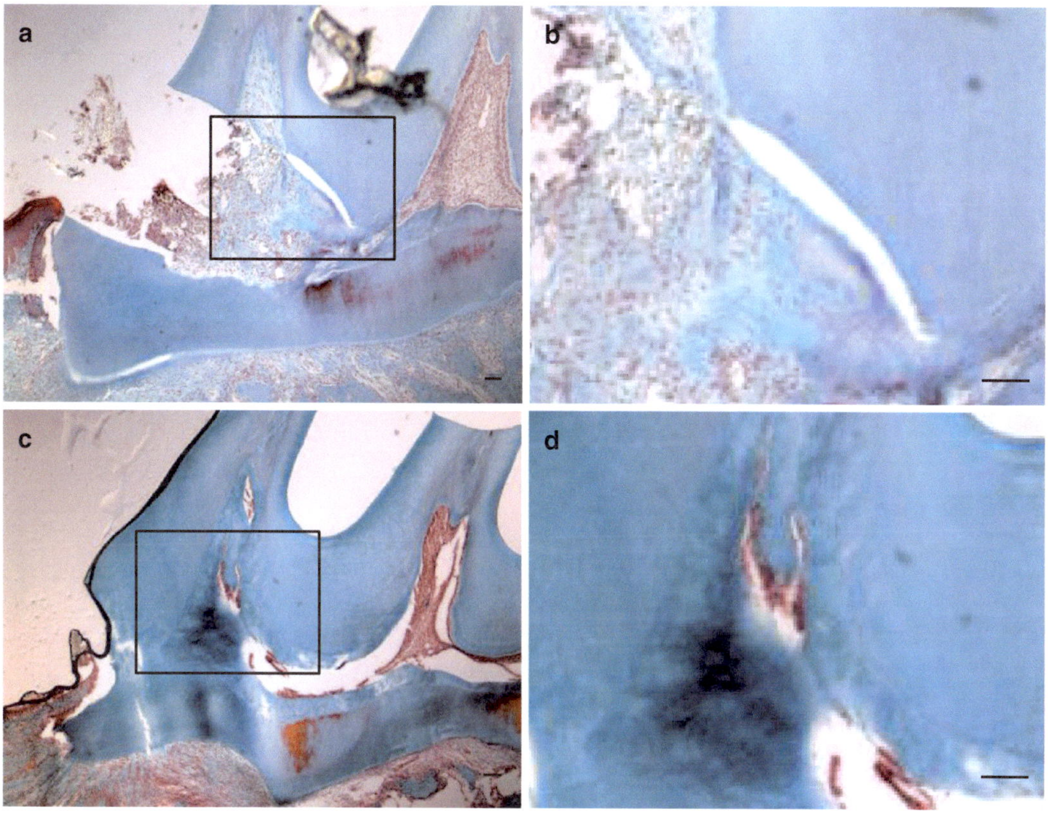

Fig. 11.21 Pulp exposure without bead implantation (control molars) contributes to the formation of a fibrous tissue. Implantation of A4 cells in the mesial pulp horn initiates 28 days after the formation of a thick reparative dentin bridge, beneath a calciotraumatic line

Fig. 11.20 Implantation of cell lines (agarose beads acting as carrier) in the dental pulp of the mouse incisor produces thick mineralized osteodentin aggregates

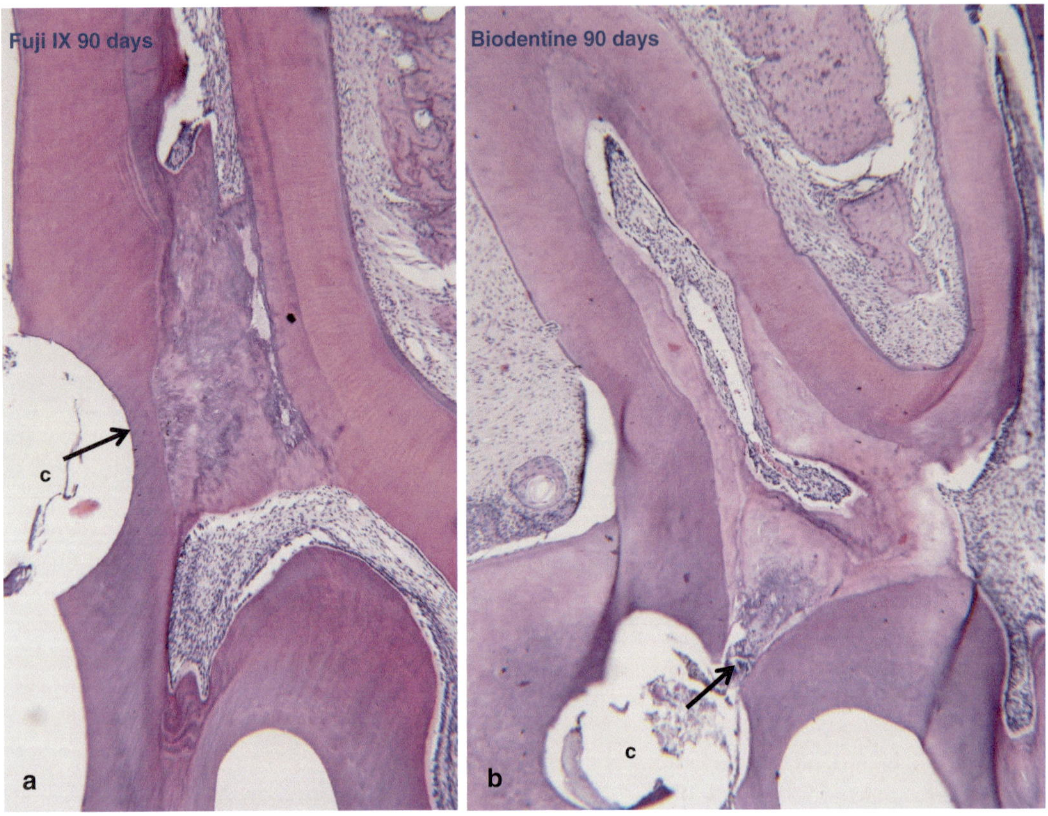

Fig. 11.22 (**a**) 90 days after filling a cervical cavity with a glass-ionomer cement (Fuji IX), reactionary dentin and a thick pulp stone obliterate the lumen of the root canal. (**b**) Direct pulp capping after 90 days with a tricalcium silicate-based cement (Biodentine) shows reparative dentin formation inside the mesial horn and root. *C* cavity. *Arrow*: pulp capping

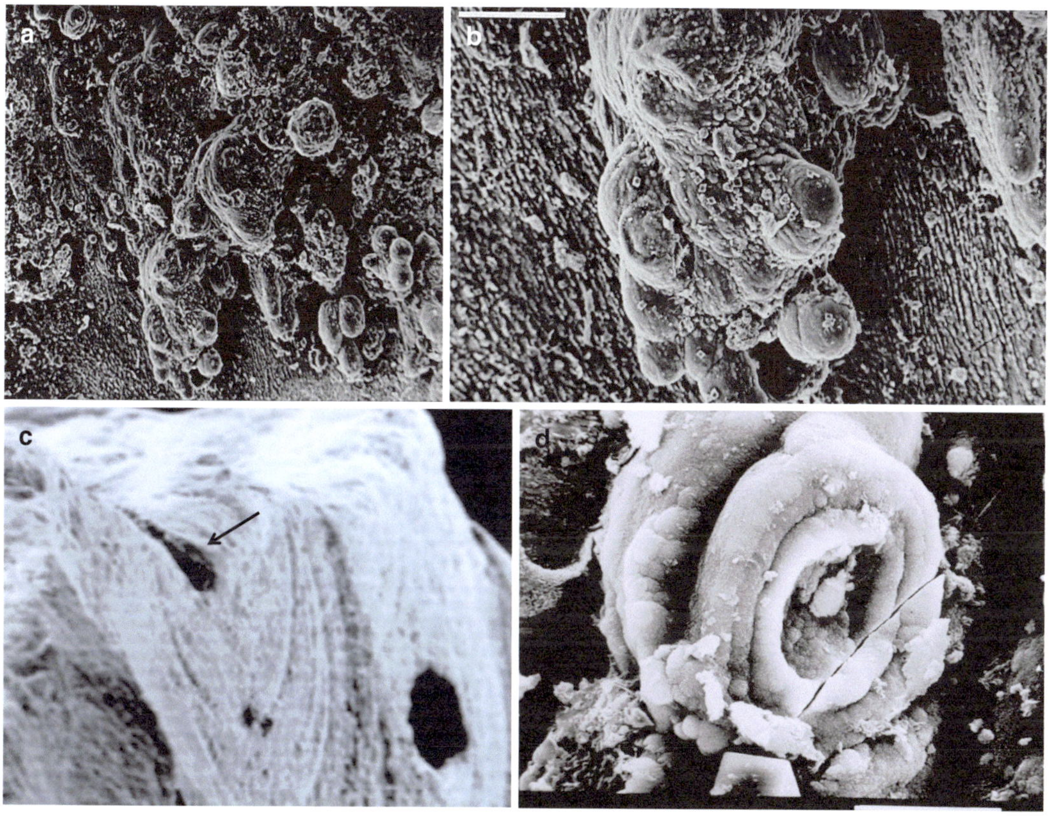

Fig. 11.23 (**a**, **b**) Reactionary dentin formed at the dentin surface. Globular structures merge with the walls of the dental pulp. (**c**) The section of a pulp stone displays the gradual increase in thickness of the pulpolithe. A clear relationship may be established between an isolated pulp stone formation and vascular initiation of the pulp mineralization. (**d**) Along the pulp surface, adherent mineralization is seen

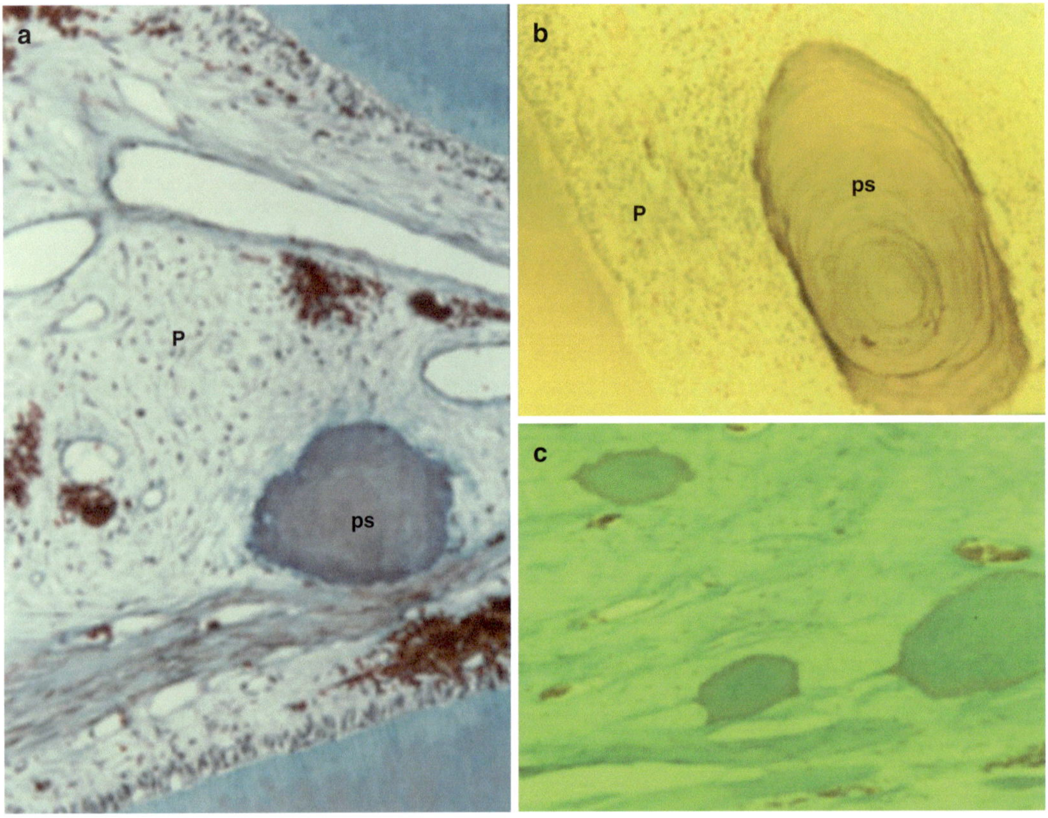

Fig. 11.24 (**a**) Isolated pulp stones (*ps*) within the dental pulp (*P*). (**b**) Lamellar growth contributes to the increase in size of the pulp stone. (**c**) Diffuse mineralization in the pulp

References

Aguiar MC, Arana-Chavez V. Ultrastructural and immunocytochemical analyses of osteopontin in reactionary and reparative dentine formed after extrusion of upper rat incisor. J Anat. 2007;210:418–27.

Aguiar MC, Arana-Chavez VE. Immunocytochemical detection of dentine matrix protein 1 in experimentally induced reactionary and reparative dentine in rat incisor. Arch Oral Biol. 2010;55:210–4.

Almushayt A, Narayanan K, Zaki AE, George A. Dentin matrix protein 1 induces cytodifferentiation of dental pulp stem cells into odontoblasts. Gene Ther. 2006;13:611–20.

Andelin WE, Shabahang S, Wright K, Torabinejad M. Identification of hard tissue after experimental pulp capping using dentin sialoprotein (DSP) as a marker. J Endod. 2003;29:646–50.

Bjorndal L. The caries process and its effect on the pulp: the science is changing and so is our understanding. J Endod. 2008;34:52–9.

Caviedes J, Munoz HR, Azueros-Holguin MM, Ulate E. Neuropeptides in dental pulp: the silent protagonists. J Endod. 2008;34:773–88.

Cox CF, Subay RK, Ostro E, Suzuki S, Suzuki SH. Tunnel defects in dentin bridges: their formation following direct pulp capping. Oper Dent. 1996;21:4–11.

Decup F, Six N, Palmier B, Buch D, Lasfargues JJ, Salih E, Goldberg M. Bone sialoprotein-induced reparative dentinogenesis in the pulp of rat's molar. Clin Oral Investig. 2000;4:110–9.

Di Nicolo R, Guedes-Pinto AC, Carvalho YR. Histopathology of the pulp of primary molars with active and arrested dentinal caries. J Clin Pediatr Dent. 2000;25:47–9.

Dimitrova-Nakov S, Baudry A, Harichane Y, Kellermann O, Goldberg M. Pulp stem cells: implication in reparative dentin formation. J Endod. 2014;40(4 Suppl): S13–8.

Fanchon S, Bourd K, Septier D, Everts V, Beertsen W, Menashi S, Goldberg M. Involvement of matrix metalloproteinases in the onset of dentin mineralization. Eur J Oral Sci. 2004;112:171–6.

Gaudin A, Renard E, Hill M, Bouchet-Delbos L, Bienvenu-Louvet G, Farges J-C, Cuturi M-C, Alliot-Licht B. Phenotypic analysis of Immunocompetent cells in healthy human dental pulp. J Endod. 2015. doi.org/10.1016/j.joen.2015.01.005.

Goldberg M. Dentin, pulp, and tooth pain. Chapter 5. In: Hand AR, Frank ME. Fundamentals of oral histology and physiology. Wiley Blackwell & Sons, Inc.; 2014. p. 85–112.

Goldberg M, Septier D, Rapoport O, Iozzo RV, Young MF, Ameye LG. Targeted disruption of two small leucine-rich proteoglycans, biglycan and decorin, excerpt divergent effects on enamel and dentin formation. Calcif Tissue Int. 2005;77:297–310.

Goldberg M, Septier D, Oldberg A, Young MF, Ameye LG. Fibromodulin-deficient mice display impaired collagen fibrillogenesis in predentin as well as altered dentin mineralization and enamel formation. J Histochem Cytochem. 2006;54:525–37.

Graham L, Cooper PR, Cassidy N, Nor JE, Sloan AJ, Smith AJ. The effect of calcium hydroxide on solubilisation of bio-active dentin matrix component. Biomaterials. 2006;27:2865–73.

Han N, Zhang Y, Li R, Li X, Zhou M, Niu Y, Zhang G. β-catenin enhances odontoblastic differentiation of dental pulp cells through activation of Runx2. PLoS One. 2014;9(2):e88890.

Huang GT-J, Potente AP, Kim J-W, Chugal N, Zhang X. Increased interleukin-8 expression in inflamed human dental pulps. Oral Surg Oral Med Oral Pathol Oral Radiol Endod. 1999;88:214–20.

Kuboki Y, Ohgushi K, Fusayama T. Collagen biochemistry of the two layers of carious dentin. J Dent Res. 1977;56:1233–7.

Kuratate M, Yoshiba K, Shigetani Y, Yoshiba N, Ohshima H, Okiji T. Immunohistochemical analysis of nestin, osteopontin, and proliferating cells in the reparative process of exposed dental pulp capped with mineral trioxide aggregate. J Endod. 2008;34:970–4.

Linde A. The extracellular matrix of the dental pulp and dentin. J Dent Res. 1985;64 Spec issue:523–9.

Massler M, Pawlak J. The affected and infected pulp. Oral Surg Oral Med Oral Pathol. 1977;43:929–47.

Mjör IA. Dentin permeability: the basis for understanding pulp reactions and adhesive technology. Braz Dent J. 2009;20:3–16.

Muromachi K, Kamio N, Matsumoto T, Matsushima K. Role of CTGF/CCN2 in reparative dentinogenesis in human dental pulp. J Oral Sci. 2012;54:47–64.

Neto LN, Marques NC, Fernandes AP, Rodini CO, Sakai VT, Abdo RC, Machado MA, Santos CF, Oliveira TM. Immunolocalization of dentin matrix protein-1 in human primary teeth treated with different pulp capping materials. J Biomed Mater Res B Appl Biomater. 2016;104(1):165–9.

Paula-Silva FWG, Ghosh A, Silva LAB, Kapila YL. The TNF-α promotes an odontoblastic phenotype in dental pulp cells. J Dent Res. 2009;88:339–44.

Rahamtulla F. Proteoglycans of oral tissues. Crit Rev Oral Biol Med. 1992;3:135–62.

Schröder U. Effects of calcium hydroxide-containing pulp capping on pulp cell migration, proliferation, and differentiation. J Dent Res. 1985;64(Spec Iss):541–8.

Sela J, Tamari I, Hirschfeld Z, Bab I. Transmission electron microscopy of reparative dentin in rat molar pulps. Primary mineralization via extracellular matrix vesicles. Acta Anat. 1981;109:247–51.

Shibata S, Yoneda S, Yanagishihta M, Yamashita Y. Isolation of proteoglycan (versican) aggregate from rat dental pulp. Arch Oral Biol. 2000;45:563–8.

Shuttleworth CA, Ward JL, Hirschmann PN. The presence of type III collagen in the developing tooth. Biochem Biophys Acta. 1978;535:348–55.

Sone S, Nakamura M, Maruya Y, Takahashi I, Mizoguchi I, Mayanagi H, Sasano Y. Expression of versican and ADAMTS during tooth eruption. J Mol Histol. 2005;36:281–8.

Stanley HR, Pereira JC, Spiegel E, Broom C, Schultz M. The detection and prevalence of reactive and physiologic sclerotic dentin, reparative dentin and dead tracts beneath various types of dental lesions according to tooth surface and age. J Oral Pathol. 1983;12:257–89.

Sulkala M, Paakkonen V, Larmas M, Salo T, Tajderhane L. Matrix metalloproteinase-13 (MMP-13) is highly expressed in human tooth pulp. Connect Tissue Res. 2004;45:231–7.

Tomson PL, Grover LM, Lumley PJ, Sloan AJ, Smith AJ, Cooper PR. Dissolution of bioactive matrix components by mineral trioxide aggregate. J Dent. 2007;35:636–42.

Tsuzaki M, Yamauchi M, Mechanic GL. Bovine dental pulp collagens: characterization of types III and V collagen. Arch Oral Biol. 1990;35:195–2000.

Tziafas D, Veis A, Alvanou A. inability of calcium hydroxide to induce reparative dentinogenesis at non-peripheral sites of dog dental pulp. Eur J Oral Sci. 1996;104:623–6.

Wisithphrom K, Windsor J. The effects of Tumor Necrosis Factor α, Interleukin-1β, Interleukin-6, and Transforming Growth Factor-β1 on pulp fibroblast mediated collagen degradation. J Endod. 2006;32:853–61.

Yamamoto R, Oida S, Yamakoshi Y. Dentin sialophosphoprotein-derived proteins in the dental pulp. J Dent Res. 2015;94(8):1120–7.

Yasuda Y, Izumikawa M, Okamoto K, Tsukuba T, Saito T. Dentin phosphophoryn promotes cellular migration of human dental pulp cells. J Endod. 2008;34:575–8.

Yoshiba K, Yoshiba N, Nakamura H, Iwaku M, Ozawa H. Immunolocalization of fibronectin during reparative dentinogenesis in human teeth after pulp capping with calcium hydroxide. J Dent Res. 1996;75:1590–7.

Yuan G, Yang G, Song G, Chen Z, Chen S. Immunohistochemical localization of the NH2-terminal and COOH-terminal fragments of dentin sialoprotein in mouse teeth. Cell Tissue Res. 2012;349:805–14.

Part III

Cervical Erosions

Ultrastructure of the Enamel-Cementum Junction

12

Michel Goldberg

Abstract

Procollagen is synthesized by secretory odontoblasts and transformed by N-terminal and C-terminal procollagen peptidases into native collagen. Lateral aggregation of collagen fibrils and end-to-end fusion allow fibrils thickening and elongation. Interfibrillar cross-links stabilize the collagen network. Smooth or pitted enamel surfaces play a role in one of the four cemento-enamel junctions (CEJ) detected in the cervical area: (1) the cementum overlapping enamel, (2) the enamel overlapping cementum, (3) the edge-to-edge relationship between enamel and cementum, and finally, (4) a gap between cementum and enamel, the exposed dentin being uncovered. Abrasion, attrition, and erosion at the cervical level lead to the formation of cervical non-carious and carious lesions. In addition, enamel perikymata and dentin sclerosis are structures implicated in tooth wear. Accumulation of cariogenic plaque in the cervical area may contribute to the formation of class V carious lesions. In addition, cervical non-carious surfaces take place in the exposed DCJ.

12.1 Procollagen Fibrillogenesis in Dentinogenesis

The cemento-enamel junction (CEJ) represents the anatomical limit between the crown and the root. It is located in the cervical region. It is used to measure the periodontal destruction by measuring the cementum-dentin junction to bone crest distance.

The formation of the CDJ starts with the bone, alveolo-dental ligament and dentin formation, and the synthesis and secretion of collagen.

The conversion of procollagen to collagen results from the activity of procollagen metalloproteinases (Fig. 12.1). Collagen fibrils have a distinct 67 nm axial periodicity and a diameter from a few nanometers to ~500 nm. The trimeric molecules comprise a Gly-X-Y triplet in which X and Y are usually proline and hydroxyproline, respectively. Collagen accumulates through a 3D network and self-assembles in the extracellular

M. Goldberg
University Paris Descartes, Sorbonne, Paris Cité and INSERM UMR-S1124, 45 rue des Saints Pères, Cedex 06, 75270 Paris, France
e-mail: mgoldod@gmail.com

M. Goldberg (ed.), *Understanding Dental Caries*, DOI 10.1007/978-3-319-30552-3_12

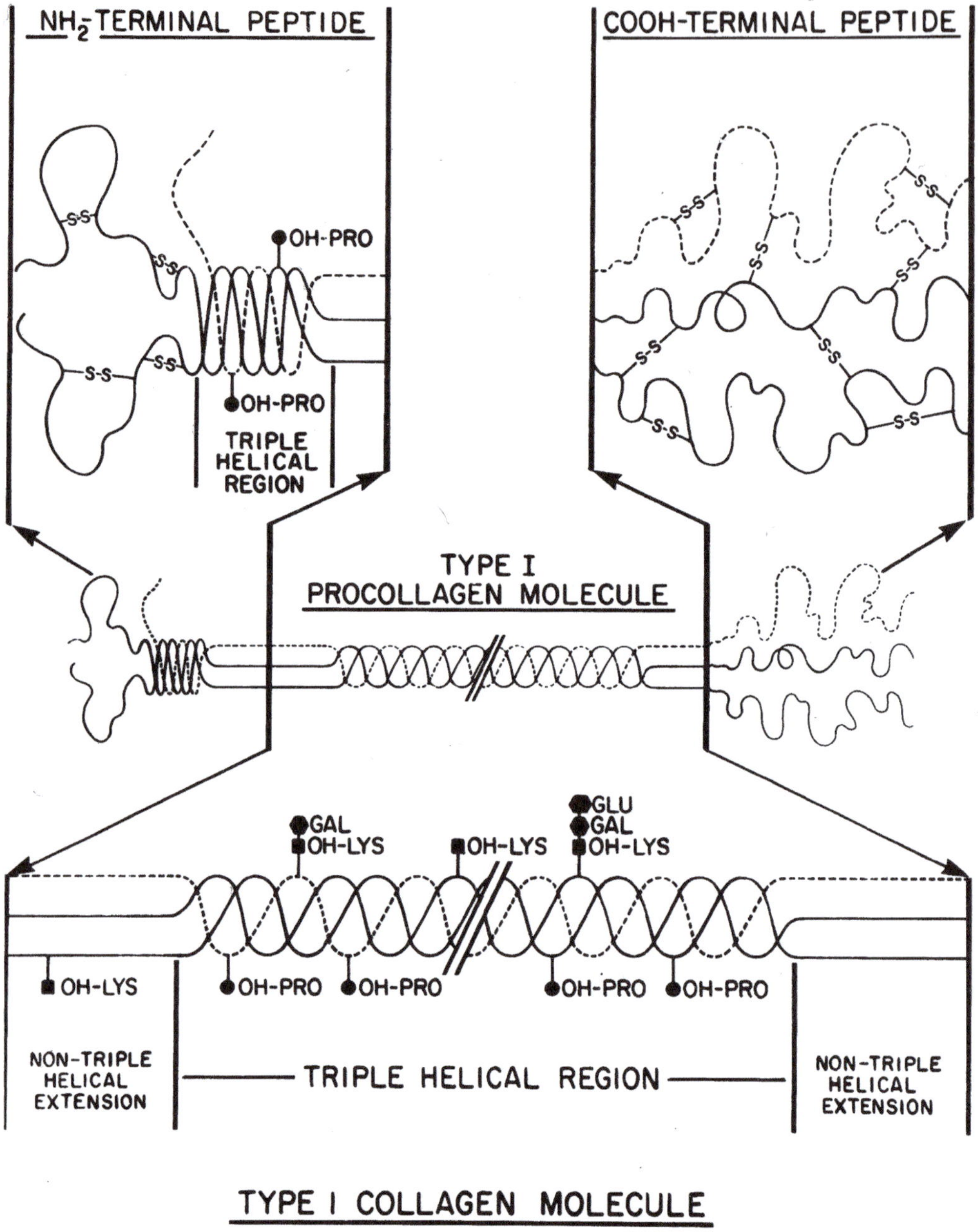

Fig. 12.1 Schematic transition between procollagen chains, nucleated under the influence of the C-propeptide. The procollagen trimer is transformed into collagen, a process followed by collagen fibrillation (Linsennnmayer 1981)

matrix. Procollagen is translocated in the lumen of the endoplasmic reticulum. Molecular chaperones and enzymes regulate foldings and trimerization. C-propeptides and N-propeptides are related to the surrounding proteins. They migrate to the Golgi apparatus, traverse the polarized stack of cisternae, and become secretory proteins, the globular N- and C-propeptides being removed by procollagen N- and C-proteinases. C-proteinase is a member of the Tolloïd family of zinc metalloproteinases (bone morphogenetic protein-1, BMP-1). The furin-like proprotein convertases are also implicated in the conversion of latent BMP-1 and ADAMTS2 to a wide variety of substrates. These events occur first intracellularly and then at the periphery of the plasma membrane. Collagen fibril assembly occurs on the cell surface and is mediated by interactions with cell-surface integrins (α5β1). Fibril-associated molecules are added at the surface of collagen fibrils, and they regulate the diameter and interactions between the fibrils. The initial stage of collagen deposition results in arrays of thin fibrils, which increase in length and diameter. Lateral association and end-to-end fusions of collagen fibrils occur and enhanced by the formation of intra- and inter-cross-links resulting from the action of lysyl oxidase enzymes (Canty and Kadler 2005). Proteoglycans such as decorin, fibromodulin, and lumican affect also fibrillogenesis (Goldberg et al. 2005).

12.2 Enamel Surface

Smooth (bands of smooth enamel prisms) or pitted (associated with the end of prisms reaching the enamel surface) surfaces are seen in enamel. They are associated with perikymata, where the crystals are radially oriented. Circadian rhythms and approximately an 8-day periodicity are apparent (Newman and Poole 1974) (Figs. 12.2 and 12.3).

12.3 Morphology of the Cemento-Enamel Junction

At the cemento-enamel junction (CEJ), the following tissue interrelationships were observed:

- Pattern I: The cementum overlaps the enamel (42–60 %); the cementoblasts produce an afibrillar cementum, dense and laminated, devoid of collagen fibrils with a 64 nm periodicity.
- Pattern II: Edge-to-edge interrelationship between cementum and enamel (situation seen in 30–41 % of the teeth).
- Pattern III: There is a gap between root cementum with exposed dentin (10–12 %) (Arambawatta et al. 2009).
- Pattern IV: The enamel overlaps cementum (1.6–2 %), (Vandana and Haneet 2014) (Figs. 12.2 and 12.4).

The intermediate cementum is a narrow zone of highly calcified tissue. It is located between the most external layer of dentin (granular Tomes' layer) and the layer of acellular cementum. It is referred to as "the hyaline layer of Hopewell-Smith." The intermediate cementum layer contains enamel matrix proteins and is a product of Hertwig's epithelial root sheath. A possible role in wound healing is hypothesized (Harrison and Roda 1995).

The cemento-enamel junction and cementum act as stress damper, decreasing stresses in the periodontal ligament (PDL) and alveolar bone under loading. It influences the stress distribution within the tooth supporting structure.

12.4 Erosive Tooth Wear (Figs. 12.4 and 12.5)

The clinical diagnosis "erosion" is made from characteristic deviations from the original anatomical tooth morphology, thus distinguishing acid-induced tissue loss from other forms of wear (Ganss and Lussi 2014). Tooth wear results from four pathologies: *abrasion*, due to the interaction between teeth and other materials; *attrition*, due to tooth-tooth contact; *erosion*, due to hard tissue dissolution by acidic substances; and *abfraction*, which intensifies wear by abrasion and/or erosion (Shellis and Addy 2014) (Figs. 12.3 and 12.4). Engineering analyses demonstrate theoretical stress concentration at the cervical areas of the teeth. Abfractions present primarily at the cervical region have typically wedge-shaped, with sharp internal and external angles. They are C-shaped lesions with rounded floors, V-shaped lesions, and Mixed-shaped lesions with flat cervical and semi-circular occlusal walls (Levrini et al. 2014). Usually observed on the buccal surface at the cemento-enamel junction, its prevalence varies between 27 and 85 % (Sarode and Sarode 2013). Excessive horizontal tooth brushing can also cause the V-shaped lesion. Occlusal stress produces

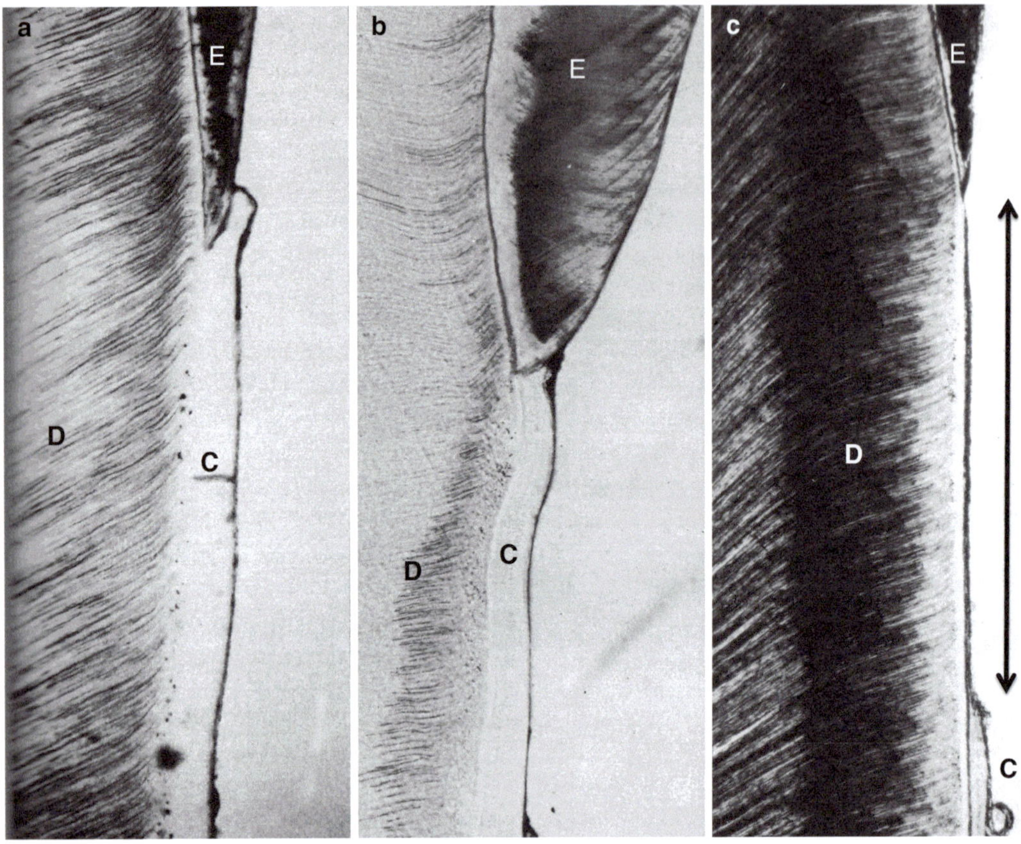

Fig. 12.2 In the cemento-enamel junction, the cementum is overlapping enamel (**a**). In (**b**) cement and enamel are continuous, forming an edge-to-edge structure. In (**c**), gaps are obvious between root cementum and exposed dentin. The 4th missing figure would be related to enamel overlapping dentin, a very seldom case

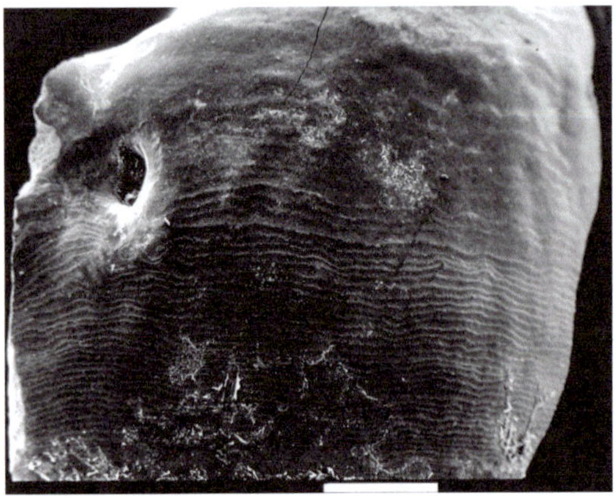

Fig. 12.3 After cleaning the enamel surface, perikymata are visible. They form alignments

cervical cracks that predispose the surface to erosion and abrasion. Most data from the literature shed lights on the different possibilities, although still hypothetical. Extrinsic factors (acid vitamin C supplements, acid foods and drinks) and intrinsic factors (gastrointestinal reflux, eating disorders such as bulimia and anorexia) contribute to cause erosion. The lesions were characterized as being unrelated to bacteria. The characteristics of abfractions are the following: in erosion, characteristic pitting is seen on enamel. In abfraction the form of wedge-shaped lesion is clearly located at the cervical level. Dental and non-dental disorders induce specific morphology and mechanisms that differ from acid etching and bonding.

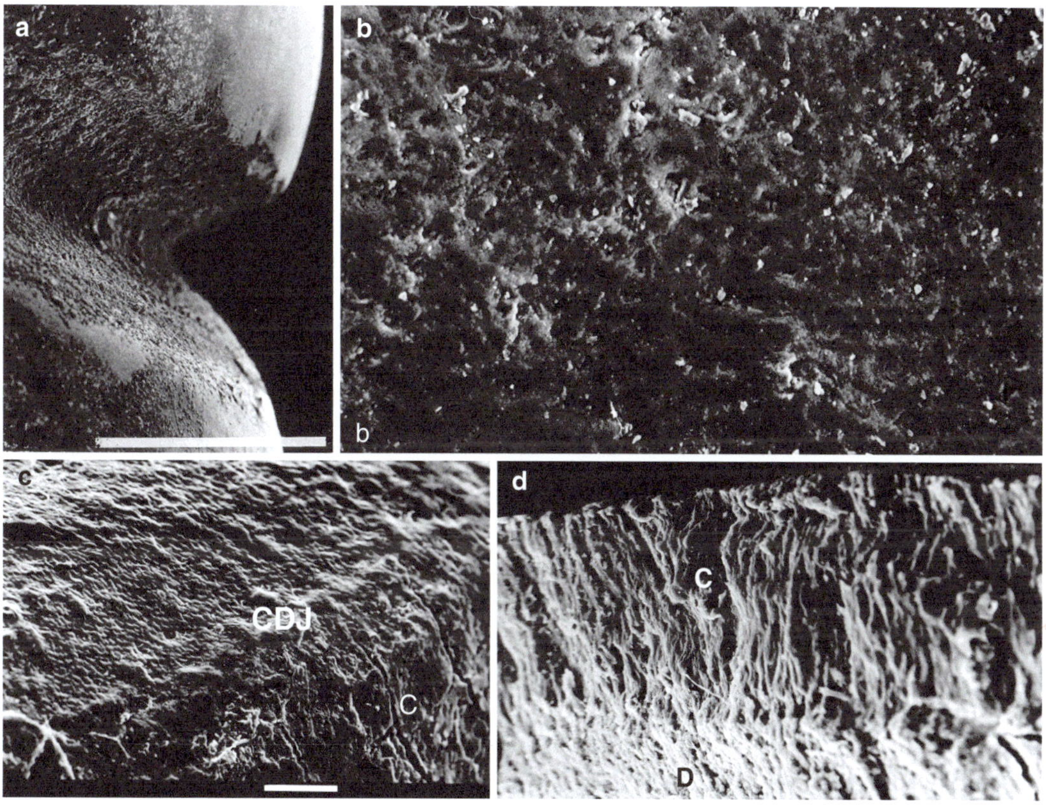

Fig. 12.4 (**a**) Abfraction at the collar region. (**b**) prints of distal ameloblasts at the surface of enamel. (**c**) lower part of a cemento-dentin junction (CDJ). *C* cementum, (**d**) *C* cementum, *D* dentin

12.5 Root Caries

Root dentin invasion shows great similarities to coronal dentin caries. The prevalence range varies from 7.3 % to 69.7 % of the population with root decay. In root caries, initial demineralization and exposure of the collagen fibrils of the ECM is exposed to bacterially derived enzymes leading to eventual cavitation and breakdown of dentin in the tooth root. The evolution of root caries is dependent of processes that enhance remineralization or inhibit demineralization (Featherstone 2004). Protective factors include saliva flow and components, proteins, antibacterial, fluoride, calcium, phosphate, dietary components, and non-cariogenic sweeteners. By contrast, pathogenic factors involve acidogenic bacteria, frequency of carbohydrate ingestion, and reduced salivary function (Featherstone 1999).

The bacterial composition of root caries flora confirms the identification of *Streptococcus mutans* and *Actinomyces viscosus*. On the basis of the presence or absence of *S. mutans*, in group I plaques, *S. mutans* comprised 30 % of the total cultivable flora. In group II plaques, *S. mutans* was not detected and *S. sanguis* formed 48 % of the total plaque flora. *A. viscosus* was the predominant organism of all plaque samples, accounting for 47 % of group I isolates and 41 % of the group II isolates (Syed et al. 1975).

Earliest lesions appear as small clefts traversing cementum and extending into the peripheral dentin that is sclerosed and tubule-free. Dentinal tubules were sclerosed passively, due to

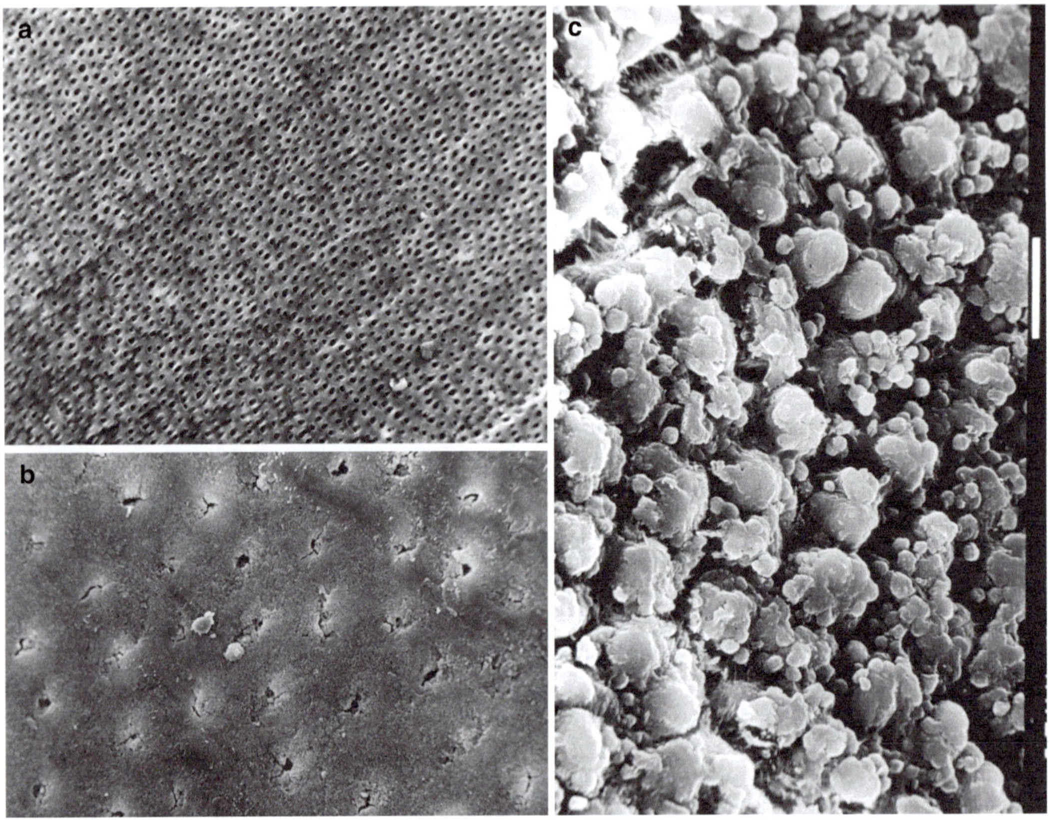

Fig. 12.5 (**a**) Circumpulpal dentin with open tubuli; (**b**) sclerotic dentin. Tubules are filled by intratubular mineral precipitations. (**c**) Globular structures of cement along the root surface

precipitation or re-precipitation of Ca and PO_4 ions. Demineralization of dentin precedes the degradation of organic matrix. In some cases, a hypermineralized layer is present both in cementum and exposed dentin. This layer is not located at the anatomical surface.

Sclerosed tubules containing rhombohedral crystals are present in the deep layers. Tubular lumens and lateral side branches having lost their peritubular dentin are filled with gram-positive microorganisms. Diffuse destruction of intertubular dentin presents crossbanded collagen fibrils. The confluence of enlarged dentinal tubules led to large bacterial zones with complete destruction of root dentin (Frank et al. 1989). The evolution of arrested carious lesions depends on the degree of active sclerosis of dentinal tubules, the degree of bacterial infection of the lesion, and the location of lesions on the various tooth surfaces. Altogether, this supports the concept of noninvasive treatment of root caries lesions without cavitation (Schüpbach et al. 1990).

Intertubular mineral crystallites decrease in size as carious lesion progresses. In the intratubular and intertubular zones, nano-size apatitic crystallites are smaller in the intertubular zones. Dissolution and precipitation mechanisms are important in the process induced by the carious attack (Zavgorodniy et al. 2008)

The dentin caries does not spread along the enamel-dentin junction (Bjorndal and Thylstrup 1995; Ekstrand et al. 1998).

In addition to the gram-positive predominant facultative anaerobic species (*Streptococcus*, *Staphylococcus*, *Lactobacillus*, and *Actinomyces*), gram-negative anaerobes, predominantly *Bacteroides*, *Prevotella*, *Selenomonas*, *Fusobacterium*, *Leptotrichia*, and *Capnocytophaga* showed the highest isolation frequencies. On all surfaces *Actinomyces* spp. are predominated with

Streptococci and *Lactobacilli* forming a minor part of the microbiota. With respect to the detected proportions of anaerobes, microaerophiles (*Actinomyces naeslundii*, *Prevotella buccae*, and *Selenomonas dianae*), significant differences were observed between the three categories of root surfaces. The total bacteria on both caries-free and caries-active surfaces were significantly higher than on arrested lesions. In general, a polymicrobial etiology for caries initiation was detected on root surfaces, with *A. naeslundii*, *Capnocytophaga* spp., and *Prevotella* spp. making specific contributions to the processes of cementum and dentin breakdown (Schüpbach et al. 1995).

References

Arambawatta K, Peiris R, Nanayakkara D. Morphology of the cemento-enamel junction in premolar teeth. J Oral Sci. 2009;51:623–7.

Bjorndal L, Thylstrup A. A structural analysis of approximal enamel caries lesions and subjacent dentin reactions. Eur J Oral Sci. 1995;103:25–31.

Canty EG, Kadler KE. Procollagen trafficking, processing and fibrillogenesis. J Cell Sci. 2005;118:1341–53.

Ekstrand KR, Ricketts DN, Kidd EAM. Do occlusal carious lesions spread laterally at the enamel-dentin junction? A histopathological study. Clin Oral Invest. 1998;2:15–20.

Featherstone JDB. Prevention and reversal of dental caries: role of low level fluoride. Community Dent Oral Epidemiol. 1999;27:31–40.

Featherstone JDB. The continuum of dental caries-evidence for a dynamic disease process. J Dent Res. 2004;83(Spec Iss C):C39–42.

Frank RM, Steuer P, Hemmerle J. Ultrastructural study on human root caries. Caries Res. 1989;23:2009–217.

Ganss C, Lussi A. Diagnosis of erosive tooth wear. Monogr Oral Sci. 2014;25:22–31.

Goldberg M, Septier D, Rapoport O, Iozzo RV, Young MF, Ameye LG. Targeted disruption of two small leucine-rich proteoglycans, biglycan and decorin, excerpts divergent effects on enamel and dentin formation. Calcif Tissue Int. 2005;77:297–310.

Harrison JW, Roda RS. Intermediate cementum-development, structure, composition, and potential functions. Oral Surg Oral Med Oral Pathol. 1995;79:624–33.

Levrini L, Di Benedetto G, Raspanti M. Dental wear: a scanning electron microscope study. BioMed Res Int. 2014; Article ID 340425.

Linsennnmayer TF. Collagen in Cell Biology of Extracellular Matrix. ED Haay ed. Chapter 1, Plenum Press. New York & London. 1981; 5–37.

Newman HN, Poole DFG. Observations with scanning and transmission electron microscopy on the structure of human surface enamel. Arch Oral Biol. 1974;19:1135–40.

Sarode GS, Sarode SC. Abfraction: a review. J Oral Maxillofac Pathol. 2013;17:222–7.

Schüpbach P, Guggenheim B, Lutz F. Histopathology of root surface caries. J Dent Res. 1990;69:1195–204.

Schüpbach P, Osterwalder V, Guggenheim B. Human root caries: microbiota in plaque covering sound, carious and arrested carious root surfaces. Caries Res. 1995;29:382–95.

Shellis RP, Addy M. The interactions between attrition, abrasion and erosion in tooth wear. Monogr Oral Sci. 2014;25:32–45.

Syed SA, Loesche WJ, Pape Jr HL, Grenier E. Predominant cultivable flora isolated from human root surface caries plaque. Infect Immun. 1975;11:727–31.

Vandana KL, Haneet RK. Cemento-enamel junction: an insight. J Indian Soc Periodontol. 2014;18:549–54.

Zavgorodniy AV, Rohanizadeh R, Swain MV. Ultrastructure of dentine carious lesions. Arch Oral Biol. 2008;53:124–32.

Cervical Erosions: Morphology and Restoration of Cervical Erosions

13

Wolfgang H. Arnold

Abstract

Cervical dentin is covered by a thin layer of acellular-afibrillar cement which develops during the early odontogenesis. The cervical cement layer is only about 100 μm thick (Fig. 13.1) and therefore vulnerable to mechanical (i.e., toothbrushing (Wiegand and Schlueter, Monogr Oral Sci 25:215–219, 2014)), chemical (i.e., soft drink consumption (Pinto et al., BMC Res Notes 6:67, 2013; Zimmer et al., PLoS One 10:e0129462, 2015; Shellis et al., Monogr Oral Sci 25:163–179, 2014)), and microbiological (i.e., gingival recession and plaque accumulation (Bignozzi et al., J Esthet Restor Dent 25:371–382, 2013; Pikdoken et al., J Oral Rehabil 38:95–100, 2011)) influences. The etiology of dental erosion is a multifactorial and complicated process (Lussi and Carvalho, Monogr Oral Sci 25:1–15, 2014). With increasing life expectancy and effective oral prevention, more patients retain their teeth. An increased prevalence of periodontal diseases such as gingival recession leaves the cervical cement uncovered in these patients. Repeated erosive stress challenges to cervical cement result in a loss of the cementum layer (Fig. 13.2a) and open dentin tubules which in turn may be the cause for dental hypersensitivity (West, Monogr Oral Sci 20:173–189, 2006). Another major risk factor is plaque accumulation on the eroded dentin surface which results in in-surface demineralization (Fig. 13.4) and finally in root caries lesions (Fig. 13.4). Iatrogenic cervical dentin erosions as a result of cervical root scaling during periodontal treatment are frequently occurring.

13.1 Morphology of Cervical Dentin Erosion

Cervical dentin erosion has to be distinguished from cervical caries lesions. Dentin erosion is a nonbacterial superficial destruction caused by acid attacks and is restricted to the cervical

W.H. Arnold
Department of Biological and Material Sciences in Dentistry, School of Dentistry, Faculty of Health Witten/Herdecke University, Alfres Herrhausenstrasse 44, Witten 58455, Germany
e-mail: Wolfgang.Arnold@uni-wh.de

M. Goldberg (ed.), *Understanding Dental Caries*, DOI 10.1007/978-3-319-30552-3_13

surface, and therefore, it is also called "near-surface demineralization" (Lussi and Carvalho 2014). Beginning cervical dentin erosion is morphologically characterized by softened surface dentin with a thin demineralized layer (Figs. 13.1 and 13.2b). Further progression of the demineralizing process leads to an increased outflow of ions from the dental hard tissue toward the surface. Precipitation of these ions is the cause for the development of a small hypermineralized surface layer (Fig. 13.3). This can be a transitory stage before the erosion may be covered by dental plaque and develops into a root caries lesion with progressing subsurface demineralization

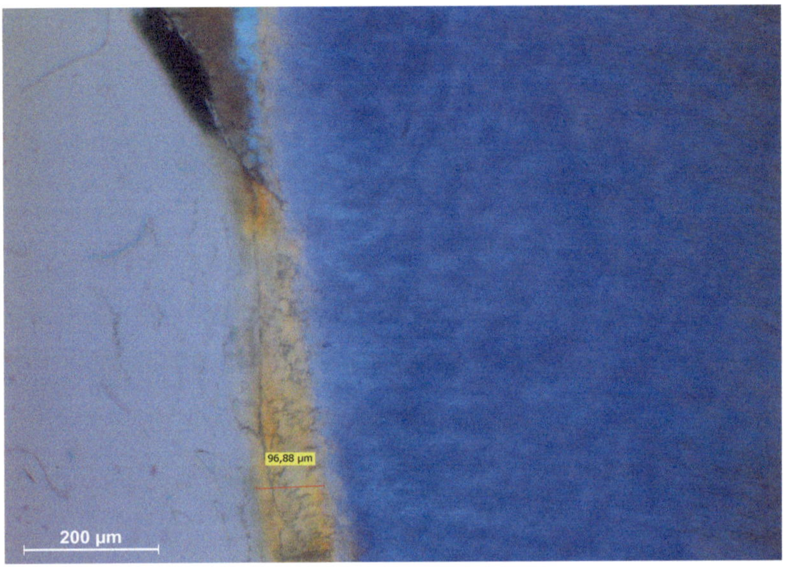

Fig. 13.1 Non-eroded healthy cervical dentin which is covered by a thin layer of acellular-afibrillar cement

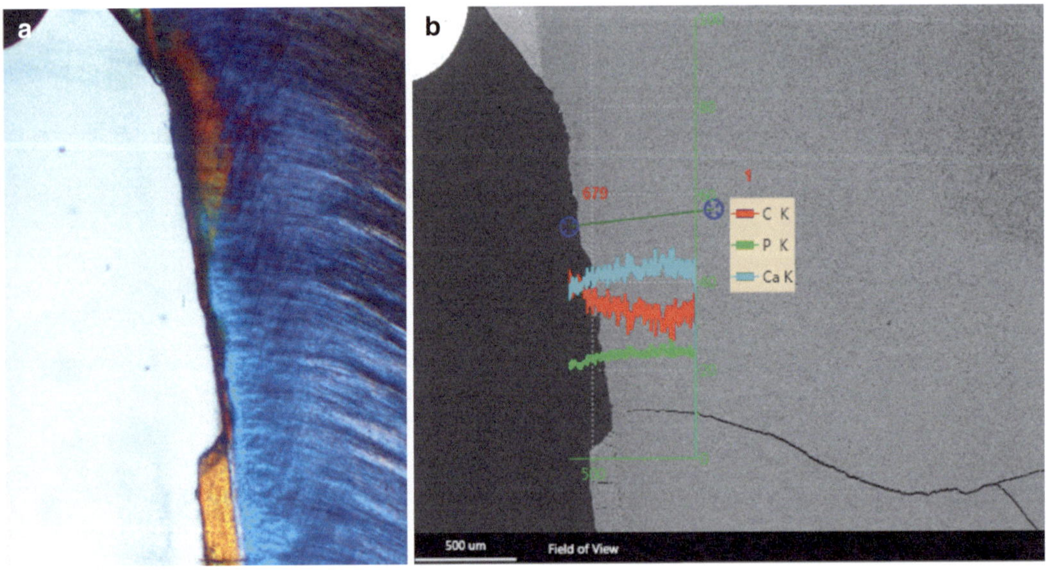

Fig. 13.2 Eroded cervical dentin with complete destruction of the cement layer; (**a**) polarized light microcopy; (**b**) EDS line scan of the same lesion. There is a light decrease of the mineral content of the surface

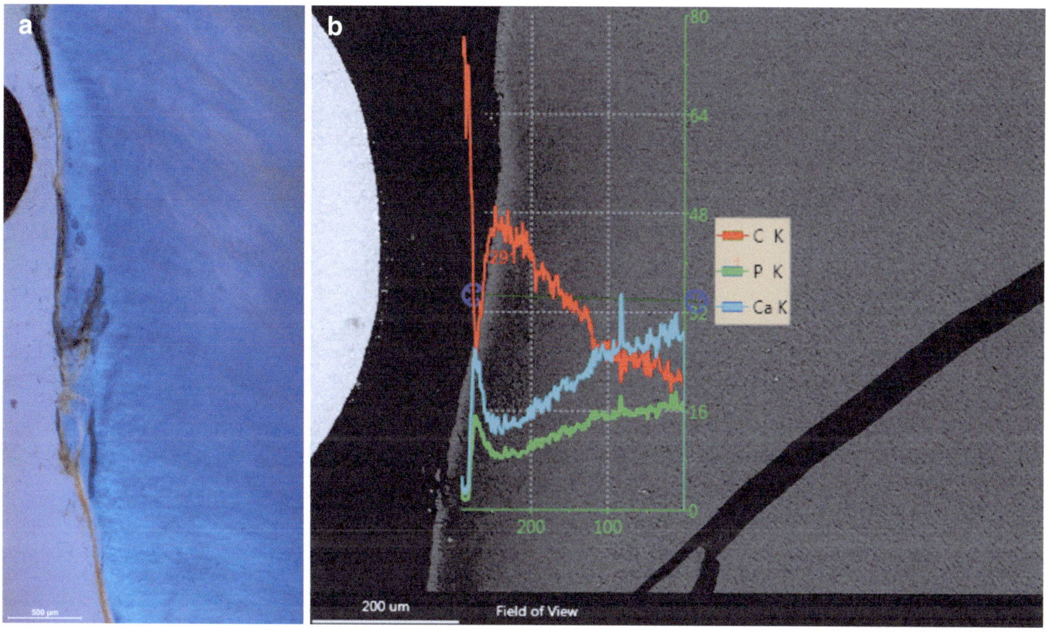

Fig. 13.3 Eroded cervical dentin with beginning demineralization; (**a**) polarized light microscopy which shows a small hypermineralized superficial layer and a small demineralized zone underneath; (**b**) EDS line scan through the eroded lesion demonstrating the superficial hypermineralized layer and the demineralized area

(Fig. 13.4). Due to the loss of cervical cement, the dentin tubules are opened (Fig. 13.5). Acids which are penetrating into these open dentin tubules dissolve peritubular dentin. As a consequence the tubule diameter is becoming wider which in turn might increase dentin hypersensitivity.

The superficial erosive demineralization results in dissolution of the mineral, but the dentin collagen fibers are remaining (Breschi et al. 2002) and protect the underlying dentin from further demineralization as this collagenous matrix is a diffusion barrier (Shellis et al. 2010). The superficial layer of eroded dentin is a spongelike relative stable structure, and the superficial cervical contour is preserved. However, eroded cervical dentin is vulnerable to mechanical influences like toothbrushing. The surface morphology of eroded dentin varies from irregular ragged surface (Fig. 13.5) to a rather smooth surface. The progression of cervical dentin erosion depended from the oral health of the host, lifestyle, and eating habits (Ganss et al. 2014).

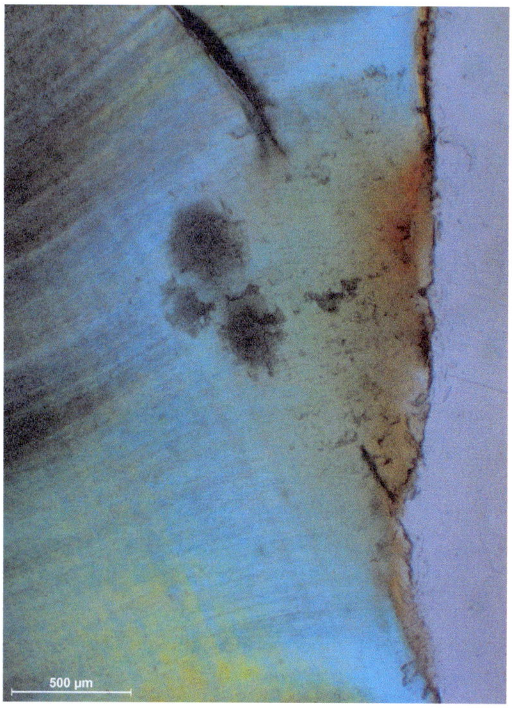

Fig. 13.4 Initial cervical root caries lesion

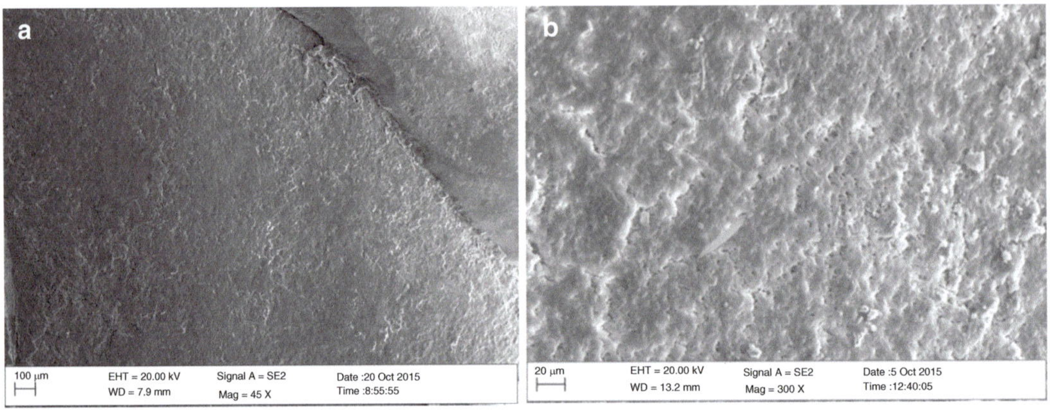

Fig. 13.5 Eroded cervical dentin area; (**a**) SEM overview of an eroded cervical area beneath the enamel – cementum junction. The surface appears to be rough; (**b**) higher magnification of the eroded area. The surface has a rugged structure. Dentin tubules are opened

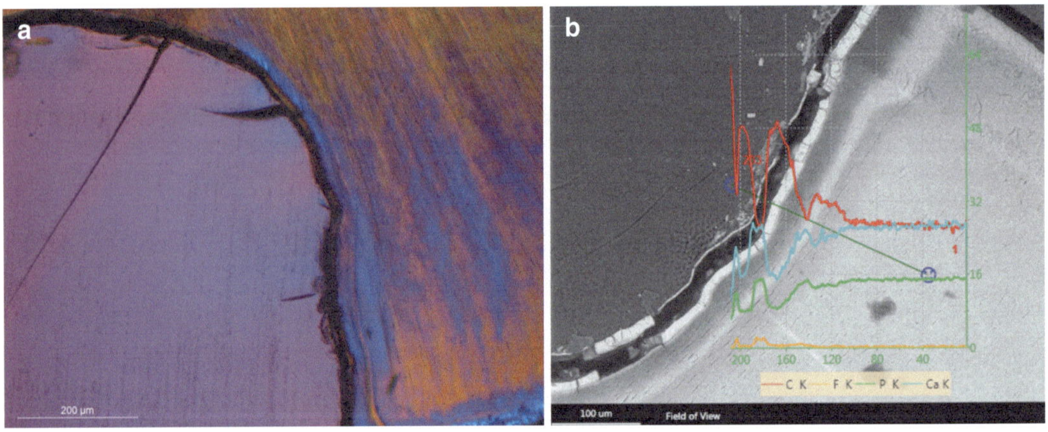

Fig. 13.6 Cervical demineralized dentin after incubation with artificial saliva and 10 ppm NaF. (**a**) A rather thick remineralized surface layer can be seen on top of the lesion. (**b**) EDS line scan through the same lesion demonstration a higher Ca, P, and F content within the superficial dentin layer

13.2 Restoration of Cervical Dentin Erosions

Generally, like enamel, dentin is capable to remineralize. Prerequisite for remineralization is a sufficient supply of Ca^{2+} and PO_4^{3-} ions. The natural supply derives from the hyper-saturated saliva. Fluoride promotes remineralizaion of hydroxyapatite and is widely used in the prevention and restoration of dentin erosions. The mechanism of the action of fluoride on remineralization of dentin is still not fully understood. Experimental studies demonstrated a positive effect of fluoride on root dentin remineralization (Addy 2005; Arnold et al. 2014; Nyvad and Fejerskov 1982) (Fig. 13.6). Fluorides are widely used for therapeutic interventions of dentin erosions. The majority are fluoridated self-care oral hygiene products. Fluoridated toothpastes for the use of remineralization of cervical dentin have two functions. Fluoride should promote dentin remineralization, whereas other ingredients like pro-arginin or hydroxyapatite are aimed to occlude open dentin tubules for diminishing dentin hypersensitivity (Arnold et al. 2015). However, a newly published meta-analysis showed that the evidence for an effectiveness of these products is rather low (Twetman 2015).

There are numerous other products available like mouthrinses, pastes, and gels. The effectiveness of fluoridated milk on dentin remineralization has been investigated in an experimental model which has shown that there is a benefit of fluoridated milk in dentin remineralization (Arnold et al. 2014).

In office varnishes are containing higher concentrations of fluoride (up to 12,000 ppm, Elmex Fluid, CB GABA, Hamburg, Germany) and are more effective in the reduction of dentin hypersensitivity (Hamlin et al. 2012). However, not much is known about their effect on the remineralization of cervical dentin erosion.

References

Addy M. Tooth brushing, tooth wear and dentine hypersensitivity – are they associated? Int Dent J. 2005;55:261–7.

Arnold WH, Heidt BA, Kuntz S, Naumova EA. Effects of fluoridated milk on root dentin remineralization. PLoS One. 2014;9, e104327. doi:10.1371/journal.pone.0104327.g005.

Arnold WH, Prange M, Naumova EA. Effectiveness of various toothpastes on dentine tubule occlusion. J Dent. 2015;43:440–9. doi:10.1016/j.jdent.2015.01.014.

Bignozzi I, Littarru C, Crea A, Vittorini Orgeas G, Landi L. Surgical treatment options for grafting areas of gingival recession association with cervical lesions: a review. J Esthet Restor Dent. 2013;25:371–82. doi:10.1111/jerd.12058.

Breschi L, et al. High resolution SEM evaluation of dentin etched with maleic and citric acid. Dent Mater. 2002;18:26–35.

Ganss C, Lussi A, Schlueter N. The histological features and physical properties of eroded dental hard tissues. Monogr Oral Sci. 2014;25:99–107. doi:10.1159/000359939.

Hamlin D, et al. Comparative efficacy of two treatment regimens combining in-office and at-home programs for dentin hypersensitivity relief: a 24-week clinical study. Am J Dent. 2012;25:146–52.

Lussi A, Carvalho TS. Erosive tooth wear: a multifactorial condition of growing concern and increasing knowledge. Monogr Oral Sci. 2014;25:1–15. doi:10.1159/000360380.

Nyvad B, Fejerskov O. Root surface caries: clinical, histopathological and microbiological features and clinical implications. Int Dent J. 1982;32:311–26.

Pikdoken L, Akca E, Gurbuzer B, Aydil B, Tasdelen B. Cervical wear and occlusal wear from a periodontal perspective. J Oral Rehabil. 2011;38:95–100. doi:10.1111/j.1365-2842.2010.02137.x.

Pinto SC, et al. Erosive potential of energy drinks on the dentine surface. BMC Res Notes. 2013;6:67. doi:10.1186/1756-0500-6-67.

Shellis RP, Barbour ME, Jones SB, Addy M. Effects of pH and acid concentration on erosive dissolution of enamel, dentine, and compressed hydroxyapatite. Eur J Oral Sci. 2010;118:475–82. doi:10.1111/j.1600-0722.2010.00763.x.

Shellis RP, Featherstone JD, Lussi A. Understanding the chemistry of dental erosion. Monogr Oral Sci. 2014;25:163–79. doi:10.1159/000359943.

Twetman S. The evidence base for professional and self-care prevention – caries, erosion and sensitivity. BMC Oral Health. 2015;15 Suppl 1:S4. doi:10.1186/1472-6831-15-s1-s4.

West NX. Dentine hypersensitivity. Monogr Oral Sci. 2006;20:173–89. doi:10.1159/000093362.

Wiegand A, Schlueter N. The role of oral hygiene: does toothbrushing harm? Monogr Oral Sci. 2014;25:215–9. doi:10.1159/000360379.

Zimmer S, Kirchner G, Bizhang M, Benedix M. Influence of various acidic beverages on tooth erosion. Evaluation by a new method. PLoS One. 2015;10, e0129462. doi:10.1371/journal.pone.0129462.

Cervical Regeneration

14

Michel Goldberg

Abstract

In different reports, cervical lesions are named erosion, abrasion, chemical abrasion, and denudation. The leading concept is that occlusal loading could be implicated in cervical stress and consequently may induce a loss of cervical tooth structure. Cervical lesion has gained over all the other terminology. Excessive occlusal biomechanical forces seem to cause loss of superficial root dentin, causing thermo-sensitivity that is mediated by dentinal fluid shifts that activate potassium ion channel receptors in pulpal nerves innervating such dentin. Carious cervical lesions may be restored after etching by adhesives combined with resin composites or by glass ionomer cements. They may influence the subjacent living pulp. Inflammation and formation of tertiary dentin are the principal evidences, detectable only after histological investigation on demineralized sections. Caries lesions may be active or inactive. About 60 % of the elderly had one or more active lesions, whereas 70 % had more than eight filled carious inactive or active surfaces (Fejerskov et al., Caries Res 25:385–391, 1991). Non-carious cervical lesions (NCCL) are predominant lesions at the junction between the crown and root. In addition, these erosions may also spontaneously remineralize. Tissue regeneration may result from reprecipitation due to salivary minerals.

14.1 Abfraction: Non-carious Cervical Lesions

Abfraction lesions are typically shaped as a wedge-shaped tissue defect (Grippo 1991). The lesion is also designated in different reports under the name of erosion, abrasion, chemical abrasion, and denudation. The concept that occlusal loading could cause cervical stress and consequently may induce a loss of cervical tooth structure has

M. Goldberg
University Paris Descartes, Sorbonne, Paris Cité and INSERM UMR-S1124, 45 rue des Saints Pères, Cedex 06, 75270 Paris, France
e-mail: mgoldod@gmail.com

M. Goldberg (ed.), *Understanding Dental Caries*, DOI 10.1007/978-3-319-30552-3_14

gained over all the other terminology. Some data demonstrate that theoretical stress concentration occurs at cervical areas of the teeth (Shetty et al. 2013). In addition, the term of toothbrush abrasion or toothbrush abuse should be the best and preferred to bruxism (Sarode and Sarode 2013).

Non-carious cervical lesions (NCCL) are caused by occlusal biomechanical forces. Using an appropriate computer program (the finite element method), the authors came to the conclusion that action of occlusal forces, especially paraxial ones, leads to significant stress in the cervical part of the tooth. Abfraction lesions result from the stress in the cervical subsuperficial enamel layer, which is almost five times higher compared with the superficial enamel (Jakupovic et al. 2014). However, brushing is also an important factor associated with NCCL, whereas the occlusal wear seems to play a minor role (Sadaf and Ahmad 2014).

The exposed cervical dentin often displays hypersensitivity (West et al. 2013). The current pain mechanism of dentin hypersensitivity (DHS) seems to be the hydrodynamic theory. Evidence demonstrates odontoblasts express mechano- and/or thermosensitive transient receptor potential ion channels (TRPV1, TRPV2, TRPV3, TRPV4, TRPM3, KCa, and TREK-1). Movements of dentinal fluids within tubules may represent a unique mechano-sensory system with odontoblast acting as sensor cells.

14.2 Pulpal Regeneration

The strategy is to use the intact ECM of pulp cells to induce the specific differentiation of bone marrow-derived mesenchymal stem cells. Tissue engineering requires a triad of cells, scaffolds, and growth factors, leading to pulp regeneration. Pulp vascularization and specialized innervation are considered as crucial for serving as mechanotransducer, providing immediate bacterial response to bacterial insult. Structural proteins and growth factors have been identified in the dental pulp including glucose-regulated protein 78 and TGF-β receptor interacting protein 1, displaying extracellular and intracellular functions. Biomimetic scaffolds induce the differentiation and regeneration of pulp tissue. Vascular endothelial growth factor (VEGF) implanted subcutaneously in nude mice promotes vascularization (Ravindran and George 2015).

14.3 Dental Pulp Engineering and Regeneration: Advancement and Challenge

Caries destroys enamel and dentin and leads to infection of the dental pulp. Regeneration starts with a blood clot used as a source of growth factors to help tissue repair (Ostby 1961). Vascularization of teeth with open apices is the best candidate for pulp tissue regeneration (Huang 2012). Morphogens (polypeptide mitogens) in conjunction with extracellular matrix molecules may have applications for dentin regeneration. Growth factors such as TGF-beta, bone morphogenetic proteins (BMP-2, BMP-4, BMP-7), and insulin-like growth factor-1 (IGF-1) play a key role in the induction of odontoblast-like cell differentiation of pulpal progenitor cells. Scaffolds such as collagen sponges, bioceramics, and polymers contribute to create a tissue construct. Derivatives of the extracellular matrix may be used (collagen, fibrin, chitosan, glycosaminoglycans, biodegradable polymers, polylactic and/or polyglycolic acids (PLGA)) and may be applied by controlled release, influencing the cell phenotype expression. Scaffold needs to be biocompatible and nontoxic, bioresorbable, and bioactive and have biomechanical properties. Altogether cells, bioactive molecules, and scaffold used as carrier contribute to revascularization of the pulp, pending an actual effective disinfection therapy (Kundabala et al. 2010).

14.4 Tooth Resorption

Invasive cervical resorption is a term used in the clinic to describe an uncommon, insidious, and often aggressive form of external tooth resorption. It may arise through an enamel defect in the tooth crown and therefore may be termed *invasive coronal resorption*. In the more apical source, it is termed *invasive radicular resorption*. Some teeth included teeth showing “pink spots.” The etiology of this disorder requires further molecular biology, enzyme histochemical or microbiological investigations. The clinical classification is the following:

Class 1 appears as a small invasive resorptive lesion near the cervical area with shallow penetration into dentin.

Class 2 denotes a well-defined invasive resorptive lesion that has penetrated close to the coronal pulp showing little or no extension into the radicular dentin.

Class 3 displays a deeper invasion of dentin by resorbing tissue, attending into the coronal third of the root.

Class 4 shows a deeper invasive resorptive process that has extended beyond the coronal third of the root.

The histopathologic appearance of such resorption showed that there is a mass of fibrous tissue, numerous blood vessels, and clastic resorbing cells adjacent to the dentin surface (Heithersay 2004).

14.5 Cervical Regeneration

Cervical regeneration may be accomplished by resin composites, glass ionomer cements, and the adhesive properties associated to these restorative materials. It cannot regenerate spontaneously in the absence of cells. Tartar deposits can reduce the depth of the lesion, and toothpastes contribute to fill the lumens of dentinal tubules, when sclerotic intraluminal mineralizations are not occluding the lumens. Changes in the brushing habits may stabilize the evolution of cervical resorption, but never restore the acquired loss of substance interfering altogether with enamel defects, the outer dentin layers (namely, the granular hyaline layers), and deeper circumpulpal dentin lesions.

When oral hygiene instruction (OHI) was applied to chlorhexidine varnish, sodium fluoride varnish, and silver diamine fluoride repeated every 3–12 months, they prevent new root caries in institutionalized elders. These preventive therapies contribute to stop the evolution of the lesion and to cervical regeneration.

References

Fejerskov O, Luan WM, Nyvad B, Budtz-Jorgensen E, Holm-Pedersen P. Active and inactive root surface caries lesions in a selected group of 60–80-year-old danes. Caries Res. 1991;25:385–91.

Grippo JO. Abfractions: a new classification of hard tissue lesions of teeth. J Esthetic Dent. 1991;3:14–9.

Heithersay GS. Invasive cervical resorption. Endodontic Topics. 2004;7:73–92.

Huang GT-J. Dental pulp and dentin tissue engineering and regeneration: advancement and challenge. Front Biosci. 2012;3:788–800.

Jakupovic S, Cerjakovic E, Topcic A, Ajanovic M, Konjhodzic-Prcic A, Vukovic A. Analysis of the abfraction lesions formation mechanisms by the finite element method. Acta Inform Med. 2014;4:241–5.

Kundabala M, Parolia A, Shetty N. Regenerative endodontics: a review. Malaysiona Dent J. 2010;31:94–100.

Ostby BN. The role of the blood clot in endodontic therapy. An experimental histologic study. Acta Odontol Scand. 1961;19:324–53.

Ravindran S, George A. Biomimetic extracellular matrix mediated somatic stem cell differentiation: application in dental pulp tissue regeneration. Front Physiol. 2015;6:118.

Sadaf D, Ahmad Z. Role of brushing and occlusal forces in non-carious cervical lesions (NCCL). Int J Biomed Sci. 2014;10:265–8.

Sarode GS, Sarode SC. Abfraction: a review. J Oral Maxillofac Pathol. 2013;17:222–7.

Shetty SM, Shetty RG, Mattigatti S, Managoli NA, Rairam SG, Patil AM. No carious cervical lesions: abfraction. J Int Oral Heath. 2013;5:143–6.

West NX, Lussi A, Seong J, Hellwig E. Dentin hypersensitivity: pain mechanisms and aetiology of exposed cervical dentin. Clin Oral Invest. 2013;17(Suppl1):S9–19.

Part IV

Fluoride

Fluoride

15

Pam Denbesten, Robert Faller, and Yukiko Nakano

Abstract

It is known that fluoride helps to prevent tooth decay, however an excess of fluoride can cause enamel fluorosis. In this chapter, we will discuss current knowledge about fluoride and its effect on teeth, including dental fluorosis, fluoride and caries prevention, and enamel remineralizing agents.

15.1 Dental Fluorosis

Dental fluorosis is a developmental condition that affects the teeth. It is caused by overexposure to fluoride during the first 7–8 years of life, the period when most of the permanent teeth are being formed.

The potential for dental fluorosis increases with the level of systemic fluoride intake. Dental fluorosis resulting from high fluoride levels in underground water is an issue in specific regions of the world. Drinking water is usually the major source of the daily fluoride intake. However, in some parts of Africa, China, the Middle East, and Southern Asia (India, Sri Lanka), as well as some areas in the Americas and Japan, high amounts of fluoride are found in vegetables, fruit, tea, and other crops (WHO/UNICEF Joint Water Supply and Sanitation Monitoring Programme 2005). The atmosphere in these areas may have high levels of fluoride from dust in areas with fluoride-containing soils and gas, released from industries, underground coal fires, and volcanic activities (WHO/UNICEF Joint Water Supply and Sanitation Monitoring Programme 2005).

Teeth with mild dental fluorosis are more resistant to dental decay; however, severely fluorosed teeth are more susceptible to decay, most likely because of the uneven surface or loss of the outer protective layer (Ockerse and Wasserstein 1955). The primary pathological finding of fluorosed enamel is a subsurface porosity, along with hyper- and hypomineralized bands within the forming enamel (Fejerskov et al. 1974, 1975,

P. Denbesten (✉)
Department of Orofacial Sciences, School of Dentistry, University of California, San Francisco, 513 Parnassus Ave, San Francisco, CA 94143, USA
e-mail: Pamela.DenBesten@ucsf.edu

R. Faller
Department of Pediatric Dentistry and Community Oral Health Sciences, Maurice H. Kornberg School of Dentistry, Temple University, Philadelphia, PA, USA
e-mail: robert.faller@yourencore.com

Y. Nakano
Center for Children's Oral Health Research, School of Dentistry, University of California, San Francisco, 513 Parnassus Ave, San Francisco, CA 94143, USA

M. Goldberg (ed.), *Understanding Dental Caries*, DOI 10.1007/978-3-319-30552-3_15

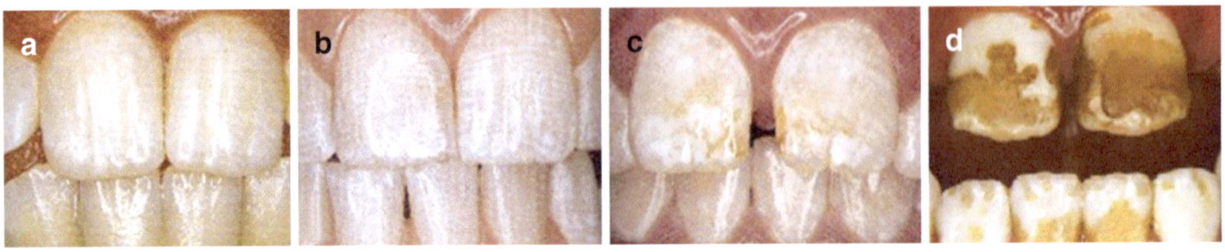

Fig. 15.1 Dental fluorosis. (**a**) Mild fluorosis with slight accentuation of the perikymata, (**b**) moderate fluorosis, showing a white opaque appearance, (**c**) moderate, white opaque enamel with some discoloration and pitting, (**d**) severe fluorosis [with permission from a reference (Denbesten and Li, 2011), Fig. 1] DENBESTEN, P. & LI, W. 2011. Chronic fluoride toxicity: dental fluorosis. Monogr Oral Sci, 22, 81–96

1977, 1979, 1991; Kidd et al. 1981; Kierdorf et al. 1993). Clinically, mild cases of dental fluorosis are characterized by a white opaque appearance of the enamel, caused by increased subsurface porosity. The earliest sign is a change in color, showing many thin white horizontal lines running across the surfaces of the teeth, with white opacities at the newly erupted incisal end. The white lines run along the "perikymata," a term referring to transverse ridges on the surface of the tooth, which correspond to the incremental lines in the enamel known as Striae of Retzius (Moller 1982; Kroncke 1966). At higher levels of fluoride exposure, the white lines in the enamel become more and more defined and thick. Some patchy cloudy areas and thick opaque bands also appear on the involved teeth. With increased dental fluorosis, the entire tooth can be chalky white and lose transparency (Moller 1982; Smith 1985). With higher fluoride doses or prolonged exposure, deeper layers of enamel are affected; the enamel becomes less well mineralized. Damage to the enamel surface, sometimes with subsequent staining of the porous enamel and exposed dentin, occurs in patients with moderate to severe degrees of enamel fluorosis (McKay 1952; Mottled Enamel. Am J Public Health Nations Health 1933) (Fig. 15.1).

15.1.1 Mechanisms of Enamel Fluorosis

Studies to determine the mechanisms by which fluoride results in dental fluorosis have used animal models. The most frequently used model to study fluorosis mechanisms is the rodent incisor, as it is not possible to do similar studies using human teeth. Fluoride can be given in drinking water beginning at 21 days, when rodents are weaned. At this time, the incisors are fully erupted; however, because the rodent incisor is a continuously erupting tooth, all stages of enamel formation are present, so that the effect of fluoride at each stage of enamel formation can be investigated.

Models to Study the Fluorosis Mechanisms Should Be Based on Comparable Concentrations to Those Found in Human Serum A difference between rodents and humans, which sometimes results in confusion as to the relevance of studies of fluoride mechanisms, is the fact that rodents must consume approximately 10 times the amount of fluoride in drinking water than humans to result in the same serum fluoride level and degree of fluorosis. For example, humans drinking 3–5 ppm fluoride in water (1 ppm F=52.6 μM) have serum fluoride levels of 3–5 μM (Guy et al. 1976) which form fluorosed enamel. For a mouse to have similar serum fluoride levels, the mouse must ingest drinking water containing approximately 50 ppm F (Zhang et al. 2014). It is not known why rodents require 10 times the concentration of fluoride in their drinking water to have serum fluoride levels similar to humans. However, the fact remains that comparable serum fluoride levels should be used to assess the biological relevance of an animal model. Much confusion has resulted in interpretation of studies on fluorosis mechanisms because of these concentration differences in fluoride ingested in water by rodents as compared to humans. Because of this, the relevance of rodent studies to fluorosis mechanisms in humans has been questioned and their relevance not clearly understood.

Similar issues relating to the relevance of the fluoride concentration used occur in vitro of fluoride mechanisms. Many in vitro studies expose cells to fluoride levels found in drinking water, which are in fact 50 times higher than would be found in serum. For example, 1 ppm F, which is equivalent to 52.6 μM F, ingested by humans in drinking water, results in serum fluoride levels of approximately 1 μM serum F. This suggests that the use of 1 ppm fluoride cell culture in vitro would actually represent fluoride levels approximately 50 times that likely are to be found at the cellular level in vivo, and the results obtained are not likely to be relevant to in vivo fluoride exposure to humans. Therefore, to understand the mechanisms by which fluoride may affect both enamel formation and other cells and tissues, experiments conducted and the interpretation of their results must be done with an understanding of biological relevance.

Fluoride Exposure Causes Both Hyper- and Hypomineralization of the Enamel Matrix Fluoride is a highly electronegative anion and, as such, enhances mineral formation. This local hypermineralization in the enamel matrix depletes the local reservoir or free calcium ions and then may also act as a physical barrier, impairing diffusion of ions and peptides, to result in a subsequent band of hypomineralized enamel (Guo et al. 2015). Therefore, within the matrix, it is possible that a more rapid mineral precipitation in the presence of fluoride may result in the presence of hypermineralized bands followed by hypomineralized bands in the enamel matrix (Bronckers et al. 2009).

Fluoride Exposure May Increase Acidification of the Developing Enamel Matrix Formation of hydroxyapatite biominerals (HAP) results in the formation of protons ($10Ca^{2+} + 6\ HPO_4^{2-} + 2H_2O \rightarrow Ca_{10}\ (PO_4)_6\ (OH)_2 + 8H^+$), which acidify the enamel matrix. Therefore, regulation of matrix pH by ameloblasts is crucial for sustained crystal growth. In the presence of fluoride, increased mineral formation may result in local acidification, which is buffered by amelogenin proteins in the enamel matrix at the secretory stage (Guo et al. 2015).

At the maturation stage, where the most of the enamel HAP mineralization occurs, the pH in the enamel matrix changes periodically between acidic (pH 5.8) and neutral (pH 7.2) (Sasaki et al. 1991; Smith 1998). Protons generated during HAP formation in the maturation stage are neutralized by bicarbonate secreted from the apical end of ruffled-ended maturation ameloblasts through anion exchangers of the Slc26a family (Jalali et al. 2014). Transmembrane proteins, including cystic fibrosis transmembrane conductance regulator, anion exchanger-2, carbonic anhydrase-2, and sodium hydrogen exchanger-1, are involved in this pH regulation mechanism (Guo et al. 2015; Lyaruu et al. 2008; Alper 2009; Concepcion et al. 2013). In the fluorosed enamel matrix, retention of amelogenin protein may also buffer pH changes in the matrix, secondary to mineral formation, thereby reducing the acidification of the matrix under ruffle-ended ameloblasts (Guo et al. 2015).

Bicarbonate is exchanged for chloride (Cl-) in the matrix, and with increased secretion of bicarbonate, the amount of chloride in the mineralizing enamel matrix is decreased. The reduced amount of Cl found in the fluorosed enamel matrix supports the hypothesis that increased enamel matrix acidification and subsequent neutralization occurs in the presence of increasing amounts of fluoride (Bronckers et al. 2015). Recent evidence has shown that maturation stage ameloblast modulation depends on Cl- (Bronckers et al. 2015), and therefore reduced Cl in the enamel matrix may be responsible for the fewer number of ameloblast modulations from ruffle-ended to smooth-ended ameloblasts, found in the presence of fluoride.

Amelogenins Are Retained in Fluorosed Maturation Stage Enamel Fluorosed maturation stage enamel is characterized by a delay in the removal of amelogenin matrix proteins (DenBesten and Crenshaw 1984; Wright et al. 1996). It is possible that this delay in removal of amelogenins is due to altered ameloblast modulation (DenBesten et al. 1985; Smith et al. 1993). Other factors that may contribute to the retention of amelogenins in fluorosed enamel include increased binding of amelogenins to the fluoride-containing HAP crystals (Tanimoto et al. 2008), which may delay the removal of amelogenins from the enamel matrix. Recent studies in mice have also shown a reduced expression of KLK4, the proteinase responsible for hydrolyzing amelogenins and other matrix proteins in the maturation stage (Suzuki et al. 2014). A reduction in KLK4 could also delay the hydrolysis of amelogenins and their removal from the enamel matrix, resulting in less final mineral formation and a more hypomineralized enamel matrix. These effects of fluoride at the maturation are consistent with the observation that fluoride-induced subsurface hypomineralization can independently occur in the maturation stage, even without prior exposure to secretory stage enamel. However, fluorosis is most severe with fluoride exposure to all stages of enamel formation (DenBesten et al. 1985; Richards et al. 1985; Suckling et al. 1988).

Fluoride Can Alter Cell Function Amelogenesis is a dynamic interaction between the differentiating ameloblasts and the self-assembling mineralized matrix. The primary mechanisms responsible for the formation of fluorosed enamel appear to be related to effects on matrix mineralization. However, it is possible that fluoride may, to a lesser extent, directly affect cell function, though it is difficult to differentiate direct cellular effects from those caused by changes in the mineralizing matrix. Some studies have found that fluoride appears to alter the timing of gene expression in ameloblasts overlying fluorosed as compared to control enamel, possibly related to a fluoride-related enhancement of $G\alpha q$ activity in secretory ameloblasts (Zhang et al. 2014).

15.1.2 Fluoride Effects on Dentin Formation

The dentin matrix is far less mineralized than the enamel matrix and is comparatively unaffected by fluoride. However, in vitro studies of mildly and moderately fluorosed human dentin, showing increased caries susceptibility (Waidyasekera et al. 2007), suggest that fluoride also alters dentin biomineralization. In support of this possibility, reduced dentin microhardness and increased dentin fluoride were shown to correlate enamel fluorosis severity (Vieira et al. 2005). Fluorosed dentin has been characterized as having increasingly disorganized dentin crystals (Kierdorf et al. 1993; Vieira et al. 2004, 2005; Nelson et al. 1989; Yaeger 1966; Waidyasekera et al. 2010), and structurally, severely fluorosed human dentin is described as the distinct layering of hypomineralized lines and extensive areas of interglobular dentin (Fejerskov et al. 1977), with the irregular and densely arranged dentinal tubules (Rojas-Sanchez et al. 2007). These studies indicate that fluoride-related changes can occur while primary dentin is formed.

15.2 Fluoride in Food and Water

Water Fluoridation One of the first attempts to provide effective caries control on a population basis was through the use of artificial water fluoridation programs. By the 1940s, there was a substantial body of literature comparing the prevalence and severity of dental caries among populations living in communities with differing levels of fluoride in the water. These studies showed that dental caries levels dropped sharply as water fluoride levels rose to 1.0 ppm. This was also the concentration at which prevalence of dental fluorosis began to increase in these same populations (Dean 1938). As a result of this work, 1 ppm F was determined to be the point at which one could expect to receive an optimal benefit with minimal side effects of dental fluorosis.

On January 25, 1945, Grand Rapids, Michigan, USA, became the first city in the world to adjust its water fluoride concentration to a level expected to reduce dental caries, and 10 years later, the study found that though mild forms of dental fluorosis were increased, dental caries was significantly decreased (Arnold et al. 1956). Other studies have continued to confirm the benefits of water fluoridation, though more recently the overall rates of caries were found to be dropping in the population at large (Brunelle and Carlos 1990). Caries rates throughout the world have followed similar trends, and interestingly, caries rates have decreased whether or not the local water supplies are fluoridated, most likely related primarily to the widespread worldwide expansion of the use of fluoride toothpaste after 1970. Recently, a Cochrane systematic review that evaluated the effectiveness of water fluoridation for the prevention of caries suggested the need to evaluate all sources of fluoride before such systems should be considered. The review concluded, "The decision to implement a water fluoridation programme relies upon an understanding of the population's oral health behavior (e.g., use of fluoride toothpaste), the availability and uptake of other caries prevention strategies, their diet and consumption of tap water and the movement/migration of the population." However, there was a significant association between dental fluorosis and level of exposure to fluoride (Iheozor-Ejiofor et al. 2015). In spite of the issues raised regarding fluoride, the use of fluoridated water has provided significant anticaries benefits. The American Dental Association, the US Center for Disease Control, and the World Health Organization all support water fluoridation. According to the (http://www.who.int/water_sanitation_health/oralhealth/en/index2.html), "Fluoridation of water supplies, where possible, is the most effective public health measure for the prevention of dental decay."

Salt Fluoridation A key objection to community water fluoridation is that it fails to provide consumers with a choice, as the only alternative is for consumers to purchase bottled water that is not fluoridated. One alternative to water fluoridation is salt fluoridation. To some, the use of salt fluoridation over water fluoridation is an attractive option. Fluoridated salt is generally sold side by side on grocery shelves with non-fluoridated salt; the choice is up to the individual consumer as to which one they prefer.

Originally introduced in 1955 in Switzerland as an extension of programs that utilized iodized salt for the prevention of thyroid conditions (Burgi and Zimmermann 2005), the fluoridation of table salt has been demonstrated to provide caries reductions on par with water fluoridation programs (Marthaler 2005) when the majority of the salt consumed is fluoridated. Fluoride concentrations in salt ranging from 90 mg/kg up to 350 mg/kg have been tested, with some studies suggesting the level of 250–300 mg/kg as being optimal. One study demonstrated that salivary fluoride levels after eating a meal prepared with salt fluoridated at 250 mg/kg were similar to those of individuals exposed to water fluoride levels of 1 mg/l (Hedman et al. 2006). A level of 200 mg/kg is considered the minimum level necessary to provide a reasonable caries benefit (Sampaio and Levy 2011), suggesting that salt fluoridation can result in increased salivary fluoride.

Human studies that assessed the effectiveness of salt fluoridation in Columbia, Hungary, and Switzerland confirmed the effectiveness of this approach, demonstrating results that were not unlike those seen with early water fluoridation programs (Marthaler and Petersen 2005; Jones et al. 2005). Fluoridated salt is relatively easy to deliver to consumers through a range of channels, including the use of domestic salt, participation in school meal programs, and bread made in local bakeries. One of the advantages to the use of salt fluoridation is its availability in areas where fluoridated toothpastes are not broadly available or are considered to be too expensive. However, when combined with the use of fluoridated toothpastes, fluoride exposures may reach above optimal levels (Baez et al. 2010).

One example that highlights the effectiveness of fluoridated salt comes from Jamaica, where virtually all salt intended for human consumption has been fluoridated since 1987 (Jones et al. 2005). Although fluoride toothpastes have been available there since 1972, an oral health survey conducted in 1984 showed extremely high caries rates in Jamaican children, with the assumption being that toothpastes were generally not used on a regular basis (Table 15.1). In 1986, the Jamaica Parliament approved a salt fluoridation program, as water fluoridation was deemed to be technically unfeasible in the region. The natural concentration of fluoride in the water was less than 0.3 mg/ml. At the time, Jamaica had only one supplier of salt, which made salt fluoridation a viable option. Salt was fluoridated at 250 mg/kg, using potassium fluoride, with technical guidance provided by the Pan American Health Organization (PAHO). Urinary excretion studies, which are commonly used to monitor excessive ingestion of fluoride (Marthaler and Schulte 2005) conducted at baseline and after 20 months of Jamaica's salt fluoridation program indicated fluoride concentrations were no greater than those that would be expected for a temperate climate where water fluoridation programs were in place. A follow-up survey in 1995 confirmed the effectiveness of the program, with dramatic reductions in caries noted in each of the age groups measured (Table 15.1).

Salt fluoridation is broadly available in many Latin American countries, with the exception of Brazil, Chile, and Panama, where fluoride toothpastes are commonly used. One issue regarding the exclusive use of fluoridated salt is the potential for erratic exposure; usage can vary significantly from one individual to another. Another issue is the lack of standardized processes for fluoridated salt in countries where there are multiple producers of salt, with no effective surveillance mechanisms in place. From an economic viewpoint, salt fluoridation appears to be a cost-effective measure, with one report indicating the per capita costs average between 0.015 and 0.030 (USD) per year (Gillespie and Marthaler 2005). However, recent reviews point to the lack of available, randomized clinical trials comparing salt fluoridation to other methods of caries prevention (Espelid 2009; Cagetti et al. 2013).

Table 15.1 Mean number of decayed, missing, or filled permanent teeth (DMFT) in Jamaican children, 1984 and 1995

Age (years)	Mean number of DMFT		Percent decrease in DMFT
	1984	1995	
6	1.71	0.22	87 %
12	6.72	1.08	84 %
15	9.60	3.02	68 %

Adapted from: Jones et al. (2005)

Milk Fluoridation In addition to salt and water fluoridation programs, milk fluoridation is another approach that is used in some geographic areas. Like water fluoridation, this approach does not require a change in consumer behaviors in order to provide an anticaries benefit. The basic premise is that ingestion of fluoridated milk will maintain salivary fluoride levels at levels similar to those achieved in individuals living in areas of optimally fluoridated water systems.

While individual trials have suggested significant benefits associated with milk fluoridation programs (Rusoff et al. 1962; Stephen et al. 1984), systematic reviews of fluoridated milk have concluded that there is a lack of well-controlled randomized clinical trials to confirm the effectiveness of this approach (Espelid 2009; Cagetti et al. 2013; Yeung et al. 2005, 2015). Though some effectiveness has been shown for primary teeth (Cagetti et al. 2013), as noted in a recent Cochrane review: "There is low quality evidence to suggest fluoridated milk may be beneficial to schoolchildren, contributing to a substantial reduction in dental caries in primary teeth. Additional randomized clinical trials of high quality are needed before we can draw definitive conclusions about the benefits of milk fluoridation"(Yeung et al. 2015).

15.3 Fluoride and Remineralizing Agents

Fluoride in the Biofilm Dental caries occurs when bacteria in a biofilm produce lactic acid by saccharolytic fermentation. This acid can penetrate through to the tooth surface that is protected by pellicle, a natural protective protein barrier, and dissolve the hydroxyapatite crystals in subsurface enamel, resulting in the formation of subsurface lesions (Levine 2011; Amaechi and van Loveren 2013; Buzalaf et al. 2011). If fluoride is present in the plaque fluid when bacteria produce acids, it will penetrate along with the acids through the plaque subsurface and adsorb to apatite crystal surfaces. When the pH returns to pH 5.5 or above, the saliva, which is supersaturated with calcium and phosphate, provides calcium and phosphate to bind to the fluoride ions and form fluorapatite mineral, which is relatively less acid soluble than the carbonated hydroxyapatite mineral of a natural tooth (Amaechi and van Loveren 2013; Buzalaf et al. 2011; Stoodley et al. 2008).

Fluoride, which is a single, highly electronegative ion, operates via two primary mechanisms: inhibiting enamel demineralization and enhancing the natural process of enamel remineralization (ten Cate and Featherstone 1991). In addition, fluoride can be incorporated into bacterial biofilms and, if present at high enough concentrations, can inhibit enolase (Qin et al. 2006). Enolase catalyzes the production of phosphoenolpyruvate, a precursor of lactic acid from 2-phosphoglycerate, during glycolysis. Oral bacteria utilize the phosphoenolpyruvate transport system to transfer mono- and disaccharides into the cytosol. Fluoride not only inhibits lactic acid production but also the phosphoenolpyruvate transport system-mediated uptake of saccharide substrates.

Of importance to both of the primary mechanisms of action for fluoride is the transport of fluoride through the biofilm to the enamel surface. Studies of the transport of fluoride through the biofilm are conflicting. One group of researchers showed that exposure of enamel to NaF (1000 ppm F-) for 30 or 120 s (equivalent to toothbrushing) or for 30 min, resulted in increased plaque fluoride concentrations near the saliva interface, while concentrations near the enamel surface remained low. Fluoride penetration increased with duration of NaF exposure, and removal of exogenous fluoride resulted in fluoride loss and redistribution. The authors concluded that penetration of fluoride into plaque biofilms during brief topical exposure is restricted, which may limit anticaries efficacy (Watson et al. 2005). However, another study showed that following the use of a 0.2% fluoride rinse, fluoride penetrated through the biofilm, causing some effect on the viability of the biofilm mass (Rabe et al. 2015). Although there are questions that still need to be answered with respect to how fluoride impacts the biofilm, it is clear that both the application and the retention of fluoride in plaque, plaque fluids, and oral tissue reservoirs play important roles in overall effectiveness of fluoride (Zero 2006).

15.3.1 Fluoride Delivered from Oral Care Products

Fluoride is widely used by oral healthcare providers to help prevent dental caries. Fluoride is available in different preparations ranging from low (0.25–1 mg per tablet; 1000–1500 mg fluorine per kg in toothpaste) to high concentrations (liquids containing 10,000 mg/L, gels containing 4000–6000 mg/kg), and varnishes (most of which contain 22,600 mg/kg) may be used for local topical applications (Slooff et al. 1988). In the USA, where fluoride products are regulated by the US Food and Drug Administration as drugs, only three sources of fluoride are allowed for inclusion in oral care products, as defined by the US caries monograph (Federal Register 1995). These include stannous fluoride (SnF_2), sodium fluoride (NaF), and sodium monofluorophosphate (Na_2FPO_3). In the European Union, where fluoride products are regulated as cosmetics, a much broader range of fluoride sources and combinations are allowed (Lippert 2013), though some of these have never been proven effective in well-controlled caries clinical trials.

The anticaries efficacy of fluoride is dependent not only on the fluoride compound used but also on the concentration and contact time of fluoride on oral surfaces, the method of delivery of the agent itself, and the bioavailability of fluoride in the mouth after use. Simply delivering fluoride from an oral care product is not as important as the ability of the agent to react with exposed tooth surfaces and to be retained in oral fluids post application (Zero 2006). The anticaries benefits of fluoride toothpaste have been confirmed in numerous well-controlled clinical trials. Clinically effective fluoride toothpaste formulations, which are used all over the world as a primary means of delivering effective caries control, have been credited with the dramatic decline in caries in multiple geographies (Zero 2006). Multiple reviews have confirmed that other approaches to deliver fluoride, such as rinses, gels, and varnishes, are also effective at providing caries control. The effectiveness of fluoride products may be affected by individual susceptibility to caries, fluoride source and level, frequency of use, and overall oral hygiene. In addition, some improvement in caries protection may be provided through the combined use of fluoride toothpastes with another topical fluoride therapy, particularly for high-risk patients (Marinho 2009).

15.3.2 Other Remineralizing Agents

Calcium and phosphate from saliva provide a natural means for remineralization processes to occur. After a cariogenic acid challenge, salivary flow results in buffering to a more neutral pH, which encourages the natural replacement of lost minerals back into the tooth surfaces. In some instances, and with extended duration of challenges, the natural remineralization processes are insufficient to maintain an effective level of mineral balance. Fluoride aids in this process by enhancing the deposition of both calcium and phosphate, along with the fluoride, into demineralized regions of the tooth surface (ten Cate and Featherstone 1991; ten Cate 1999).

Newer remineralization therapies are intended to enhance the natural remineralization process by providing elevated levels of calcium and phosphate to supplement the levels provided by saliva (Pfarrer and Karlinsey 2009; Cochrane et al. 2010). The goal of these therapies is to increase subsurface diffusion of calcium and phosphate into the tooth surface, without increasing calculus formation, and to have remineralization effects at least equivalent to those of fluoride. Various approaches have been suggested, including combining remineralization agents with fluoride to enhance the efficacy of fluoride, using remineralization agent in combination with lower levels of fluoride to decrease the potential for dental fluorosis in younger children, and using remineralization agents alone, with only background exposure to fluoride (Zero 2006). Vehicles proposed for the delivery of remineralization agents have included not only toothpastes but also mouth rinses, gels, lozenges, chewing gums, and various foods and beverages. A number of remineralization therapies have been incorporated into commercial products and are currently being sold in the market. These include Recaldent™ (CPP-ACP – GC Corporation, Alsip, IL., USA), NovaMin® (GlaxoSmithKline, Brentford, UK), and Tricalcium Phosphate (TCP – 3M ESPE, St Paul, MN, USA). All of these approaches are based on the delivery of calcium and phosphate to the tooth surface.

Recaldent™ combines casein phosphopeptide (CPP) from milk with amorphous calcium phosphate (ACP), to stabilize ACP in the dental plaque biofilm. CPP-ACP is claimed to provide a reservoir of calcium and phosphate ions to maintain a state of supersaturation with respect to tooth enamel, to buffer plaque pH, and to provide ions necessary for remineralization of subsurface lesions.

NovaMin® is an inorganic amorphous calcium sodium phosphosilicate (CSPS), belonging to a class of materials which are known as "bioactive glasses." In the presence of water or saliva, NovaMin® releases sodium ions, which is intended to increase the local pH and initiate the release of calcium and phosphate. The calcium-phosphate complexes crystallize into a carbonated hydroxyapatite, which is chemically and structurally similar to biological apatite.

Tricalcium phosphate (TCP) is a bioactive formulation of β-tricalcium phosphate that is claimed to work synergistically with fluoride to enhance mineralization of subsurface lesions when compared to using fluoride alone. When used in toothpaste formulations, a protective barrier is created around the calcium, allowing it to coexist with the fluoride ions. During toothbrushing, TCP comes into contact with saliva, causing the barrier to dissolve and release calcium and phosphate.

Another approach, CaviStat™, was a technology that combined calcium carbonate with arginine bicarbonate. A published clinical study compared the effectiveness of a dentifrice formulated with these ingredients, showing the product was more effective than the fluoride control (Acevedo et al. 2005). However, the study was poorly controlled, with the test product being used under supervised conditions and the F-control product being used under ad-lib conditions, and had not been repeated. The technology has recently been marketed under the trade name Pro-Argin™ and is currently sold outside the USA in combination with fluoride.

In addition to direct remineralization therapies, agents such as xylitol are reported to work indirectly to promote remineralization by decreasing bacteria and bacterial function. This approach is intended to create an environment where reparative remineralization is optimized. Xylitol is a 5-carbon sugar alcohol that is commonly found in birch tree sap and naturally occurring in some fruits and vegetables. Like all of the sugar alcohols, it is noncariogenic. However, much research has focused on whether or not it is also anticariogenic. It is believed that xylitol works to prevent cavities in multiple ways. Bacteria cannot break down xylitol into acid as they do from other fermentable sugars (i.e., sucrose, glucose, fructose, dextrose, etc.). When bacteria ingest xylitol, they do not consume as much of other fermentable sugars, which reduces acid production. Xylitol can help control the number of acid-producing bacteria in the mouth, which can in turn help prevent cavities. It is available in many commercial product forms, such as gums, mints, toothpastes, and mouth rinses. Xylitol is usually measured in grams, and studies show the recommended therapeutic dose is 6–11 g per day. Ingestion of more than 25–30 g in one day may result in an upset stomach and/or diarrhea. Xylitol can be very harmful, even potentially fatal, to dogs, as they cannot metabolize it like people can.

Unfortunately, in order for xylitol to be effective, it is necessary to essentially remove all other sources of fermentable sugar that the oral bacteria are likely to ingest. The most successful product studies using xylitol have come from chewing gum studies, and in those study subjects had to use 5–6 sticks per day in order to demonstrate effectiveness (Marinho 2009). Other studies were those such as the Turku sugar studies, in which xylitol was shown to be effective; however, the trial involved essentially complete substitution of sucrose with xylitol over the course of the 2-year clinical study (Scheinin et al. 1976). A recent Cochrane review (Riley et al. 2015) concluded that fluoride toothpaste containing xylitol may provide a slight improvement in anticaries benefits compared to fluoride alone; however, there is little evidence to support a significant anticaries benefit for products formulated only with xylitol.

In theory, the use of remineralization therapies makes technical sense, and both in vitro and in situ studies have suggested these approaches may provide enhanced mineralization benefits (Pfarrer and Karlinsey 2009; Reynolds 2009; Karlinsey et al. 2010). However, at present, there is little clinical evidence available to confirm that these approaches provide any greater benefit than fluoride, working in combination with natural levels of calcium and phosphate in saliva. For now, fluoride remains the most well-established remineralization therapy available.

References

Acevedo AM, Machado C, Rivera LE, Wolff M, Kleinberg I. The inhibitory effect of an arginine bicarbonate/calcium carbonate CaviStat-containing dentifrice on the development of dental caries in Venezuelan school children. J Clin Dent. 2005;16(3):63–70.

Alper SL. Molecular physiology and genetics of Na+-independent SLC4 anion exchangers. J Exp Biol. 2009;212(Pt 11):1672–83.

Amaechi BT, van Loveren C. Fluorides and non-fluoride remineralization systems. Monogr Oral Sci. 2013;23:15–26.

Arnold Jr FA, Dean HT, Jay P, Knutson JW. Effect of fluoridated public water supplies on dental caries prevalence. Public Health Rep. 1956;71(7):652–8.

Baez RJ, Marthaler TM, Baez MX, Warpeha RA. Urinary fluoride levels in Jamaican children in 2008, after 21 years of salt fluoridation. Schweiz Monatsschr Zahnmed. 2010;120(1):21–8.

Bronckers AL, Lyaruu DM, DenBesten PK. The impact of fluoride on ameloblasts and the mechanisms of enamel fluorosis. J Dent Res. 2009;88(10):877–93.

Bronckers AL, Lyaruu D, Jalali R, Medina JF, Zandieh-Doulabi B, DenBesten PK. Ameloblast modulation and transport of Cl-, Na+, and K+ during amelogenesis. J Dent Res. 2015;94(12):1740–7.

Brunelle JA, Carlos JP. Recent trends in dental caries in U.S. children and the effect of water fluoridation. J Dent Res. 1990;69 Spec No:723–7; discussion 820–3.

Burgi H, Zimmermann MB. Salt as a carrier of iodine in iodine deficient areas. Schweiz Monatsschr Zahnmed. 2005;115(8):648–50.

Buzalaf MA, Pessan JP, Honorio HM, ten Cate JM. Mechanisms of action of fluoride for caries control. Monogr Oral Sci. 2011;22:97–114.

Cagetti MG, Campus G, Milia E, Lingstrom P. A systematic review on fluoridated food in caries prevention. Acta Odontol Scand. 2013;71(3–4):381–7.

Cochrane NJ, Cai F, Huq NL, Burrow MF, Reynolds EC. New approaches to enhanced remineralization of tooth enamel. J Dent Res. 2010;89(11):1187–97.

Concepcion AR, Lopez M, Ardura-Fabregat A, Medina JF. Role of AE2 for pHi regulation in biliary epithelial cells. Front Physiol. 2013;4:413.

Dean HT, United States Public Health Service: Endemic fluorosis and its relation to dental caries. Washington: U.S. Govt. print. off.; 1938. 1 p.l., 10 p. incl. tables. p.

DenBesten PK, Crenshaw MA. The effects of chronic high fluoride levels on forming enamel in the rat. Arch Oral Biol. 1984;29(9):675–9.

DenBesten PK, Crenshaw MA, Wilson MH. Changes in the fluoride-induced modulation of maturation stage ameloblasts of rats. J Dent Res. 1985;64(12):1365–70.

Espelid I. Caries preventive effect of fluoride in milk, salt and tablets: a literature review. Eur Arch Paediatr Dent. 2009;10(3):149–56.

Fejerskov O, Johnson NW, Silverstone LM. The ultrastructure of fluorosed human dental enamel. Scand J Dent Res. 1974;82(5):357–72.

Fejerskov O, Silverstone LM, Melsen B, Moller IJ. Histological features of fluorosed human dental enamel. Caries Res. 1975;9(3):190–210.

Fejerskov O, Thylstrup A, Larsen MJ. Clinical and structural features and possible pathogenic mechanisms of dental fluorosis. Scand J Dent Res. 1977;85(7):510–34.

Fejerskov O, Larsen MJ, Josephsen K, Thylstrup A. Effect of long – term administration of fluoride on plasma fluoride and calcium in relation to forming enamel and dentin in rats. Scand J Dent Res. 1979;87(2):98–104.

Fejerskov O, Yanagisawa T, Tohda H, Larsen MJ, Josephsen K, Mosha HJ. Posteruptive changes in human dental fluorosis – a histological and ultrastructural study. Proc Finn Dent Soc. 1991;87(4):607–19.

Gillespie GM, Marthaler TM. Cost aspects of salt fluoridation. Schweiz Monatsschr Zahnmed. 2005;115(9):778–84.

Guo J, Lyaruu DM, Takano Y, Gibson CW, DenBesten PK, Bronckers AL. Amelogenins as potential buffers during secretory-stage amelogenesis. J Dent Res. 2015;94(3):412–20.

Guy WS, Taves DR, Brey WS. Organic fluorocompounds in human plasma: prevalence and characterization. Biochemistry involving carbon-fluorine bonds. ACS symposium series. 28: American Chemical Society; 1976. p. 117–34.

Hedman J, Sjoman R, Sjostrom I, Twetman S. Fluoride concentration in saliva after consumption of a dinner meal prepared with fluoridated salt. Caries Res. 2006;40(2):158–62.

Iheozor-Ejiofor Z, Worthington HV, Walsh T, O'Malley L, Clarkson JE, Macey R, et al. Water fluoridation for the prevention of dental caries. Cochrane Database Syst Rev. 2015;6, CD010856.

Jalali R, Guo J, Zandieh-Doulabi B, Bervoets TJ, Paine ML, Boron WF, et al. NBCe1 (SLC4A4) a potential pH regulator in enamel organ cells during enamel development in the mouse. Cell Tissue Res. 2014;358(2):433–42.

Jones S, Burt BA, Petersen PE, Lennon MA. The effective use of fluorides in public health. Bull World Health Organ. 2005;83(9):670–6.

Karlinsey RL, Mackey AC, Walker ER, Frederick KE. Surfactant-modified beta-TCP: structure, properties, and in vitro remineralization of subsurface enamel lesions. J Mater Sci Mater Med. 2010;21(7):2009–20.

Kidd EA, Thylstrup A, Fejerskov O. The histopathology of enamel caries in fluorosed deciduous teeth. Caries Res. 1981;15(5):346–52.

Kierdorf U, Kierdorf H, Fejerskov O. Fluoride-induced developmental changes in enamel and dentine of European roe deer (Capreolus capreolus L.) as a result of environmental pollution. Arch Oral Biol. 1993;38(12):1071–81.

Kroncke A. Perikymata. Dtsch Zahnarztl Z. 1966;21(12):1397–401.

Levine M. Susceptibility to dental caries and the salivary proline-rich proteins. Int J Dent. 2011;2011:953412.
Lippert F. An introduction to toothpaste – its purpose, history and ingredients. Monogr Oral Sci. 2013; 23:1–14.
Lyaruu DM, Bronckers AL, Mulder L, Mardones P, Medina JF, Kellokumpu S, et al. The anion exchanger Ae2 is required for enamel maturation in mouse teeth. Matrix Biol J Int Soc Matrix Biol. 2008;27(2):119–27.
Marinho VC. Cochrane reviews of randomized trials of fluoride therapies for preventing dental caries. Eur Arch Paediatr Dent. 2009;10(3):183–91.
Marthaler TM. Increasing the public health effectiveness of fluoridated salt. Schweiz Monatsschr Zahnmed. 2005;115(9):785–92.
Marthaler TM, Petersen PE. Salt fluoridation-an alternative in automatic prevention of dental caries. Int Dent J. 2005;55(6):351–8.
Marthaler TM, Schulte AG. Monitoring salt fluoridation programs through urinary excretion studies. Schweiz Monatsschr Zahnmed. 2005;115(8):679–84.
McKay FS. The study of mottled enamel (dental fluorosis). J Am Dent Assoc. 1952;44(2):133–7.
Moller IJ. Fluorides and dental fluorosis. Int Dent J. 1982;32(2):135–47.
Mottled Enamel. Am J Public Health Nations Health. 1933;23(1):47–8.
Nelson DG, Coote GE, Vickridge IC, Suckling G. Proton microprobe determination of fluorine profiles in the enamel and dentine of erupting incisors from sheep given low and high daily doses of fluoride. Arch Oral Biol. 1989;34(6):419–29.
Ockerse T, Wasserstein B. Stain in mottled enamel. J Am Dent Assoc. 1955;50(5):536–8.
Pfarrer AM, Karlinsey RL. Challenges of implementing new remineralization technologies. Adv Dent Res. 2009;21(1):79–82.
Qin J, Chai G, Brewer JM, Lovelace LL, Lebioda L. Fluoride inhibition of enolase: crystal structure and thermodynamics. Biochemistry. 2006;45(3):793–800.
Rabe P, Twetman S, Kinnby B, Svensater G, Davies JR. Effect of fluoride and chlorhexidine digluconate mouthrinses on plaque biofilms. Open Dent J. 2015;9:106–11.
Reynolds EC. Casein phosphopeptide-amorphous calcium phosphate: the scientific evidence. Adv Dent Res. 2009;21(1):25–9.
Richards A, Kragstrup J, Nielsen-Kudsk F. Pharmacokinetics of chronic fluoride ingestion in growing pigs. J Dent Res. 1985;64(3):425–30.
Riley P, Moore D, Ahmed F, Sharif MO, Worthington HV. Xylitol-containing products for preventing dental caries in children and adults. Cochrane Database Syst Rev. 2015;3, CD010743.
Rojas-Sanchez F, Alaminos M, Campos A, Rivera H, Sanchez-Quevedo MC. Dentin in severe fluorosis: a quantitative histochemical study. J Dent Res. 2007;86(9):857–61.
Rusoff LL, Konikoff BS, Frye Jr JB, Johnston JE, Frye WW. Fluoride addition to milk and its effect on dental caries in school children. Am J Clin Nutr. 1962;11:94–101.
Sampaio FC, Levy SM. Systemic fluoride. Monogr Oral Sci. 2011;22:133–45.
Sasaki S, Takagi T, Suzuki M. Cyclical changes in pH in bovine developing enamel as sequential bands. Arch Oral Biol. 1991;36:227–31.
Scheinin A, Makinen KK, Ylitalo K. Turku sugar studies. V. Final report on the effect of sucrose, fructose and xylitol diets on the caries incidence in man. Acta Odontol Scand. 1976;34(4):179–216.
Slooff W, Janssen PJCM, Janus JA, Knaap AGAC. Basisdocument fluoriden. Bilthoven: Rijksinstituut voor Volksgezondheid en Milieuhygiëne; 1988.
Smith GE. Fluoride, teeth and bone. Med J Aust. 1985;143(7):283–6.
Smith CE. Cellular and chemical events during enamel maturation. Crit Rev Oral Biol Med Off Publ Am Assoc Oral Biol. 1998;9(2):128–61.
Smith CE, Nanci A, Denbesten PK. Effects of chronic fluoride exposure on morphometric parameters defining the stages of amelogenesis and ameloblast modulation in rat incisors. Anat Rec. 1993;237(2):243–58.
Stephen KW, Boyle IT, Campbell D, McNee S, Boyle P. Five-year double-blind fluoridated milk study in Scotland. Community Dent Oral Epidemiol. 1984;12(4):223–9.
Stoodley P, Wefel J, Gieseke A, Debeer D, von Ohle C. Biofilm plaque and hydrodynamic effects on mass transfer, fluoride delivery and caries. J Am Dent Assoc. 2008;139(9):1182–90.
Suckling G, Thurley DC, Nelson DG. The macroscopic and scanning electron-microscopic appearance and microhardness of the enamel, and the related histological changes in the enamel organ of erupting sheep incisors resulting from a prolonged low daily dose of fluoride. Arch Oral Biol. 1988;33(5):361–73.
Suzuki M, Shin M, Simmer JP, Bartlett JD. Fluoride affects enamel protein content via TGF-beta1-mediated KLK4 inhibition. J Dent Res. 2014;93(10):1022–7.
Tanimoto K, Le T, Zhu L, Chen J, Featherstone JD, Li W, et al. Effects of fluoride on the interactions between amelogenin and apatite crystals. J Dent Res. 2008;87(1):39–44.
ten Cate JM. Current concepts on the theories of the mechanism of action of fluoride. Acta Odontol Scand. 1999;57(6):325–9.
ten Cate JM, Featherstone JD. Mechanistic aspects of the interactions between fluoride and dental enamel. Crit Rev Oral Biol Med Off Publ Am Assoc Oral Biol. 1991;2(3):283–96.
Vieira AP, Hancock R, Limeback H, Maia R, Grynpas MD. Is fluoride concentration in dentin and enamel a good indicator of dental fluorosis? J Dent Res. 2004;83(1):76–80.

Vieira A, Hancock R, Dumitriu M, Schwartz M, Limeback H, Grynpas M. How does fluoride affect dentin microhardness and mineralization? J Dent Res. 2005;84(10):951–7.

Waidyasekera PG, Nikaido T, Weerasinghe DD, Wettasinghe KA, Tagami J. Caries susceptibility of human fluorosed enamel and dentine. J Dent. 2007;35(4):343–9.

Waidyasekera K, Nikaido T, Weerasinghe D, Watanabe A, Ichinose S, Tay F, et al. Why does fluorosed dentine show a higher susceptibility for caries: an ultra-morphological explanation. J Med Dent Sci. 2010;57(1):17–23.

Watson PS, Pontefract HA, Devine DA, Shore RC, Nattress BR, Kirkham J, et al. Penetration of fluoride into natural plaque biofilms. J Dent Res. 2005;84(5):451–5.

WHO/UNICEF Joint Water Supply and Sanitation Monitoring Programme. Water for life, making it happen. Geneva: World Health Organization/UNICEF; 2005.

Wright JT, Chen SC, Hall KI, Yamauchi M, Bawden JW. Protein characterization of fluorosed human enamel. J Dent Res. 1996;75(12):1936–41.

Yaeger JA. The effects of high fluoride diets on developing enamel and dentin in the incisors of rats. Am J Anat. 1966;118(2):665–83.

Yeung CA, Hitchings JL, Macfarlane TV, Threlfall AG, Tickle M, Glenny AM. Fluoridated milk for preventing dental caries. Cochrane Database Syst Rev. 2005;3, CD003876.

Yeung CA, Chong LY, Glenny AM. Fluoridated milk for preventing dental caries. Cochrane Database Syst Rev. 2015;8, CD003876.

Zero DT. Dentifrices, mouthwashes, and remineralization/caries arrestment strategies. BMC Oral Health. 2006;6 Suppl 1:S9.

Zhang Y, Kim JY, Horst O, Nakano Y, Zhu L, Radlanski RJ, et al. Fluorosed mouse ameloblasts have increased SATB1 retention and Galphaq activity. PLoS One. 2014;9(8), e103994.

Part V

Invasive and Non-invasive Therapies

Brushing, Toothpastes, Salivation, and Remineralization

16

Robert Faller and Agnes Bloch-Zupan

Abstract

Having clean, healthy teeth has been a desired outcome of numerous approaches that have been devised over the course of civilization. However, it has not been until that past few decades that we have seen incredible progress toward actually achieving this goal. The development of safe, modern toothpastes, coupled with active ingredients that target oral diseases, has had a dramatic impact on controlling many of these diseases. As a result, the longevity of teeth has been significantly improved. In order to properly care for our dentition over the longer term, improved cleaning instruments, such as specially designed manual brushes and oscillating-rotating power brushes, have also been developed. Key to a clean, healthy mouth is not only the teeth themselves but also the entire oral environment, including saliva, gingiva, and the tongue. As older populations now find their teeth remain viable into their senior years, they are sometimes faced with challenges that previous populations have not had to encounter, such as salivary dysfunction resulting as an outcome of other health-related treatments. Even here, there has been significant progress from an oral care standpoint, with new technologies being developed to safely and effectively address these issues. The progress that dental researchers have made over the past few decades toward achieving the goal of healthy hard and soft tissues is multi-faceted. Results have been significant. Having clean, healthy teeth for a lifetime is now achievable.

R. Faller (✉)
Department of Pediatric Dentistry and Community Oral Health Sciences, Maurice H. Kornberg School of Dentistry, Temple University, Philadelphia, USA
e-mail: robert.faller@yourencore.com

A. Bloch-Zupan
Faculté de Chirurgie Dentaire, Université de Strasbourg, Centre de Référence des maladies odontologiques de maladies rares, Strasbourg, France

Pôle de Médecine et Chirurgie Bucco-dentaires, Hôpitaux Universitaires Strasbourg, Hôpital Civil, Strasbourg, France

M. Goldberg (ed.), *Understanding Dental Caries*, DOI 10.1007/978-3-319-30552-3_16

16.1 Toothbrushing and Toothpaste

The importance of clean teeth, and their connection with whole body health, is not a new concept. In fact, writings by early Egyptians, Greeks, and Romans suggested the overall need for oral hygiene (Guerini 1909). The earliest utensils for cleaning teeth were cleaning sticks called miswaks (Hyson 2003), which were either used alone or in combination with crushed eggshells, powdered ash, or other similar ingredients (Forward 1991). The development of more modern versions of toothpaste began in the 1800s, where early formulations were made using other natural abrasives, such as ground cuttlefish bone, powdered coral, pumice, or sand (Gershon et al. 1957). By the 1850s, chalk was added as an abrasive. Fluoride was first introduced into toothpaste in 1914, although the earliest fluoride toothpastes provided no efficacy due to the deactivation of the fluoride with calcium-based abrasives (chalk) that were used. Early toothpastes also contained soap. By the early 1950s, soap had been replaced by surfactants, such as sodium lauryl sulfate. Surfactants provide the foaming action that many consumers like, and they also aid in the cleaning process by helping to loosen debris. Research over the last century shows the most effective cleaning and stain removal is a joint outcome of appropriately designed toothbrushes with properly formulated abrasive-containing toothpastes (Vallotton 1945; Kitchin and Robinson 1948; Tantbirojn et al. 1998; Mankodi et al. 1999).

The physical act of brushing results in a significant dilution of toothpaste during use. For this reason, the amount of active ingredient in toothpaste is generally included at concentrations that are four to five times (or more) the level of active used in mouthrinses. For example, the level of active included in a fluoride mouthrinse formulation is between 100 and 225 ppm, while the level of fluoride formulated into most toothpastes is between 1000 and 1500 ppm (Zero 2006). During brushing, salivary stimulation results in dilution of toothpaste and the formation of an active slurry that results in an effective treatment concentration of about 250 ppm F during use (Turssi et al. 2010; Stookey et al. 2011).

16.1.1 Changes in Fluoride Concentration of Saliva During Brushing

The process of brushing results in a significant rise in salivary fluoride levels, followed by a rapid drop in concentration. Salivary fluoride clearance is biphasic: a combined effect resulting from brushing, salivary stimulation, and rinsing. Normal physiological levels of fluoride range in the order of 0.01 to 0.05 ppm F. During brushing, teeth initially come into contact with toothpaste containing approximately 1100 ppm F, which is quickly diluted by saliva. In the first few minutes after product use, salivary fluoride levels are generally in the range of 10–20 ppm; by 15 min these levels are reduced to around 1 ppm F, and when measured 2–6 h after use, salivary F levels are further reduced to between 0.03 and 0.08 ppm F. In vitro studies have demonstrated that the process of demineralization can be effectively inhibited with as little as 1 ppm F, while the process of remineralization can be enhanced in the presence of only 0.03–0.08 ppm F (Featherstone 1996; Bruun et al. 1984; Duckworth and Morgan 1991; Featherstone 1999). When combined with calcium and phosphate from the saliva, these low levels of fluoride are highly effective for countering demineralization processes. While one can debate the optimum level of salivary fluoride for both enhancing remineralization and inhibiting demineralization, it is clear that the amount of fluoride in currently marketed toothpastes provides an enhancement in salivary fluoride levels that helps inhibit and even reverse the progression of caries.

In addition to dilution of the active ingredients during use, the slurry interacts with the mechanical action of the toothbrush, resulting in the dispersion of the product throughout the oral cavity. This helps ensure the active agent is thoroughly distributed in the mouth, providing both therapeutic and cosmetic benefits to as many tooth surfaces as possible. Key ingredients in toothpaste formulations, such as surfactants, help the slurry penetrate into and under plaque-covered areas, as well as help lift and loosen food debris in pits and fissures, where bacteria accumulate. The mechanical action of the toothbrush can then be more effective in the removal of the plaque and debris (Zero 2006; Lippert 2013). In fact, toothbrushing is an extremely efficient means to help remove plaque. It is also the most common form of human oral hygiene (Lippert 2013).

The removal of plaque by toothbrushing is important, since the bacteria in plaque are responsible for oral disease, such as caries and gingivitis. Caries is one of the most widespread diseases of the industrialized world, affecting the vast majority of both adults and children (World Health Organization 2015). Plaque-induced gingivitis is estimated to affect up to 80 % of adults and is also commonly found in children (World Health Organization 2015; Ainamo et al. 1997). Gingivitis, considered to be one of the most preventable diseases, is an early stage periodontal disease. It is caused by the buildup of plaque bacteria on tissues surrounding the teeth. Failure to remove plaque, which is a naturally occurring bacterial biofilm, can eventually lead to gingivitis. Gingivitis is characterized by inflammation of the gingivae, with symptoms including red, swollen, and bleeding gums. Left uncontrolled, gingivitis can lead to periodontitis and chronic bad breath. For some people, there may be no pain or apparent signs of infection, which can leave these individuals unaware that they have gingivitis; others may be aware of the problem but believe it is "normal" and fail to ensure their oral hygiene habits are sufficient to control its progression (Beaglehole et al. 2009; Bakdash 1995).

A host of toothbrush designs, including both manual and power brushes, have been developed that provide consumers with many options for their individual oral hygiene routines. Modern toothpastes incorporate a wide range of oral benefits that are also designed for individual users. The combined use of modern toothpastes with modern toothbrush designs enables users to decide on an individual basis which option works best for them.

16.1.2 Modern Toothpastes

Although the regular use of toothpastes in the Western world was not common early in the twentieth century (Saxer and Yankell 1997), by the middle of the century, this began to change. It was at this time that researchers began to recognize the potential for the use of specially formulated toothpastes to promote either therapeutic or cosmetic benefits or both. The clinical confirmation that stannous fluoride-containing toothpaste could provide dramatic reductions in caries (Muhler et al. 1954; Muhler and Radike 1957; Muhler 1958) initiated a new age in dental research that continues to this day. Within the next few decades, manufacturers began to test and add a range of new ingredients, such as various fluoride agents, pyrophosphate, specially prepared abrasives, potassium nitrate, peroxide, triclosan, and others, to toothpaste formulations in order to enhance and expand upon the list of benefits that could be delivered from properly formulated products (Fischman et al. 1992; White 1995). Since the introduction of therapeutic toothpastes, most Western countries have experienced a marked decline in dental caries (Marthaler et al. 1994) and periodontal disease (Cobb et al. 2009). Many factors have undoubtedly contributed to this improvement, but it is widely accepted that better home oral hygiene and the use of modern toothpastes are major contributors (Bratthall et al. 1996; Splieth and Meyer 1996; Petersson and Bratthall 1996). While all of the primary fluoride sources used in modern toothpastes provide important anticaries benefits, stabilized stannous fluoride (SnF_2) is unique among the fluoride agents due to its ability to simultaneously provide anticaries, antibacterial, antisensitivity, and erosion prevention benefits from a single active (Baig et al. 2014).

Modern toothpastes are relatively complex formulations, designed to clean, remove surface stains, freshen breath, and deliver therapeutic benefits all while being delivered to a very complex biological system that includes oral biofilms, salivary flow, and potential interactions with other product ingredients. In addition, a significant number of consumers rinse their mouths with water after use, which results in either further dilution of actives or possibly complete removal of the actives from the mouth. This necessitates that the active agents work in a highly efficient manner within the first 30–45 s of brushing or to include mechanisms that enable the active agents to be retained on oral surfaces after brushing/rinsing. Toothpastes are very different from other oral care products, such as mouthrinses, which do not contain abrasives, do not result in significant dilution during use, and are generally not rinsed out after use.

The process of caries occurs under plaque, and the penetration of fluoride through plaque and into the demineralized enamel is a time-dependent process (Watson et al. 2005). In addition to the concentration of fluoride in a toothpaste (Walsh et al. 2010), the actual brushing time and quantity of toothpaste used may be important factors related to both fluoride retention and enamel remineralization (Creeth et al. 2013). The act of rinsing after the use of toothpaste can impact both the concentration and the total contact time of fluoride with tooth surfaces. One prospective study did not find any correlation between water rinsing after the use of fluoride toothpaste and anticaries efficacy (Machiulskiene et al. 2002); however, the study was a school-based design that did not control the use of products at home. Other studies have demonstrated that subjects who rinsed thoroughly after toothpaste use resulted in a greater incidence in caries (Ashley et al. 1999; Sjögren and Birkhed 1993; Chesters et al. 1992; Chestnutt et al. 1998). For adolescents and adults, where the potential for dental fluorosis is not an issue, a recommendation to brush and spit, rather than brush, rinse, and spit, may be a more effective option for toothpaste use.

16.1.3 Modern Toothpaste Components

The majority of today's modern toothpastes comprise a biologically active fluoride source incorporated into a mix of therapeutic and cosmetic ingredients as well as a host of other ingredients that include abrasives, binders, surfactants, buffering agents, humectants, preservatives, sweeteners, flavorings, and dyes (Fig. 16.1).

These components help keep the toothpaste properly mixed with a smooth consistency, and they make the product palatable to the consumer. The abrasive, humectant, and solvent ingredients typically represent about 95 % of the overall toothpaste formulation. Today's modern toothpastes represent highly sophisticated formulation science that has enabled the inclusion of a multitude of additional benefits beyond caries prevention. These include ingredients for calculus (tartar) inhibition, plaque and gingivitis control, sensitivity reduction, erosion prevention, whitening/stain removal, and oral malodor control.

16.1.4 Fluoride and Non-fluoride Mineralization Systems

In the last few decades, significant research has focused on the use of new technologies, either alone or in combination with fluoride, to enhance the remineralization potential of toothpastes beyond the level provided by fluoride. A number of approaches have been suggested, including casein phosphopeptide and amorphous calcium phosphate, tricalcium phosphate, bioglass, arginine bicarbonate, nanoapatites, etc. Although there are a limited number of clinical studies that have been conducted to assess a few of these approaches, the majority of the available data is limited to in vitro or in situ model studies rather than properly controlled caries clinical trials (Amaechi and van Loveren 2013). As such, there is insufficient data available at this point to determine if any of these approaches provide any added clinical benefits beyond what is already being delivered with conventional

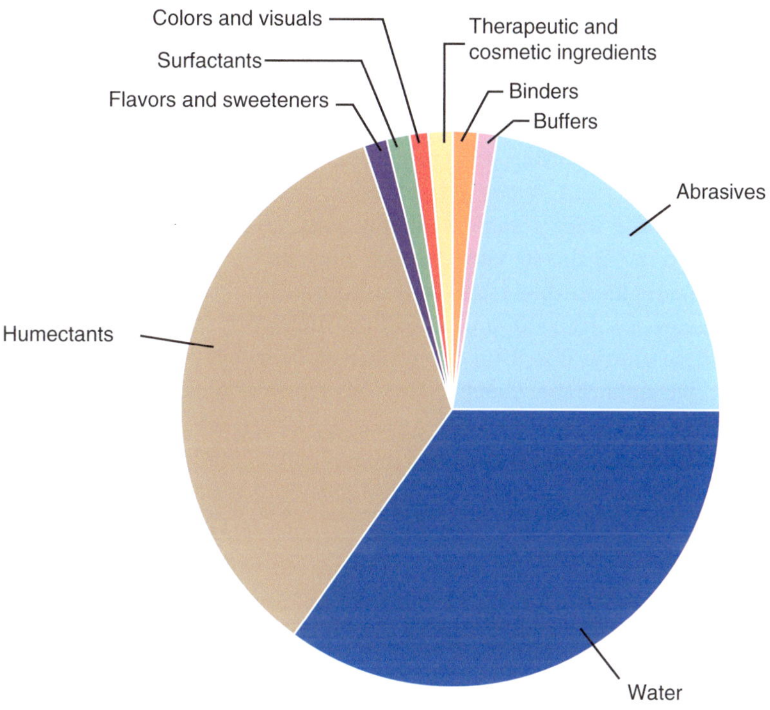

Fig. 16.1 Toothpaste ingredients. Toothpastes contain a number of ingredients that stabilize the product and/or provide esthetic benefits, in addition to the ingredients that provide therapeutic or cosmetic benefits (Adapted from Koenigs and Faller (2015). Reprinted with permission)

fluoride sources. For a more complete discussion of fluoride and other mineralization agents incorporated into and delivered from toothpastes, see Chapter 15.

Even with the significant expansion of benefits delivered by modern toothpaste formulations, it is important to remember that the most important benefit these products deliver is with regard to caries prevention. It has been known for many years that compromising fluoride availability can adversely impact toothpaste performance. The earliest clinical trials that tested NaF in toothpaste formulations that contained a calcium carbonate abrasive demonstrated no anticaries efficacy; this was a result of the NaF interaction with the calcium abrasive system, resulting in the formation of an inactive calcium fluoride (Bibby 1948). It is therefore important to ensure that new additives do not compromise the anticaries effectiveness of any new formulation. For example, upon the introduction of a triclosan/PVM/MA copolymer system into a sodium fluoride toothpaste to aid in the control of plaque and gingivitis, three caries clinical trials were conducted to demonstrate the addition of the new agent did not adversely impact the caries benefit delivered by the fluoride active (Feller et al. 1996; Hawley et al. 1995; Mann et al. 1996). Although this level of clinical evaluation is not necessary for every new formulation, it highlights the issue that new ingredients may adversely impact overall product efficacy, and an appropriate evaluation is needed to ensure the caries benefit has not been compromised.

16.1.5 Toothpastes and Abrasivity

Toothpaste abrasives help keep teeth clean by removing stain that forms in the pellicle layer on exposed tooth surfaces (Addy and Moran 1995). One of the key focus areas of modern toothpaste development has been the cleaning potential of toothpastes, which is partly a function of the abrasivity of the individual products. A paper by Kitchen and Robinson in 1948 (Kitchin and Robinson 1948) asked a very important question: "How abrasive must a dentifrice be?" In this paper, the authors directly compared the clinical stain removal ability of toothpaste formulations with in vitro assessments of the abrasivity of these same formulations. In this study, the authors found that over 90 % of tooth stain could be removed in approximately 2 weeks using toothpastes that contained levels and types of abrasives that produced less than 1 mm of dentin wear, as measured using the in vitro method they had developed. This method included brushing tooth specimens for 100,000 strokes with a diluted dentifrice slurry. Based on the results of their work, the authors concluded:

> Dentifrice abrasiveness greater than that necessary to cut 1 mm per 100,000 strokes into the cervical area of teeth with the apparatus employed appears to be unnecessary even for very heavy strainers… Generally speaking, for stainers with cervical exposure, a dentifrice with a safety index as high as is consistent with prevention of stain accumulation is desirable. Reliable current information on dentifrice abrasion, determined by testing whole dentifrices on dentin, should be available (Kitchen and Robinson 1948).

Later efforts, primarily in the 1950s and 1960s, led to the development of formal abrasivity testing procedures, and these served as the basis for standards currently recommended by the American Dental Association (ADA) and the International Standards Organization (ISO). Given the growing consumer expectation for multi-benefit products, dentifrice formulations need to deliver a level of abrasiveness sufficient to control staining and plaque buildup, without risking the use of overly aggressive abrasive systems that could be deleterious to hard tissues after long-term use. Some researchers have proposed the use of a Cleaning Efficiency Index as one way to assess the cleaning/abrasion balance (Schemehorn et al. 2011). Further work in this area would be helpful, and it needs to incorporate human use studies as part of the evaluation. As a general rule, modern dentifrices are formulated to provide specific therapeutic/cosmetic benefits while delivering abrasivity levels that are well within the accepted limits, with the goal of ensuring consumers receive the best products possible for their specific oral health needs. A recently published paper on the history of the development of abrasivity standards for toothpastes provides an excellent summary of these efforts as well as technical insight into their interpretation regarding not only tooth cleaning potential but also with regard to other oral care issues such as dental erosion (St John and White 2015).

16.1.6 Toothpastes and Abrasivity Testing

The most widely used method for assessing toothpaste abrasivity is the Radioactive (also referred to as Relative) Dentin Abrasivity (RDA) method, an in vitro radiotracer method developed as an outcome of studies by Grabenstetter et al. (Grabenstetter et al. 1958) and Hefferren (1976). This method has served the industry well, establishing a limit of abrasivity of an RDA of 250, under which a dentifrice can be used safely on a daily basis for a lifetime. The industry has largely self-regulated since these standards were put in place, with dentifrices being used safely for the last half century. Although the method has been accepted across the industry and practiced for many years, there is a clear need for modern updating. The requirement for radiotracer capabilities significantly restricts the ability of many researchers to focus on the development of new abrasive technologies for toothpaste. Over the years, alternative methods have been proposed, such as profilometry (Addy 2010). Although one profilometry method has received some level of acceptance, until recently profilometry methods in general have not been thoroughly validated with regard to their ability to directly duplicate the accepted radiotracer method. A number of papers have suggested similar, but not direct, agreement between methods (Kinoshita et al. 1979; Davis and Winter 1976; Davis 1979; Sabrah et al. 2013). A recent study by White and colleagues, however, has provided the first evidence of a profilometry-based method that is both linearly and proportionally correlated with the conventional RDA method (White et al. 2015).

In addition to RDA measures, some researchers have suggested REA (Relative Enamel

Abrasivity) measures might also be helpful to consider. REA measures are done using essentially the same techniques as RDA, with an adjustment made in the calculations that takes into account the relative differences in hardness between dentin and enamel (Addy 2010). One of the primary issues with the use of REA measures is the lack of confirmed correlation between REA and RDA values. For example, studies have demonstrated that not all toothpastes with high RDA values also have a high REA value. In fact, some toothpastes with high RDA values have been shown to provide low REA values, and others with low RDA have demonstrated high REA (Joiner et al. 2004). While dentin wear has been correlated to RDA values in the laboratory (White et al. 2015; Philpotts et al. 2005), no such correlation has been demonstrated with regard to REA measurements.

16.2 Toothbrush: Manual vs. Power

Once a consumer has chosen which toothpaste is best suited to meet his/her individual needs, the decision as to which toothbrush to use is also an important aspect of that person's oral hygiene routine. Although the majority of people brush their teeth with a manual toothbrush, many fail to achieve optimal gingival health. This is primarily due to the fact that most people do not brush long enough or using the proper technique, even if brushing twice-per-day (Beaglehole et al. 2009; Tedesco 1995). Numerous brushing implements are available to the consumer, including a wide range of brush head sizes and geometries and bristle filament stiffness and design (end-rounded or not) and brushes which are manually powered, battery-powered, rechargeable, sonic, oscillation-rotation, and others. Combining the range of the various toothbrush designs with individual brushing techniques provides a rather complex mix of potential brushing scenarios.

Brushing teeth properly is important for maintaining healthy teeth and gums, and it reduces the risk of developing tooth decay and gingival disease, which are the major causes of tooth loss. From the standpoint of plaque removal, better cleaning can generally be achieved with the use of power toothbrushes (see discussions that follow). There are a number of differences between manual and power brushes, and each user must decide which option best meets their individual needs (Table 16.1).

Table 16.1 Each individual user must evaluate the key differences and options provided by the various types of toothbrushes available

Benefits of manual and powered toothbrushes
Manual brush
Inexpensive
Widely available in retail outlets
Wide variety of designs available
Power brush
Certain technologies provide more effective plaque removal and gingivitis reduction than manual brushes
Some models have compliance-enhancing features (e.g., timer, pressure sensor, different brushing modes)
Advanced models with Bluetooth technology provide real-time feedback, track brushing sessions, and allow the patient and oral health professional to customize the brushing session based on the patient's individual needs

16.2.1 Brushing Techniques

To brush properly with a manual toothbrush, oral health professionals generally recommend the use of fluoride toothpaste along with a soft-bristled brush, which should be replaced about every three months. Most dental health professionals recommend brushing for at least two minutes, twice per day using a standard brushing technique. This includes brushing all tooth surfaces (buccal, lingual, and occlusal) in each of the four quadrants of the mouth, for 30 s per quadrant, morning and night. With regard to the position of the brush, hold the brush at a 45-degree angle to the gumline and use short, half-tooth wide strokes, making sure to reach the back teeth. On the lingual surfaces of the anterior teeth, the brush should be placed vertically and gentle up-and-down strokes can be used. On the occlusal surfaces of the teeth, the brush should be held flat, using back and forth strokes along these surfaces. Finally, the tongue should be brushed using a back-to-front sweeping motion. This helps remove food particles and odor-causing bacteria which contribute to malodor if not removed.

Although manual toothbrushes are not able to provide many of the features that are being incorporated into many power brushes, they still are able to provide important benefits for people who prefer these types of brushes. For example, some brushes incorporate angled, extra-long or multilevel bristle tufts, all of which are designed to help clean in hard-to-reach areas. Cupped bristles, ergonomically designed handles with special grips, tapered or angled brush heads, gum stimulators, tongue cleaning pads, etc. are all manual toothbrush innovations designed to provide a better cleaning experience for individual users, all of which can help improve oral health. In addition to the design of the brush itself, the use of supplemental means, such as dental floss, interdental brushes, mouthrinses, etc., may further enhance the overall oral hygiene experience.

16.2.2 Clinical Brushing Studies

In addition to individual brushing technique, the number of brushing sessions per day, the duration of brushing, and the type of toothbrush used have a direct impact on the amount of plaque removed. Randomized clinical trials provide an important means for demonstrating the effectiveness of various toothbrush designs with regard to plaque reduction. A recent systematic review evaluating manual brush designs found that angled bristle designs demonstrate greater plaque removal efficacy compared to those with flat-trim or multilevel bristles (Slot et al. 2012). Since the introduction of power brushes, well-designed and controlled clinical trials have measured the relative ability of power vs. manual brush designs with regard to plaque removal. In a recent historical review of clinical studies, the independent, not-for-profit Cochrane Collaboration concluded that oscillating-rotating technology was the only type of power brush that consistently reduced plaque and gingivitis more effectively than a manual toothbrush in both the short and long term (Yaacob et al. 2014). In addition, a recent review by Grender and colleagues, in which 6 clinical trials were assessed with regard to the ability of oscillating-rotating brushes to remove plaque from specific tooth surfaces, found that oscillating-rotating brushes resulted in significantly greater plaque removal on lingual, approximal, and gingival areas compared to either sonic or manual brushes included in the studies (Grender et al. 2013).

16.2.3 Power Brush Options

Power toothbrushes currently on the market include battery-powered as well as rechargeable electric brushes. Rechargeable electric toothbrushes are more sophisticated, and these differ significantly in the type of cleaning technology used. Many different types and designs are available, with various modes of action, including side-to-side, ultrasonic, counter-oscillation, circular, and oscillation-rotation. A 2011 Cochrane review compared the efficacy of various power technologies (Deacon et al. 2010). Three hundred and ninety-eight studies were included; 17 trials with 1369 subjects met selection criteria and were ultimately evaluated. Seven studies compared rotation-oscillation and side-to-side (sonic) technologies. The review found, "Brushes with a rotation oscillation action reduced plaque and gingivitis more than those with a side-to-side (sonic) action in the short term (4–12 weeks)."

One of the benefits of electric toothbrushes is the amount of technology and features that can be integrated into their design. Brushing techniques vary, depending on the type of toothbrush used. Some of the currently available models incorporate multiple brushing modes that are specifically designed for sensitive teeth, provide whitening benefits, or even to massage gums. Some models include sensors that signal when too much pressure is applied, timers to help ensure a sufficient duration of brushing, and digital reminders to replace the brush head at regular intervals, among others. Most recently models have been introduced with Bluetooth technology to provide real-time brushing feedback, track brushing sessions, and allow the patient and oral health professional to customize brushing areas based on the patient's individual needs. Importantly, all of these features can help consumers improve their routine brushing habits (Walters et al. 2007).

16.3 Saliva and Saliva Substitutes

Saliva is necessary, not only for lubrication of the mouth but also for buffering bacterial acids, providing proteins that deposit onto tooth surfaces and form the protective pellicle, delivering key minerals required for remineralization processes, providing protection against a range of microbes that we are constantly exposed to through our mouths, and other key oral functions that are critical to long-term oral health. Saliva is also important for the dispersion of actives in toothpaste during the process of brushing (Turssi et al. 2010; Stookey et al. 2011). A reduction in salivary flow, often the result of salivary gland hypofunction or xerostomia, is a common occurrence. This is particularly true in the elderly, as a result of the intake of a wide range of routine medications. Significant reduction in salivary flow can lead to discomfort, difficulty in eating, and an increase in oral diseases, such as caries (Deng et al. 2015). While the diagnosis of salivary gland hypofunction and xerostomia is relatively easy to make, treatment of these conditions can be rather difficult. The primary objective, beyond ensuring proper medical treatment, is to provide as much hydration as possible, to reduce all unnecessary medications, and to provide topical remedies, such as saliva substitutes when possible. When salivary flow is severely diminished, as is often the case with head-and-neck radiation patients, parasympathomimetic drugs are sometimes used to help alleviate the problem. The increased caries incidence in individuals suffering from hyposalivation is often the result of a reduced buffer capacity, compromised ability to clear the mouth of debris, and a reduced potential for remineralization, coupled with a diet that may be high in carbohydrates and cariogenic salivary stimulants (Kielbassa et al. 2006; Dreizen et al. 1977; Vissink et al. 2003). Fluoride mouthrinses, as well as high fluoride concentration toothpastes, are often recommended in cases where saliva flow is restricted (Meyerowitz et al. 1991; Su et al. 2011).

While some saliva substitutes have been demonstrated to have a demineralization potential, others have been shown to exhibit remineralization potential and should be a desired approach to help control caries progression (Kielbassa et al. 2001; Meyer-Lueckel et al. 2002; Smith et al. 2001). These products incorporate key minerals required for mineralization, such as fluoride, calcium, and phosphate. It has been recommended that a preferred approach is the use of saliva substitutes supersaturated with respect to octacalcium phosphate (OCP), as this form is less likely to form complexes with polymer ingredients included in artificial saliva formulas (Zandim et al. 2011). Although this approach makes excellent technical sense, there are few well-controlled studies available that provide confirmation of benefits. For the time being, the use of fluoride with saliva substitutes that have at least been demonstrated to exhibit some level of remineralization potential should be preferred over those that fail to provide such potential.

Saliva substitutes alone, however, should make up only a portion of an overall treatment plan for those in need of such care. According to the American Dental Association Council on Scientific Affairs, "Comprehensive management of xerostomia and hyposalivation should emphasize patient education and lifestyle modifications. It also should focus on various palliative and preventive measures, including pharmacological treatment with salivary stimulants, topical fluoride interventions and the use of sugar-free chewing gum to relieve dry-mouth symptoms and improve the patient's quality of life" (Plemons et al. 2014).

Interesting Papers Sälzer S, Rosema NA, Martin EC, Slot DE, Timmer CJ, Dörfer CE, van der Weijden GA. The effectiveness of dentifrices without and with sodium lauryl sulfate on plaque, gingivitis and gingival abrasion-a randomized clinical trial. Clin Oral Investig. 2015 Aug 22. [Epub ahead of print].

References

Addy M. Determination of relative dentifrice abrasivity to enamel and dentine by a surface profile method. J Clin Dent. 2010;21(Suppl):13–4.

Addy M, Moran J. Mechanisms of stain formation on teeth, in particular associated with metal ions and antiseptics. Adv Dent Res. 1995;9:450–6.

Ainamo J, Xie Q, Ainamo A, Kallio P. Assessment of the effect of an oscillating/rotating electric toothbrush on oral health: a 12 month longitudinal study. J Clin Periodontol. 1997;24:28–33.

Amaechi BT, van Loveren C. Fluorides and non-fluoride remineralization systems. Monogr Oral Sci. 2013;23:15–26.

Ashley PF, Attrill DC, Ellwood RP, Worthington HV, Davies RM. Toothbrushing habits and caries experience. Caries Res. 1999;33:401–2.

Baig AA, Faller RV, Yan J, Ji N, Lawless M, Eversole SL. Protective effects of SnF2 – part I. Mineral solubilisation studies on powdered apatite. Int Dent J. 2014;64 Suppl 1:4–10.

Bakdash B. Current patterns of oral hygiene product use and practices. Periodontol 2000. 1995;8:11–43.

Beaglehole, R, Benzian H, Crail J, Mackay I, King J (ed), Lacey C (ed), Wyse E (ed). The oral health atlas: mapping a neglected global health issue. 1st ed. FDI World Dental Education Ltd & Myriad Editions, Switzerland; 2009.

Bibby BG. Fluoride mouthwashes, fluoride dentifrices, and other uses of fluorides in control of caries. J Dent Res. 1948;27(3):367–75.

Bratthall D, Hänsel-Petersson G, Sundberg H. Reasons for the caries decline: what do the experts believe? Eur J Oral Sci. 1996;104(4 (Pt 2)):416–22; discussion 423–5, 430–2.

Bruun C, Givskov H, Thylstrup A. Whole saliva fluoride after toothbrushing with NaF and MFP dentifrices with different F concentrations. Caries Res. 1984;18(3):282–8.

Chesters RK, Huntington E, Burchell CK, Stephen KW. Effect of oral care habits on caries in adolescents. Caries Res. 1992;26:299–304.

Chestnutt IG, Schafer F, Jacobson AP, Stephen KW. The influence of toothbrushing frequency and post-brushing rinsing on caries experience in a caries clinical trial. Community Dent Oral Epidemiol. 1998;26:406–11.

Cobb CM, Costerton JW, Van Dyke TE. Have we become so focused on inflammation and host response that we have neglected the role of bacteria in initiating periodontal disease? Compend Contin Educ Dent. 2009;30(1):46, 48.

Creeth J, Zero D, Mau M, Bosma ML, Butler A. The effect of dentifrice quantity and toothbrushing behaviour on oral delivery and retention of fluoride in vivo. Int Dent J. 2013;63 Suppl 2:14–24.

Davis WB. A comparison of dentine abrasion data generated by radiotracer and surface profilometer methods. J Oral Rehabil. 1979;6:1977–81.

Davis WB, Winter PJ. Measurement in vitro of enamel abrasion by dentifrice. J Dent Res. 1976;55:970–5.

Deacon SA, Glenny AM, Deery C, Robinson PG, Heanue M, Walmsley AD, Shaw WC. Different powered toothbrushes for plaque control and gingival health. Cochrane Database Syst Rev. 2010;(12):CD004971. Accessed as up-to-date: 24 Mar 2011. doi:10.1002/14651858.CD004971.pub2.

Deng J, Jackson L, Epstein JB, Migliorati CA, Murphy BA. Dental demineralization and caries in patients with head and neck cancer. Oral Oncol. 2015;51(9): 824–31. doi:10.1016/j.oraloncology.2015.06.009. Epub 2015 Jul 18.

Dreizen S, Brown LR, Daly TE, Drane JB. Prevention of xerostomia-related dental caries in irradiated cancer patients. J Dent Res. 1977;56:99–104.

Duckworth RM, Morgan SN. Oral fluoride retention after use of fluoride dentifrices. Caries Res. 1991;25(2):123–9.

Featherstone JD. Modeling the caries-inhibitory effects of dental materials. Dent Mater. 1996;12(3):194–7.

Featherstone JD. Prevention and reversal of dental caries: role of low level fluoride. Community Dent Oral Epidemiol. 1999;27(1):31–40.

Feller RP, Kiger RD, Triol CW, Sintes JL, Garcia L, Petrone ME, Volpe AR, Proskin HM. Comparison of the clinical anticaries efficacy of an 1100 NaF silica-based dentifrice containing triclosan and a copolymer to an 1100 NaF silica-based dentifrice without those additional agents: a study on adults in California. J Clin Dent. 1996;7(4):85–9.

Fischman SL, Truelove RB, Hart R, Cancro LP. The laboratory and clinical safety evaluation of a dentifrice containing hydrogen peroxide and baking soda. J Clin Dent. 1992;3:104–10.

Forward G. Role of toothpastes in the cleaning of teeth. Int Dent J. 1991;41:164–70.

Gershon S, Pokras H, Rider T. Dentifrices. In: Sagarin E, editor. Cosmetics-science and technology. New York: Interscience Publishers, Inc.; 1957. p. 296–360.

Grabenstetter RJ, Broge RW, Jackson FL, Radike AW. The measurement of the abrasion of human teeth by dentifrice abrasives: a test utilizing radioactive teeth. J Dent Res. 1958;37:1060–8.

Grender J, Williams K, Walters P, Klukowska M, Reick H. Plaque removal efficacy of oscillating-rotating power toothbrushes: review of six comparative clinical trials. Am J Dent. 2013;26:68–74.

Guerini V. A history of dentistry from the most ancient times until the end of the eighteenth century. Philadelphia: Lea & Febiger; 1909.

Hawley GM, Hamilton FA, Worthington HV, Davies RM, Holloway PJ, Davies TG, Blinkhorn AS. A 30-month study investigating the effect of adding triclosan/copolymer to a fluoride dentifrice. Caries Res. 1995;29:163–7.
Hefferren JJ. A laboratory method for assessment of dentifrice abrasivity. J Dent Res. 1976;55(4):563–73.
Hyson Jr JM. History of the toothbrush. J Hist Dent. 2003;51(2):73–80.
Joiner A, Pickles MJ, Tanner C, Weader E, Doyle P. An in situ model to study the toothpaste abrasion of enamel. J Clin Periodontol. 2004;31(6):434–8.
Kielbassa AM, Shohadai SP, Schulte-Mönting J. Effect of saliva substitutes on mineral content of demineralized and sound dental enamel. Support Care Cancer. 2001;9:40–7.
Kielbassa AM, Hinkelbein W, Hellwig E, Meyer-Lückel H. Radiation-related damage to dentition. Lancet Oncol. 2006;7:326–35.
Kinoshita S, Arai T, Uraguchi R. Abrasive properties of commonly used dentifrices. Bull Tokyo Med Dent Univ. 1979;26:225–42.
Kitchen PC, Robinson HBG. The abrasiveness of dentifrices as measured on the cervical areas of extracted teeth. J Dent Res. 1948;27:195–200.
Kitchin PC, Robinson HBG. How abrasive need a dentifrice be? J Dent Res. 1948;27:501–6.
Koenigs PM, Faller RV. Fundamentals of dentifrice: oral health benefits in a tube, course number: 410; www.dentalcare.com. Accessed 15 Dec 2015.
Lippert F. An introduction to toothpaste – its purpose, history and ingredients. Monogr Oral Sci. 2013;23:1–14.
Machiulskiene V, Richards A, Nyvad B, Baelum V. Prospective study of the effect of post-brushing rinsing behaviour on dental caries. Caries Res. 2002;36:301–7.
Mankodi S, Sowinski J, Davies R, Ellwood R, Bradshaw B, Petrone M, DeVizio W, Chaknis P, Volpe A, Proskin H. A six-week clinical efficacy study of a tooth whitening tartar control dentifrice for the removal of extrinsic tooth stain. J Clin Dent. 1999;10:99–102.
Mann J, Karniel C, Triol CW, Sintes JL, Garcia L, Petrone ME, Volpe AR, Proskin HM. Comparison of the clinical anticaries efficacy of a 1500 NaF silica-based dentifrice containing triclosan and a copolymer to a 1500 NaF silica-based dentifrice without those additional agents: a study on adults in Israel. J Clin Dent. 1996;7(4):90–5.
Marthaler TM, Steiner M, Menghini G, Bandi A. Caries prevalence in Switzerland. Int Dent J. 1994;44(4 Suppl 1):393–401.
Meyer-Lueckel H, Schulte-Mönting J, Kielbassa AM. The effect of commercially available saliva substitutes on predemineralized bovine dentin in vitro. Oral Dis. 2002;8:192–8.
Meyerowitz C, Featherstone JDB, Billings RJ, Eisenberg AD, Fu J, Shariati M, Zero DT. Use of an intra-oral model to evaluate 0.05% sodium fluoride mouthrinse in radiation-induced hyposalivation. J Dent Res. 1991;70(5):894–8.
Muhler JC. The effect of a modified stannous fluoride-calcium pyrophosphate dentifrice on dental caries in children. J Dent Res. 1958;37:448–50.
Muhler JC, Radike AW. Effect of a dentifrice containing stannous fluoride on dental caries in adults II. Results at the end of two years of unsupervised use. J Am Dent Assoc. 1957;55:196–8.
Muhler JC, Radike AW, Nebergall WH, Day HG. The effect of a stannous fluoride-containing dentifrice on caries reduction in children. J Dent Res. 1954;33(5):606–12.
Petersson GH, Bratthall D. The caries decline: a review of reviews. Eur J Oral Sci. 1996;104(4 (Pt 2)):436–43.
Philpotts CJ, Weader E, Joiner A. The measurement in vitro of enamel and dentine wear by toothpastes of different abrasivity. Int Dent J. 2005;55(3 Suppl 1):183–7.
Plemons JM, Al-Hashimi I, Marek CL, American Dental Association Council on Scientific Affairs. Managing xerostomia and salivary gland hypofunction: executive summary of a report from the American Dental Association Council on Scientific Affairs. J Am Dent Assoc. 2014;145(8):867–73. doi:10.14219/jada.2014.44.
Sabrah AHA, Lippert F, Kelly AB, Hara AT. Comparison between radiotracer and surface profile methods for the determination of dentifrice abrasivity. Wear. 2013;306:73–9.
Saxer UP, Yankell SL. Impact of improved toothbrushes on dental diseases. I. Quintessence Int. 1997;28:513–25.
Schemehorn BR, Moore MH, Putt MS. Abrasion, polishing, and stain removal characteristics of various commercial dentifrices in vitro. J Clin Dent. 2011;22(1):11–8.
Sjögren K, Birkhed D. Factors related to fluoride retention after toothbrushing and possible connection to caries activity. Caries Res. 1993;27:474–7.
Slot DE, Wiggelinkhuizen L, Rosema NA, van der Weijden GA. The efficacy of manual toothbrushes following a brushing exercise; a systematic review. Int J Dent Hyg. 2012;10:187–97.
Smith G, Smith AJ, Shaw L, Shaw MJ. Artificial saliva substitutes and mineral dissolution. J Oral Rehabil. 2001;28:728–31.
Splieth C, Meyer G. Factors for changes of caries prevalence among adolescents in Germany. Eur J Oral Sci. 1996;104(4 (Pt 2)):444–51.
St John S, White DJ. History of the development of abrasivity limits for dentifrices. J Clin Dent. 2015;26(2):50–4.
Stookey GK, Featherstone JDB, Rapozo-Hilo M, Schemehorn BR, Williams RA, Baker RA, Barker ML, Kaminski MA, McQueen CM, Amburgy JS, Casey K, Faller RV. The Featherstone laboratory pH cycling model – a prospective multi-site validation exercise. Am J Dent. 2011;24:322–8.
Su N, Marek CL, Ching V, Grushka M. Caries prevention for patients with dry mouth. J Can Dent Assoc. 2011;77:b85.

Tantbirojn D, Ko C, Douglas W. Stain removal efficacy: an in vitro evaluation using quantitative image analysis. Quintessence Int. 1998;29:28.

Tedesco LA. Behavioral research related to oral hygiene practices: a new century model of oral health promotion. Periodontol 2000. 1995;8:15–23.

Turssi CP, Messias DC, Hara AT, Hughes N, Garcia-Godoy F. Brushing abrasion of dentin: effect of diluent and dilution rate of toothpaste. Am J Dent. 2010;23(5):247–50.

Vallotton CF. An acquired pigmented pellicle of the enamel surface. J Dent Res. 1945;24:161–9.

Vissink A, Jansma J, Spijkervet FK, Burlage FR, Coppes RP. Oral sequelae of head and neck radiotherapy. Crit Rev Oral Biol Med. 2003;14:199–212.

Walsh T, Worthington HV, Glenny AM, Appelbe P, Marinho VCC, Shi X. Fluoride toothpastes of different concentrations for preventing dental caries in children and adolescents. Cochrane Database of Systematic Reviews 2010, Issue 1. Art. No.: CD007868. DOI: 10.1002/14651858.CD007868.pub2.

Walters PA, Cugini M, Biesbrock AR, Warren PR. A novel oscillating-rotating power toothbrush with SmartGuide: designed for enhanced performance and compliance. J Contemp Dent Pract. 2007; 8(4):1–9.

Watson PS, Pontefract HA, Devine DA, Shore RC, Nattress BR, Kirkham J, Robinson C. Penetration of fluoride into natural plaque biofilms. J Dent Res. 2005;84:451–5.

White DJ. A "return" to stannous fluoride dentifrices. J Clin Dent. 1995;(Spec No 6):29–36.

White DJ, Schneiderman E, Colon E, St John S. A profilometry based dentifrice abrasion method for V8 brushing machines Part I: the RDA-PE method and correlation to conventional RDA. J Clin Dent. 2015;26:1–6.

World Health Organization. What is the burden of oral disease? Retrieved 14 Dec 2015 from http://www.who.int/entity/oral_health/disease_burden/global/en/.

Yaacob M, Worthington HV, Deacon SA, Deery C, Walmsley AD, Robinson PG, Glenny AM. Powered versus manual toothbrushing for oral health. Cochrane Database Syst Rev. 2014;(6):CD002281. doi:10.1002/14651858.CD002281.pub3.

Zandim DL, Tschoppe P, Sampaio JE, Kielbassa AM. Effect of saliva substitutes in combination with fluorides on remineralization of subsurface dentin lesions. Support Care Cancer. 2011;19(8):1143–9. doi:10.1007/s00520-010-0924-8. Epub 2010 Jun 11.

Zero DT. Dentifrices, mouthwashes, and remineralization/caries arrestment strategies. BMC Oral Health. 2006;6(Suppl 1):S9. Published online 2006 Jun 15. doi:10.1186/1472-6831-6-S1-S9.

Resin Infiltration Treatment for Caries Lesions

17

Colin Robinson

Abstract

Destruction of the teeth by bacterially produced acid, i.e. dental caries, is perhaps the most prolific of human diseases. Caries involves the dissolution of dental enamel by bacterially produced acid on the tooth surface. Enamel is a cell-free tissue comprising >95 % by volume of crystals of the mineral hydroxyapatite. The hydroxyapatite crystals are substituted with a variety of extraneous ions, which alter the chemical and physical characteristics of the crystals. Fluoride, for example, renders crystals less susceptible to acid dissolution, while carbonate increases crystal acid solubility (see review by Robinson et al. (2000)). The porosity occurring prior to this breakdown does, importantly, afford the possibility of restoring the enamel using materials which are not acid soluble and without removal of "diseased," i.e. porous tissue. This concept of "filling without drilling" was proposed some 30 years or so ago and recently reviewed. Inducing suitable material to enter the extremely small pores of the enamel lesion improves attachment and penetration of sealant resins. Etching the enamel surface with acid produced pits ~4 microns in diameter, related to enamel prisms, into which some sealant was found to enter. Resin infiltration did not restore the enamel to its original state but improved mechanical properties of the lesion surface in terms of hardness and elasticity. However, the surface zone was a barrier to effective resin infiltration proved to be most problematical in terms of both attaching resins to the lesion surface and infiltrating materials into the lesion interior.

17.1 Background

A detailed consideration of caries lesion chemistry and the ultrastructure of enamel lesions has indicated that remineralisation, i.e. regrowth of crystals, occurs naturally during the course of the disease process (Johansen 1965; Silverstone 1967; Robinson et al. 2000). In this context the most

C. Robinson
Dental School, University of Leeds,
Clarendon Way, Leeds LS2 9LU, UK
e-mail: C.Robinson@leeds.ac.uk

M. Goldberg (ed.), *Understanding Dental Caries*, DOI 10.1007/978-3-319-30552-3_17

obvious way to treat the disease was to enhance this process of remineralisation, i.e. redeposition of calcium phosphate mineral to replace that which had been lost. This could take the form of regrowth of partially dissolved crystals or deposition of new crystals. Remineralisation has been approached by application of various solutions to the tooth surface, which contain calcium, phosphate and often fluoride. Ideally this would entail depositing mineral, which was less soluble than the original mineral crystals such that the tissue is less likely to be subject to further acid attack. However, if the caries dissolution process outstrips the remineralisation process, then ultimate tooth destruction can occur and other means of treatment must be sought.

Once dissolution has begun, the essential characteristic of the caries lesion is porosity and almost all current diagnostic procedures rely on detecting some aspect of this porosity (Mitropoulos 1985; Angmar-Mansson and ten Bosch 2001; Attrill and Ashley 2001). Pores between the crystals appear at the nanometre level in early stages of the lesion leading to much larger pores as dissolution proceeds. This eventually results in mechanical breakdown of the enamel. At this late stage restoration is necessary when porous tissue is removed and a restorative material placed.

The porosity occurring prior to this breakdown does, importantly, afford the possibility of restoring the enamel using materials which are not acid soluble and without removal of "diseased," i.e. porous tissue. If the small pores of the developing lesion can be infiltrated with a suitable material, then lesions can be treated from very early porosity to a stage approaching mechanical breakdown. This concept of "filling without drilling" was proposed some 30 years or so ago and recently reviewed (Robinson 2011).

17.2 Uptake of Extraneous Materials into Carious Lesions

The central question confronting infiltration of caries lesions is to what extent materials are able to enter lesion porosities. During the caries process and concurrent with diffusion of mineral ions out of caries lesions of enamel, it has become apparent that material can diffuse into the tissue. Mineral ions, mainly calcium and phosphate as well as fluoride, are able to enter the lesion and when this happens to a sufficient extent, the dissolution process is overwhelmed and repair (remineralisation) occurs. More pertinent to infiltration is the fact that relatively large organic molecules from saliva and possibly the diet can also enter the developing lesion. These include albumin and immunoglobulins (Robinson et al. 1998; Shore et al. 2000). In smooth surface lesions, penetration does not seem to be rapid, however, and is therefore presumed to occur during the demineralisation/remineralisation process (Robinson et al. 1998). The effect of such organic molecules on the progress of the lesion is unclear. Albumin, for example, can hinder apatite crystal growth (Garnette and Dieppe 1990) and may therefore hamper the remineralisation process. However, it is also possible that organic materials can protect the surface of mineral crystals by inhibiting acid dissolution (Chin et al. 1993). This raised the possibility of infiltrating organic materials into the lesion with the possible protective effects indicated above but also with the capacity to nucleate new mineral and hence remineralise the tissue (Kirkham et al. 2007).

Infiltration of organic materials into lesions does, however, highlight another possibility. If it proved possible to infiltrate materials into the lesion pores which would convert to a solid state, this would not only occlude the pores but might inhibit diffusion of acid into the tissue and dissolved mineral ions out as well as protecting the crystal surfaces from further dissolution. Solid organic material would also add mechanical strength to the porous tissue. Ideal candidates for such materials are the polymerising resins.

17.3 Infiltration of Carious Enamel with Resin Materials

17.3.1 Background

The major issue facing infiltration of caries lesions, i.e. "filling without drilling," is one of inducing suitable material to enter the extremely small pores of the enamel lesion. This is most likely to be successful by capillary action after drying the lesion. Such rapid uptake would be most suitable for the relatively short periods required for clinical treatment. The extent to which lesions can be infiltrated will depend in the first instance on the size of the pores. These will range from nanometre to micrometre sizes (Phakey et al. 1974; Johnson 1967). Pore sizes in mature enamel range from 2–10 nm between crystals and possibly slightly larger at the periphery of the prisms. Pore sizes increase from the lesion front to the body of the lesion (Johnson 1967) such that the oldest part of the lesion with largest pores and greatest porosity should be closest to the tooth surface. At the ultrastructural level, the larger pores of the lesion body exist at the periphery of prisms and can be up to a micron or so in width. They extend down into the enamel and may be of considerable length. Lateral connection of pores may occur but to a much lesser extent than that in the direction of the prism long axes. Advanced lesions are likely to exhibit even larger pores.

However, in lesions with an intact surface, an important complicating factor is the presence of an apparently intact surface zone. Subsequent work revealed that this is not in fact an intact original surface but is considerably altered chemically and structurally and results from dissolution and reprecipitation of calcium phosphate minerals. The pore volume of this surface zone is low and lies in the range of 0.1 to 1 %, i.e. very close to that of intact surface enamel. The size of pores has been difficult to ascertain but appears to be in the range of 2–10 nm between crystals (Palamara et al. 1986).

This surface zone has proved most problematical in terms of both attaching resins to the lesion surface and infiltrating materials into the lesion interior.

17.3.2 Fissure Sealing

Some of the earliest work relating to penetrating both intact enamel and lesion surfaces stems from the field of "fissure sealants" (Buonocore 1955; Simonsen 2002). Still in use today, these resins were intended to attach and/or to or penetrate slightly into the intact enamel surface. Subsequent polymerisation produced a protective coating on the tooth surface. This would smooth out fissures to reduce stagnation sites and additionally protect the surface from acid attack.

Attempts to improve attachment and to some extent penetration of sealant resins were made by etching the enamel surface with acid. Etching enamel surfaces produced pits ~ 4 microns in diameter, related to enamel prisms, into which some sealant was found to enter (Buonocore 1955). This anchored the resin to the tooth/lesion surface and offered some considerable surface protection to intact enamel surfaces and to some extent caries lesions. Penetration/infiltration of enamel lesions, however, was limited to not much more than the very surface of perhaps 4–10 microns. While this treatment was not initially designed to infiltrate the caries lesion but to adhere to and protect intact enamel, the possibility of inhibiting further acid attack by attempting to infiltrate enamel lesions was explored (Davila et al. 1975). Penetration was limited, but acid treatment of the lesion surface dramatically improved penetration compared with untreated teeth indicating that the surface zone was a barrier to effective infiltration.

17.3.3 Infiltration

A more direct approach to infiltrating lesions was made by Robinson et al. (1976) with an attempt to establish criteria for infiltrative resins as follows:

1. *The infiltration material should ideally be hydrophilic if not water based when applied and hydrophobic when finally polymerised.* Carious lesions tend to develop in relatively inaccessible parts of the dentition, e.g. molar fissures and interproximal surfaces. These regions and the porous enamel of the lesion itself are usually wet. It is thus desirable to dry lesions as much as possible to provide rapid access by capillary action, rather than

the longer processes of diffusion through lesion fluid. Since it is difficult to dry out carious enamel thoroughly, hydrophilic or water-based materials would be desirable. This would allow mixing with and diffusion through remaining endogenous water. The inclusion of water-soluble cariostatic ions such as fluoride would also be permitted. Dissolution or degradation of the final product would be less likely if the final material was also hydrophobic.

2. *The material should be surface-active and possess a low viscosity*. In view, not only of the inaccessibility of caries prone sites but also of the extremely small pores of early enamel lesions, low viscosity and ideally surface-active materials are desirable. This would permit rapid access to lesion sites and penetration of the pores of lesions by capillary action. Ultimately it could conceivably spread over the tooth surface and "seek out" porous tissue.
3. *The material should have bactericidal or at least bacteriostatic properties*. Bacteria can never be completely excluded from caries lesion sites so that their elimination or at least control is desirable. Continued antibacterial activity in the final polymerised state would continue to protect the caries prone site.
4. *The material should be tolerated by the dentin/pulp complex over the life of the tooth as well as by adjacent oral tissues*. Ideally both initial and final states should be biocompatible. If lesions communicate in any way with the dentin, unpolymerised material or other soluble components of the infiltration medium may rapidly reach the dentin/pulp complex. If polymerisation is not complete, this could continue over a prolonged period.
5. *The material should be ideally self-polymerising*. For light-cured materials, poor light penetration, for example, in deep lesions might mean that monomer could persist within the depth of the lesion reducing mechanical strength and possibly giving rise to pulpal inflammation. The problem will be exacerbated in deep fissures, interproximal sites, and, for example, leaking restorations. While current light-cured restorative resins might not present a serious problem in this respect, future new materials or those modified to improve properties, such as penetration, may do so. A *self-polymerising* system, however, would continue to polymerise even in deep lesions reducing the availability of unreacted material.
6. *The material, in its final state, should offer some mechanical support*. Because lesions consist of porous, physically weakened enamel, some mechanical support should be provided. This would be achieved by polymerisation to a solid state. Interaction with endogenous mineral and protein perhaps by cross-linking would be of considerable advantage in this respect.
7. *Full occlusion of lesion pores is desirable*. Reduction of acid access and mechanical support would be maximised by full occlusion of lesion pores. Determination of the extent of pore occlusion as well as penetration depth is therefore important. This would also permit an assessment of resin shrinkage.
8. *The material should be cosmetically acceptable*. While this is desirable, it might not be absolutely necessary since most of the sites where lesions occur are not readily visible.
9. *Convenience of application*. The material should be applied effectively and conveniently to specific intraoral sites within an acceptable time frame. Even the most recent developments in infiltration procedures require similar application times as conventional restorations (Splieth et al. 2010 ORCA Symposium). High penetration is usually accompanied by increased wettability resulting in uncontrolled spread during application so that protection of adjacent soft tissues may be an issue.
10. *Cost*. Low cost is clearly desirable. However, cost of clinical materials/treatments is usually related to demand as new means of manufacture and delivery are developed.

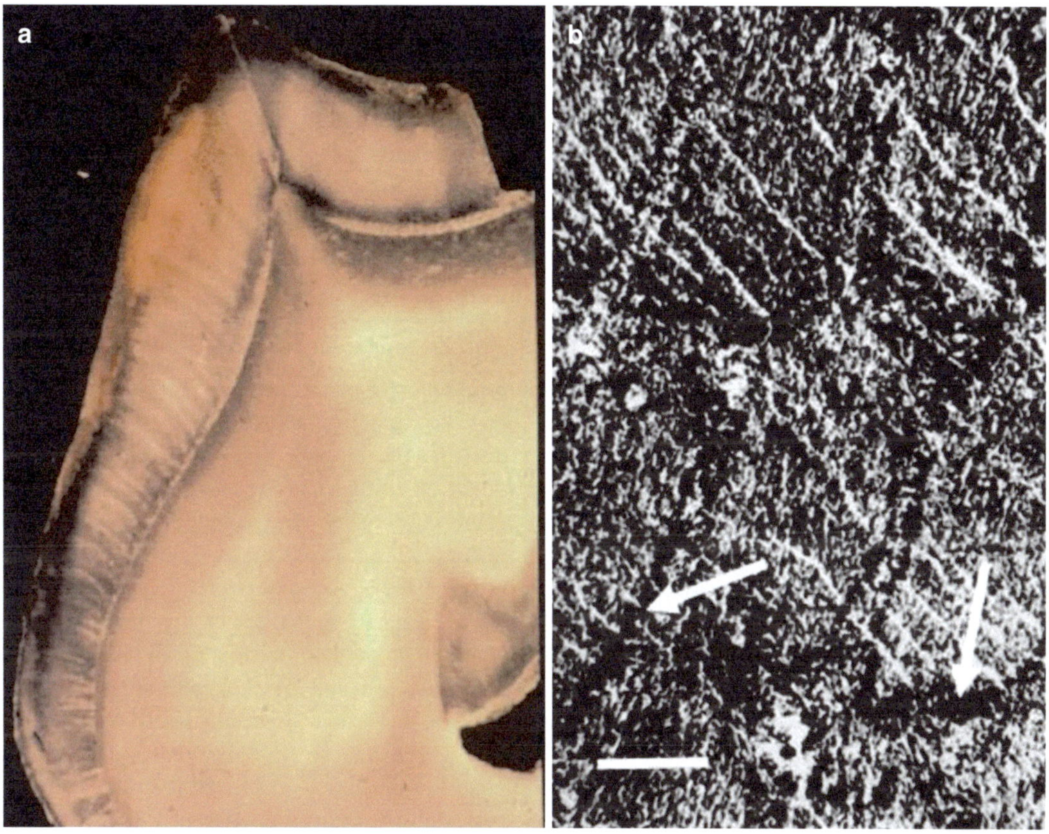

Fig. 17.1 (**a**) Mesiodistal section of premolar monkey tooth (macaque iris) after in vivo treatment using resorcinol formaldehyde resin (Robinson et al. 1976). The resin is seen as a red colouration extending from the lesion surface to the visible limit of the lesion. In this instance, this is the dark zone. (**b**) Electron microradiograph of human white spot carious enamel, ~dark zone region after infiltration with ^{14}C-labelled resorcinol formaldehyde resin in vitro (Robinson et al. 1976). The section is viewed with the radiographic film in situ. The prism outlines are visible as dense black lines (*arrows*). This may be due to fogging by the labelled phenol but, in addition, reduction by the resin itself. The image indicates penetration of resin along prism boundaries in the earliest parts of the lesion. Bar = 1 μm

17.3.4 Resins for Infiltration

17.3.4.1 Resorcinol Formaldehyde

On the basis of the above criteria, initial studies establishing proof of principle investigated a resorcinol formaldehyde resin (Robinson et al. 1976). This penetrated lesions with intact surfaces both in vitro and in vivo but with variable depths. However, when the lesion surface was etched using hydrochloric acid, effective penetration into the lesion as far as the dark zone was observed, i.e. penetration into the earliest stages of the lesion (Fig. 17.1a). Penetration into deep and narrow fissures was also reported. Since the resin was self-coloured due to oxidation, visualisation was straightforward although colour could be eliminated by using ammonium hydroxide to adjust the pH of the unpolymerised resin. Ultrastructural localisation was attempted by incorporating ^{14}C-labelled phenol into the resin prior to uptake in vitro. Electron microscope sections of the lesions were prepared and exposed to high-resolution photographic film for several days (Fig. 17.1b). Dark grains were revealed at the prism peripheries indicating penetration along prism boundaries deep within the lesions. These may be photoinduced silver grains but may also result from some reduction by the resin itself.

While not being clinically suitable, this material did establish proof of principle in terms of very effective infiltration of caries lesions of enamel with a protective effect against further acid attack. It also highlighted the issues of determining the extent of penetration and the extent to which lesion pores had been occluded.

17.3.4.2 Methacrylate-Based Resins

To date, the ubiquitous methacrylates and their derivatives have received most detailed investigation. The methacrylates present numerous advantages. They are easily available, and many are already in use in dentistry alleviating the need for extensive toxicology trials. Although not completely without risk, a great deal of work has established their biocompatibility (Hume and Gerzina 1996) and their physical properties both before and after polymerisation. They are also relatively easy to polymerise in the oral environment.

Using existing resin preparations, some lesion infiltration by methacrylate resins was reported by Davila et al. (1975). Later studies achieved almost complete penetration in some cases (Rodda and Patanapiradej 1983; Robinson et al. 2001; Gray and Shellis 2002). The more successful preparations with suitable properties are in fact adhesives. Their more effective penetration is most likely a result of lower viscosity and lower surface tension than corresponding unfilled resin preparations. Some of these have already shown potential for use with regard to infiltration of caries lesions, for example, Scotchbond, Gluma 2000, All-Bond 2 and Amalgambond plus (Robinson et al. 2001). Using artificial white spot caries, i.e. demineralised enamel, to allow direct comparisons, some products showed deep penetration throughout the observable demineralised region as well as occlusion of most lesion porosity. Preparations which were less successful tended to be more viscous. Those which showed penetration also conferred a resistance to further acid attack.

In terms of development, an advantage of methacrylate-based preparations is that their physical properties can be selected or altered to suit usage. Etching compounds can be included to open up the surface for adhesion and penetration. In addition, viscosity and surface tension can be altered to improve penetration into the extremely small pores of the lesion (Buonocore 1955; Simonsen 2002; Irinoda et al. 2000; Paris et al. 2007; Meyer-Lueckel and Paris 2010). The latter authors proceeded to develop a modified methacrylate-based resin preparation specifically designed for infiltration. This has shown good penetration of natural lesions with intact surfaces and conferred resistance to further acid attack (Paris et al. 2010, 2013). This product has also shown some success in treating lesions within narrow molar fissures (Paris et al. 2014). Subsequently a wide range of available dental products, mainly methacrylate based, have been investigated for both lesion penetration and the effect on further exposure to acid attack. These comprised both unfilled resins per se and adhesive materials. Adhesive materials seem to show more promise than most resins probably due to their lower viscosity and the fact that many include etching properties derived from incorporated acids which would assist opening up the surface zone of the lesion. Some of these are indicated below. The adhesives Xeno bond V and Single bond variants based on a hydroxyethyl methacrylate adhesive showed good penetration and considerable inhibition of further demineralisation in both cavitated and non-cavitated lesions (El-Kalla et al. 2012). In addition, methacrylate modified with triethylene glycol was also found to be very effective, supporting the view that more hydrophilic properties may facilitate infiltration (Meyer-Lueckel and Paris 2010). A combination of both adhesive (Heliobond) and resin (Icon) was studied by Schmidlin et al. (2012) and proved more effective than resin alone. All showed some protective effect compared with untreated lesions. While this may be due to protection of the crystals within the lesion, judging from the histological data, blocking of surface pores may be as important as infiltration of the entire lesion.

For individual resins, penetration was often variable particularly in the case of natural lesions. Reasons for this variation most probably lie with the state of the lesion. Differences in the extent of demineralisation of the lesion associated with variations in pore size, pore distribution and pore volume (Arnold and Gaengler 2012). For example, inactive lesions were less readily penetrated or protected by resin probably due to smaller pores especially in the outer regions of the lesion where more remineralisation would be expected (Neuhaus et al. 2013). Other components may also affect resin behaviour. Saliva contamination before resin treatment reduced the protective effect of resin against acid demineralisation. This may be due to compromised penetration of resin by salivary proteins (Gelani et al. 2014).

In addition, however, the use of acid in opening up or removing the surface zone and the way it is applied need to be considered. Acid containing gels and painting the lesion surface with acid have been used, and in this respect it was found that hydrochloric acid was more effective than phosphoric acid (Robinson et al. 1976; Paris et al. 2007). This is likely due to the fact that the use of acid gels or painting the enamel surface do not agitate the applied acid. From early work, etching enamel with poor agitation leads to local concentration of acid anions and dissolved calcium phosphate. In the case of phosphoric acid, this will not only limit dissolution but can also result in some redeposition of phosphate-containing mineral, perhaps obscuring the small pores of the enamel lesion. In support of this view, more success was achieved when gels were rubbed on to lesion surfaces when it was also reported that addition of abrasion also facilitated penetration (Lausch et al. 2015). For this reason an extremely fine localised hydrochloric acid spray was used in early experimentation (Robinson et al. 1976, 2000).

There are some disadvantages with current methacrylate preparations. The methacrylates are not self-polymerising and require light activation and/or catalytic activation. Catalytic activators may be cytotoxic, and their possible interface with live tissue, i.e. dentin or pulp, must be taken into account. In this context, light activation would be preferable. However, the stagnation sites where lesions occur, i.e. in deep molar fissures and interproximal areas between teeth, are not necessarily easily penetrated by light. This could lead to the possibility of incomplete polymerisation and a resulting weak polymer and/or of residual monomer leaching from the lesion into adjacent tissue. Long-term effects of this possibility are not yet known.

Most importantly all of the work to date concerning infiltration of caries lesions has indicated that with current materials, opening up of the surface zone and/or removing some surface enamel is an almost necessary prerequisite for successful infiltration. The removal of the lesion surface does, however, raise issues with regard to the surface integrity of the infiltrated lesion over the long term and effects on the adhesion of pellicle and plaque proteins.

17.3.5 Detection of Resin Within the Lesion and Measurement of Occluded Volume

In developing materials specifically for infiltration, the depth of penetration and the ultrastructural location of infiltrant are important parameters in assessing effectiveness. Determination of volume of lesion pores occluded, i.e. filled by resin, is also extremely important in this respect. Data on volume of pores occluded not only provides information concerning penetration effectiveness but also on resin shrinkage during treatment. If the method is nondestructive, it can be used to assess the effects of further acid attack on the treated lesions directly by measuring any increase in pore volume due to further demineralisation.

17.3.5.1 Detection of Infiltrated Resin

As far as penetration is concerned, incorporation of dye into the resin is useful for simple visualisation of penetration (Robinson et al. 2001). For greater resolution, confocal laser scanning microscopy (CLSM) is a valuable tool and has provided useful data on the extent of resin infiltration as well as some data on histological location. In those parts of the lesion infiltrated, this has demonstrated that resin appears to occupy the body of enamel prisms (Fig. 17.2) (Paris et al. 2007). It is of interest to note here that while resin (the methacrylate-based adhesive Excite) was present in the bodies of prisms, the prism boundaries, a region considered to be at least as porous as prism bodies, seemed to contain less resin. The porosity of both prism bodies and prism boundaries is clearly seen by green fluorescein staining of

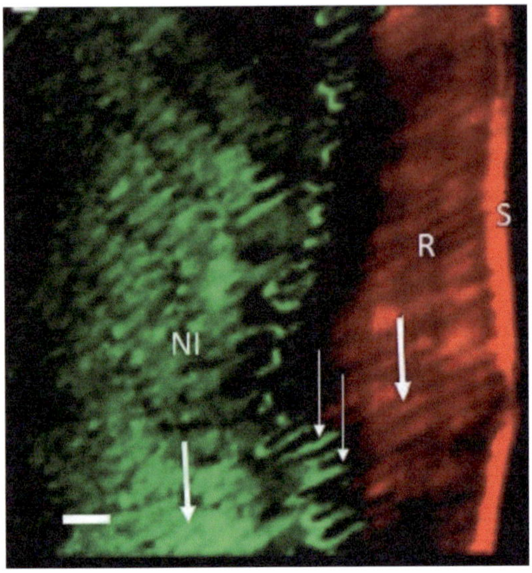

Fig. 17.2 CLSM image of an HCl-etched lesion treated with the adhesive Excite (Adapted from Paris et al. 2007 with permission). *S* surface of lesion, *R* the outermost 50–100 μm of prism cores are filled with resin (*red* fluorescence *heavy arrow*), *NI* non-infiltrated parts of the lesion body, the highly porous prism cores (*heavy arrow*) and prism boundaries (*light arrows*) show green fluorescence. Bar = ~10 μm

non-infiltrated regions of the lesion. This may be due to local variations in pore structure, but whatever the reason for this is, it raises the important question that while resin may be visibly present, it does not indicate the extent to which porosities are actually occluded. Fully occluded pores would offer maximum protection against further entry of acid and egress of dissolved mineral ions as well as conferring maximum mechanical support. See also Gelani et al. (2014). CLSM has limited penetration into enamel such that estimating penetration depth from the outer surface is limited. Currently such assessments are carried out on tooth sections after in vitro or if possible after in vivo administration. The resin must be labelled with a fluorescent probe to render it visible.

Radiographic procedures are appropriate if resins are rendered radio-opaque. This is not feasible, however, with current methacrylate-based resins since they are radiolucent. Incorporation of radio-opaque components or a radio-opaque filler would be necessary. The technology is, however, of value in assessing the protective effect of resin against further demineralisation. Autoradiography is also a useful approach for investigations in vitro and has the possibility for detailed ultrastructural location (see Fig. 17.1b).

17.3.5.2 Determination of Occluded Pore Volume

Measurement of volume occluded by resin is also an important parameter as indicated above. Partially occluded pores will offer less protection to further acid attack as well as poorer mechanical support.

Determination of occluded pore volume is not easily achieved but has been attempted in studies with resorcinol formaldehyde and some dental resin adhesives (Robinson et al. 1976, 2001). Lesion pores were infiltrated with 2-chloronaphthalene, known to penetrate even the pores of the earliest stages of lesion formation. Quantitative extraction of the 2-chloronaphthalene permitted a determination of accessible lesion pore volume. Subsequent measurement after resin infiltration provided a measurement of volume occluded by resin. This also permitted a measurement of resin shrinkage. This was up to 30 % for the resorcinol preparation but was reduced to almost zero by a second treatment indicating almost 100 % pore occlusion. The method was highly reproducible in artificial lesions (6 % standard deviation) but was less so for natural lesions. This is most likely due to more complex pore structure of natural lesions and the presence of organic material such as proteins in the lesion (Robinson et al. 1998; Shore et al. 2000).

17.3.6 Effects of Infiltration on Carious Tissue

Infiltration as a clinical treatment is still at an early stage so that there is little data on the long-term effects of infiltration on caries lesions. A systematic review has concluded that the treatment is useful for preventing caries progression in lesions with intact surfaces, but studies are required to establish durability of the treatment in terms of tooth integrity as well as caries progress (Doméjean et al. 2015). Some shorter-term investigations have been carried out mainly with regard to cosmetic acceptability of the treatment especially on lesions resulting from stagnation around orthodontic brackets.

These reported an initial improvement in lesion appearance which was sustained over a 6-month or 1-year period. This suggests that resin treatment did not result in a lesion surface which was prone to staining rendering it suitable for visible sites in the mouth (Feng and Chu 2013; Borges et al. 2014; Knösel et al. 2013). It may also suggest that the surface was not rendered more prone to plaque deposition.

Some studies have been carried out concerning physical properties of the infiltrated lesion (Tostes et al. 2014; Paris et al. 2013). These have suggested that infiltration did not restore the enamel to its original state but did result in improved mechanical properties of the lesion surface in terms of hardness and elasticity. Some additional surface treatment may therefore be desirable.

17.3.7 Application to Other Enamel Dysplasias Exhibiting Abnormal Porosity

This approach has the potential to expand into other areas. Caries lesions in which the surface has been breached could be treated if the final product were sufficiently strong mechanically and abrasive resistant to form part of the tooth surface. In such a case, a two-component/two-stage treatment could be envisaged. While current material (Icon) is not considered suitable for deeper lesions involving dentin, future developments in infiltration materials may make this possible perhaps together with treatment of exposed dentin. The main proviso will be issues relating to damaging the dentin/pulp complex.

There is also the possibility of treating marginal leakage. If infiltrants can be induced to enter the junction between restoration and tooth, then replacement of the restoration may be avoided (Tulunoglu et al. 2014).

Other enamel dysplasias with porous defects could also be treated such as severe fluorosis, amelogenesis imperfecta, epidermolysis bullosa and molar incisor hypomineralisation (MIH). Noninvasive treatment of epidermolysis bullosa would be particularly beneficial since conventional treatment of such patients is extremely traumatic with the high risk of soft tissue damage. Recent interest has centred on molar incisor hypomineralisation (MIH), a developmental defect in which erupted enamel is incompletely mineralised and contains substantial amounts of serum as well as developmental proteins. Some limited success was achieved with a current product. Such limitation is most likely due to the presence of protein in the MIH enamel obscuring lesion pores (Crombie et al. 2014; Kumar et al. 2012). This may be analogous to the effects of saliva on the effectiveness of infiltration where salivary proteins may obstruct access to lesion pores (Gelani et al. 2014). Clearly the effects of protein within the lesion are an area which would benefit from further investigation. Since it has been reported that removal of protein from the lesion can lead, for example, to improved uptake of calcium ions (Robinson et al. 1990; Iizuka et al. 2014), this may be another potential approach to improving resin uptake.

While not showing frank porosity in depth, eroded enamel has also been treated by resin infiltration with encouraging results in that infiltration inhibited further erosion without the necessity for acid etching (de Oliveira et al. 2014). In this case, however, we may be looking at something between the fissure sealing concept and infiltration. This highlights the fact that it is not easy to discern between effects generated by simply sealing the lesion surface and partially infiltrating the body of the lesion. In this context and as stated above, the pore volume occluded by resin is an important parameter since only by filling the lesion will mechanical strength be imparted to the caries lesion by infiltration.

17.3.8 Future Developments

17.3.8.1 Design of Infiltration Materials

Infiltration of caries lesions is likely to become an established approach to the treatment of non-cavitated caries lesions of enamel. Most of this work has employed methacrylate-based preparations which have worked effectively in both penetrating lesions and reducing further acid demineralisation. Further development of these materials is possible. Modification of the resins themselves perhaps could include greater penetration, lower shrinkage and self-polymerisation. Inclusion of nanoparticulate solids would add to the mechanical strength of the lesion. This could also address the problem of the lesion surface which had been etched and often removed prior to infiltration. Inclusion of other materials, for example, fluoride, calcium and phosphate, would be advantageous. However, most methacrylate preparations are essentially hydrophobic such that inclusion of water-soluble components such as fluoride is limited.

New materials need to be investigated as a guide using the criteria set out above. A water-based or at least hydrophilic material would offer the possibility of including water-soluble materials. These could include fluoride which assists in remineralisation, and the resin itself could be modified to provide initiation sites for deposition of new mineral. Antibacterial materials such as the biguanide chlorhexidine could be included to deal with bacteria in the lesion and future surface colonisation and possibly anti-inflammatory agents to reduce any effect on the dentin or dental pulp. Factors to stimulate growth of reparative dentin are also possibilities. This would require investigations, for example, of concentration of active agents and rate of delivery.

With suitable developments in materials, it is not beyond the bounds of possibility that in the future some form of self-infiltration treatments might be possible.

References

Angmar-Månsson B, ten Bosch JJ. Quantitative light-induced fluorescence (QLF™): a method for assessment of incipient caries lesions. Dentomaxillofac Radiol. 2001;30:298–307.

Arnold WH, Gaengler P. Light and electron microscope study of infiltration of resin into initial caries lesions- a new methodological approach. J Microsc. 2012;245:26–33.

Attrill DC, Ashley PF. Diagnostics: occlusal caries detection in primary teeth: a comparison of DIAGNOdent with conventional methods. Br Dent J. 2001;190:440–3.

Borges A, Caneppele T, Luz M, et al. Colour stability of resin used for caries infiltration after exposure to different staining solutions. Oper Dent. 2014;39: 433–40.

Buonocore MG. A simple method of increasing the adhesion of acrylic filling materials to enamel surfaces. J Dent Res. 1955;34:849–53.

Chin KOA, Johnsson M, Bergey EJ, et al. A constant composition kinetics study of the influence of salivary cystatins, statherin, amylase and human serum albumin on hydroxyapatite dissolution. Colloids Surf A Physicochem Eng Asp. 1993;78:229–34.

Crombie F, Manton D, Palamara J, et al. Resin infiltration of developmentally hypomineralised enamel. Int J Paediatr Dent. 2014;24:51–5. doi:10.1111/ipd.12025.

Davila JM, Buonocore MG, Greeley CB, et al. Adhesive penetration in human artificial and natural white spots. J Dent Res. 1975;54:999–1008.

de Oliveira GC, Boteon AP, Ionta FQ, et al. In vitro effects of resin infiltration on enamel erosion inhibition. Oper Dent. 2014. doi:10.2341/14-162-L.

Doméjean S, Ducamp R, Léger S, et al. Resin infiltration of non-cavitated caries lesions: a systematic review. Med Princ Pract. 2015;24:216–21.

El-Kalla IH, Saudi HI, El-Agamy RA. Effect of adhesive resin application on the progression of cavitated and non-cavitated incipient carious lesions. Am J Dent. 2012;25:176–80.

Feng CH, Chu XY. Efficacy of one year treatment of icon infiltration resin on post-orthodontic white spots. Beijing Da Xue Xue Bao. 2013;45:40–3.

Garnette J, Dieppe P. The effects of serum and human albumin on calcium hydroxyapatite crystal growth. Biochem J. 1990;266:863–8.

Gelani R, Zandona AF, Lippert F, et al. *In vitro* progression of artificial white spot lesions sealed with an infiltrant resin. Oper Dent. 2014;39:481–8. doi:10.2341/13-202-L.

Gray GB, Shellis P. Infiltration of resin into white spot caries-like lesions of enamel: an in vitro study. Eur J Prosthodont Restor Dent. 2002;10:27–32.

Hume WR, Gerzina TM. Bioavailability of components of resin-based materials which are applied to teeth. Crit Rev Oral Biol Med. 1996;7:172–9.

Iizuka J, Mukai Y, Taniguchi M, et al. Chemical alteration by tooth bleaching of human salivary proteins that infiltrated subsurface enamel lesions – experimental study with bovine lesion model systems. Dent Mater J. 2014;33:663–8.

Irinoda Y, Matsumura Y, Kito H, et al. Effect of sealant viscosity on the penetration of resin into etched human enamel. Oper Dent. 2000;25:274–82.

Johansen E. Comparison of the ultrastructure and chemical composition of sound and carious enamel from human permanent teeth. In: Stack MV, Fearnhead RW, editors. Tooth enamel. Bristol: J Wright and Sons; 1965. p. 177–81.

Johnson NW. Some aspects of the ultrastructure of early human enamel caries seen with the electron microscope. Arch Oral Biol. 1967;12:1505–21.

Kirkham J, Firth A, Vernals D, et al. Self-assembling peptide scaffolds promote enamel remineralisation. J Dent Res. 2007;86:426–30.

Knösel M, Eckstein A, Helms HJ. Durability of aesthetic improvement following Icon resin infiltration of multibracket-induced white spot lesions compared with no therapy over 6 months: a single-centre, split-mouth, randomized clinical trial. Am J Orthod Dentofacial Orthop. 2013;144:86–96. doi:10.1016/j.ajodo.2013.02.029.

Kumar H, Palamara J, Burrow MF, et al. Resin infiltration-taking the first steps to filling the holes in cheese molars. Ann R Australas Coll Dent Surg. 2012;21:120–3.

Lausch J, Paris S, Selje T, et al. Resin infiltration of fissure caries with various techniques of pretreatment *in vitro*. Caries Res. 2015;49:50–5. doi:10.1159/000366082.

Meyer-Lueckel H, Paris S. Infiltration of natural caries lesions with experimental resins differing in penetration coefficients and ethanol addition. Caries Res. 2010;44:408–14.

Mitropoulos CM. The use of fibre-optic transillumination in the diagnosis of posterior approximal caries in clinical trials. Caries Res. 1985;19:379–84.

Neuhaus KW, Schlafer S, Lussi A, et al. Infiltration of natural caries lesions in relation to their activity status and acid pretreatment *in vitro*. Caries Res. 2013;47:203–10. doi:10.1159/000345654.

Palamara J, Phakey PP, Rachinger WA, et al. Ultrastructure of the intact surface zone of white spot and brown spot carious lesions in human enamel. J Oral Pathol Med. 1986;15:28–35.

Paris S, Meyer-Lueckel H, Kielbassa AM. Resin infiltration of natural caries lesions. J Dent Res. 2007;86:662–6.

Paris S, Hopfenmuller W, Meyer-Lueckel H. Resin infiltration of caries lesions: an efficacy randomized trial. J Dent Res. 2010;89:823–6.

Paris S, Schwendicke F, Seddig S, et al. Micro-hardness and mineral loss of enamel lesions after infiltration with various resins: influence of infiltrant composition and application frequency *in vitro*. J Dent. 2013;41:543–8.

Paris S, Lausch J, Selje T, et al. Comparison of sealant and infiltrant penetration into pit and fissure caries lesions *in vitro*. J Dent. 2014;42:432–8. doi:10.1016/j.jdent.2014.01.006.

Phakey PP, Rachinger WA, Zybert JJ. Visualisation of the pore structure of human enamel. Nature. 1974;252:584–5.

Robinson C. Filling without drilling. J Dent Res. 2011;90:1261–3.

Robinson C, Hallsworth AS, Weatherell JA, et al. Arrest and control of carious lesions; a study based on preliminary experiments with resorcinol-formaldehyde resin. J Dent Res. 1976;55:812–8.

Robinson C, Hallsworth AS, Shore AS, et al. Effect of surface zone deproteinisation on the access of mineral Ions into subsurface carious lesions of human enamel. Caries Res. 1990;24:226–30. doi:10.1159/000261272.

Robinson C, Shore RC, Bonass WA, et al. Identification of human serum albumin in human caries lesions of enamel: the role of putative inhibitors of remineralisation. Caries Res. 1998;32:193–9.

Robinson C, Shore RC, Brookes SJ, et al. The chemistry of enamel caries. Crit Rev Oral Biol Med. 2000;11:481–95.

Robinson C, Brookes SJ, Kirkham J. *In vitro* studies of the penetration of adhesive resins into artificial caries-like lesions. Caries Res. 2001;35:136–41.

Rodda JC, Patanapiradej V. Penetration of dental resins into caries-like lesions. J Dent Res. 1983;62:659–659.

Schmidlin PR, Sener B, Attin T, et al. Protection of sound enamel and artificial enamel lesions against demineralisation. J Dent. 2012;40:851–6. doi:10.1016/j.jdent.07.003.

Shore RC, Kirkham J, Brookes SJ, et al. Distribution of exogenous proteins in caries lesions in relation to the pattern of demineralisation. Caries Res. 2000;34:188–93.

Silverstone LM. Observations on the dark zone in early enamel caries and in artificial caries-like lesions. Caries Res. 1967;1:261–74.

Simonsen RJ. Pit and fissure sealant: review of the literature. Pediatr Dent. 2002;24:393–414.

Splieth CH, Ekstrand KR, Alkilzy M, et al. Sealants in dentistry: outcomes of the ORCA Saturday Afternoon Symposium. Caries Res. 2010;44:3–13.

Tostes MA, Santos Jr E, Camargo Jr SA. Effect of resin infiltration on the nanomechanical properties of demineralized bovine enamel. Indian J Dent. 2014;5:116–22. doi:10.4103/0975-962X.140819.

Tulunoglu O, Tulunoglu I, Antonson S, et al. Effectiveness of an infiltrant on sealing of composite restoration margins with/without artificial caries. J Contemp Dent Pract. 2014;15:717–25.

18 Minimally Invasive Therapy: Keeping Treated Teeth Functional for Life

Jo E. Frencken and Soraya C. Leal

18.1 Introduction

In many countries around the world, the prevalence and severity of dental caries have decreased during the last three decades. This outcome should not come as a surprise as dental caries is a preventable disease. During these decades, many studies have been carried out to investigate which factors keep healthy teeth healthy and which cause tooth surfaces to demineralise. This great focus on oral health makes it difficult to accept that untreated carious cavities in permanent teeth are the number one prevalent condition out of 291 medical diseases and conditions investigated over the period 1990–2010 (Marcenes et al. 2013). The same condition, but in primary teeth, was the tenth most prevalent condition over the same period. The global economic impact of all dental diseases amounted to US$442 billion in 2010 (Listl et al. 2015). This is an astronomically high figure considering that the two major dental diseases, dental caries and periodontal diseases, are largely preventable.

J.E. Frencken (✉)
Department of Oral Function and Prosthetic Dentistry, Radboud University Medical Center, Nijmegen, P.O. Box 9101, Nijmegen 6500 HB, The Netherlands
e-mail: j.frencken@dent.umcn.nl

S.C. Leal
Department of Dentistry, Faculty of Health Sciences, University of Brasilia, Campus Darcy Ribeiro, Asa Norte, Brasilia 70670-410, Brazil

It goes without saying that the dental profession needs to take some responsibility for the findings of the above-mentioned studies. The public is also owed an explanation about how a preventable disease can end up so high in the ranking order of most prevalent diseases and conditions. What should be done to improve population oral health and to reduce the economic burden of dental diseases? What lessons can be learnt from the past? Has sufficient emphasis been given to keeping healthy teeth healthy? How appropriately have dentists managed dental caries and treated cavitated teeth? Are dentists up-to-date with modern evidence-based treatment concepts or do they still follow the outdated ideas of G.V. Black? Many questions such as these need to be answered by the world dental profession and professionals and, in particular, by the leaders of dental training institutions. These institutions are the places where young dental students receive their training and become competent to assist the public in keeping healthy teeth healthy. These are also the places where young dentists should learn that they are students for life.

This chapter briefly discusses minimal intervention dentistry (MID) as a modern concept for managing dental caries and goes on to present contemporary methods of managing dentine carious lesions. MID is a response to the outdated principles of managing dentine carious cavities developed by G.V. Black, more than 100 years ago.

M. Goldberg (ed.), *Understanding Dental Caries*, DOI 10.1007/978-3-319-30552-3_18

18.2 Minimal Intervention Dentistry

18.2.1 Its Rationale

MID is a philosophy or concept that attempts to ensure that teeth are kept functional for life (Frencken et al. 2012a). Its development was facilitated by the many studies performed on a pallet of dental caries-related topics, of which the most important contributions are presented in the next section of this chapter. But not only dental studies have contributed to the development of MID; demographic information has also played a role. For example, the proportion of 70-year-olds in Sweden who have retained their natural teeth has increased, from 13.3 in 1973 to 20.7 in 2003 (Hugoson et al. 2005) (Table 18.1). The same pattern is apparent in other European countries (Müller et al. 2007a). At the same time, life expectancy in Organisation for Economic Co-operation and Development (OECD) countries has increased, from 64.6 years in 1960 to 78.4 years in 2013 (OECD 2015). The increase in life expectancy implies that many more people reach old age. If these people aim to enjoy a good appearance, be able to eat a good meal and enjoy various types of drinks, and engage in a social life in confidence as they used to, they need to have a good set of functional natural teeth. And, in order to achieve this objective at an old age, tooth-saving actions should start when these people are young. This suggests that dentists should ask when they perform a procedure: how will what I am doing now affect the life of the tooth and the person when that person has reached old age? And, as discussed above, life expectancy is increasing year by year in most countries, as is the number of natural teeth in these increasingly elderly people.

18.2.2 Its Cornerstones

The topics that have played a major role in the development of the MID philosophy are presented below.

Fluoride: Many studies from 1940 onwards that have assessed the effect of water fluoridation and fluoride toothpaste, varnish, gel and mouth rinses on the progression of carious lesions have contributed greatly to the development of the MID philosophy. These studies have shown that the main long-term action of fluoride retards the progression of a carious lesion, rather than preventing its development (Backer-Dirks et al. 1961).

Sugar: Studies from the 1950–1970 period that assessed the effect of various forms of sugar-containing food and beverages revealed that free sugar is an aetiological factor in the onset and progression of carious lesions and that its detrimental effect can be countered by reducing sugar intake and frequency of consumption.

Dental biofilm: This topic was researched extensively in the 1960s–1980 period. The outcomes of this research resulted in the acceptance that dental biofilm, when allowed to become cariogenic, is the main cause of demineralisation of tooth surfaces. Biofilm should be at least disturbed or at best removed from tooth surfaces daily, if carious lesion development is to be minimised. In combination with fluoride toothpaste, biofilm removal with a toothbrush has become a major cornerstone in managing carious lesions for communities worldwide (Frencken et al. 2002).

Table 18.1 Mean number of existing teeth (excluding edentulous individuals) by age groups in 1973, 1983, 1993 and 2003 (Hugoson et al. 2005)

	Age group (yrs)						
Year of investigation	20	30	40	50	60	70	80
1973	27.2	25.8	23.2	21.5	18.2	13.3	
1983	27.4	26.9	24.8	22.7	18.6	15.5	13.7
1993	27.3	27.3	26.6	24.7	21.7	18.1	15.7
2003	27.4	27.2	26.5	26.1	23.3	20.7	18.4

Adhesive dental materials: With the appearance of the first research article on the use of composite resin in humans (Buonocore 1955), tooth cavities could be physically reduced in size, with the result that more healthy tooth structure could remain in place. With the appearance of the first glass-ionomer cement in 1969, a biologically based adhesive dental material was introduced (Wilson and Kent 1972), which provided preventive care (sealants) and restorative care (restorations).

Removal of carious tissue: Retaining sound tooth structure, and thus increasing the chance of maintaining tooth vitality and function, was further increased as a result of the work conducted by scholars such as Massler (1967) and Fusayama (1997) from 1960 to 1980. These authors showed that only the 'infected' ('outer carious' or 'decomposed') dentine needed to be removed as part of the cavity preparation process and that the 'affected' ('inner carious' or 'demineralised') dentine could remain. This demineralised dentine would remineralise under a well-placed, well-sealed and well-maintained restoration (Ngo et al. 2006; Alves et al. 2010; Peters et al. 2010).

Repeat restoration cycle: This important cornerstone of MID showed that 'eliminating' carious lesions to improve oral health through restorative procedures based on the G.V. Black concept does not keep teeth functional for life for all individuals. The repeat restoration cycle clearly demonstrated that preventive or nonoperative actions should go hand in hand with restorative care and that assessment of carious lesion development and progression plays a vital part in the provision of adequate oral health care (Elderton 1990).

By early 1990, research had shown that managing dental carious lesions should depart from the traditional surgical approach and move to a 'biological' or 'medical' approach. The research pointed to a completely new approach in the management of the carious lesion.

This new management approach is named minimal intervention dentistry. Its aim is to keep teeth healthy and functional for life. This is achieved through implementing the following important strategies for keeping teeth free from carious lesions: (i) early caries detection and assessment of caries activity and caries risk with validated instruments, (ii) remineralisation of demineralised enamel and dentine, (iii) optimal caries-preventive measures, (iv) minimally invasive operative interventions, and (v) repair rather than replacement of defective restorations (Tyas et al. 2000). It is evident from these strategies that MID does not exclusively equate to cutting smaller cavities than before, as many dentists had initially thought (McIntyre 1994; Burke 2008).

The aspects of the first three MID strategies 'early caries detection and caries activity and risk assessment', 'remineralisation of demineralised enamel and dentine', and 'fluoride as a caries-preventive measure' are presented in Chaps. 9, 14, 15, 16, respectively. These aspects of the strategies should be employed throughout a person's life, and only when oral health maintenance has failed and a cavity has developed should a minimally invasive operative intervention be undertaken. The effectiveness of some non-fluoride caries-preventive measures and the last MID strategy (repair versus replacement of faulty restorations) are discussed in the present chapter.

18.3 Managing Dental Caries

'Dental caries' is the name of a disease and a carious lesion is the consequence of the caries process over time. A carious lesion appears in various forms, which vary from a small demineralised area in enamel to a large cavity in dentine with or without pulpal involvement. The two major aetiological factors that govern the development and progression of a carious lesion are the supply of fermentable carbohydrates, particularly free sugars, and the inability to remove the cariogenic bacterial biofilm from a tooth surface adequately and regularly. These factors are behaviourally determined and, therefore, form the foundation for the understanding that dental caries is a behavioural and not an infectious disease as many dentists erroneously think and are being taught in many dental schools in countries around the world. One should realise that removing microorganisms cannot cure dental caries, neither is a dental carious lesion caused by specific microorganisms as was thought in the past (Chap. 5).

18.3.1 Managing Enamel Carious Lesions: Therapies Other Than Fluoride and Infiltration

As was mentioned at the start of this chapter, a significant reduction of cavitated dentine carious lesions has been observed worldwide in the last three decades (WHO 2013). Because of this positive development, the need for concentrating more on the detection and registration of early signs of dental caries has become evident. Although caries detection and assessment systems, that included enamel carious lesions, have been available since the 1950s (Backer-Dirks et al. 1961; Marthaler 1966), new caries detection systems that include enamel lesions have been developed in the last decade. These systems are distinctly different from the one usually recommended by the World Health Organization (WHO), which only records obvious cavitation in dentine. Examples of such new systems are the Nyvad criteria (Nyvad et al. 1999), ICDAS (Pitts 2004) and the CAST instrument (Frencken et al. 2011). As a consequence of this shift in approach, a variety of nonoperative approaches, tailored to avoid the progression of enamel carious lesions into frank cavitation, have been developed and investigated. The most studied therapy for controlling enamel carious lesions concerns the use of fluoride in its different presentation forms. The mode of action and effectiveness of these forms are presented in detail in Chap. 15.

More recently, a microinvasive therapy initially developed for controlling enamel carious lesions located at approximal surfaces has been proposed (Paris and Meyer-Lueckel 2010). This therapy, called resin infiltration, has received a great deal of attention from researchers and has shown promising results that are discussed in Chap. 17. Therapies other than fluoride and resin infiltration that also aim at controlling enamel carious lesions are being propagated. These therapies are presented below.

18.3.1.1 Casein Phosphopeptides-Amorphous Calcium Phosphate

Studies in vitro, in situ and in humans have shown that casein phosphopeptides (CPP) have a caries-inhibiting effect, which is explained by their ability to stabilise calcium and phosphate and keep them in a soluble amorphous state (ACP) (Reynolds 1998). When in their ionic form and in the face of a cariogenic challenge, both calcium and phosphate ions can be released, which reduces the demineralisation and stimulates the remineralisation process (Andersson et al. 2007; Yengopal and Mickenautsch 2009).

CPP-ACP is present in chewing gums, mouth washes, topical creams, and, more recently, in varnishes. Moreover, as CPP-ACP has been shown to have a synergism with fluoride, some CPP-ACP-based products to which fluoride has been added, such as topical creams, are available.

Three systematic reviews have been published with regard to CPP-ACP effectiveness in caries prevention. Two of these reviews were published before 2010 (Azarpazhooh and Limeback 2008; Yengopal and Mickenautsch 2009) and suggested that more in vivo studies with long follow-up periods were needed, specifically to compare CPP-ACP with fluoride compounds, before the clinical benefits of the product observed in some clinical trials could be generalised. More recently, a review that was aimed at assessing the effectiveness of CPP-ACP formulations of Tooth Mousse® and Tooth Mousse Plus® (which contains fluoride) in preventing and treating enamel carious lesions did not identify any significant benefit of applying Tooth Mousse® over brushing with fluoridated toothpaste. Moreover, evidence that Tooth Mousse Plus® presents any advantages over Tooth Mousse® was not observed. Similarly to the other two reviews, the authors of the most recent published review concluded that more well-designed randomised clinical trials are required before Tooth Mousse® products can be recommended for preventing and treating enamel carious lesions (Raphael and Blinkhorn 2015).

18.3.1.2 Ozone

Ozone therapy for treating carious lesions relies on the fact that ozone kills bacteria by destroying microorganism cell walls and cytoplasmatic membranes (Yamayoshi and Tatsumi 1993). From a simplistic view, one might immediately conclude that such a therapy is likely to be very effective in avoiding the occurrence of carious lesions or in arresting the lesions already present, as such lesions will not be initiated or progress in the absence of bacteria. However, controversial results regarding the effect of ozone on cariogenic bacteria have been presented. The application of ozone failed to reduce the amount of viable bacteria in infected dentine beneath demineralised enamel (Baysan and Beighton 2007) and also in cariogenic biofilm (Müller et al. 2007b). Nevertheless, it was effective in killing *Streptococcus mutans*, *Lactobacillus casei* and *Actinomyces naeslundii* in an in vitro experiment (Johansson et al. 2009).

A systematic review of the literature in which the clinical application and remineralisation potentials of ozone in dentistry were assessed concluded that, while the results of laboratory studies have shown promise for using ozone in managing dental and root caries, clinical studies have not been able to prove that ozone therapy is superior to other nonoperative therapies (Azarpazhooh and Limeback 2008). The same conclusions have been pointed out in two other reviews that recommended, in addition, that more well-designed clinical trials are needed, specifically to compare ozone with other caries-preventive therapies such as fluoride, oral hygiene control, sealants and chlorhexidine (Burke 2012; Almaz and Sönmez 2015).

18.3.1.3 Chlorhexidine-Containing Agents

Chlorhexidine is available in mouth rinses, gel and varnish. At high concentrations, chlorhexidine is bactericidal; at low concentrations, it is bacteriostatic. The dental caries prophylactic effect of chlorhexidine in its various products has been investigated in a number of systematic reviews (van Rijkom et al. 1996; Zhang et al. 2006; James et al. 2010; Slot et al. 2011), with the latest, Cochrane Review, published in 2015 (Walsh et al. 2015). The authors of the latest review found 'little evidence from the eight trials on varnishes and gels included in the review to either support or refute the assertion that chlorhexidine is more effective than placebo or no treatment in the prevention of dental caries or the reduction of mutans streptococci levels in children and adolescents'. Furthermore, evidence that in the absence of regular professional tooth cleaning and oral hygiene instruction, chlorhexidine varnish provides a beneficial effect in special needs patients is weak (Slot et al. 2011).

The overall conclusion about chlorhexidine as a carious lesion control agent is that evidence of its effectiveness in mouth rinses and gel products is not available (van Rijkom et al. 1996; James et al. 2010; Walsh et al. 2015). Chlorhexidine varnish can at best be considered a short-term option for carious lesion control in individuals at high-caries risk who have high microorganism counts (Whelton and O'Mullane 2001; Du et al. 2006; de Amorim et al. 2008) such as children suffering from severe early childhood caries, people wearing fixed orthodontic appliances (Derks et al. 2004) and elderly people with reduced salivary flow (Slot et al. 2011). Treatment by means of chlorhexidine varnish should be accompanied by biofilm removal.

18.3.1.4 Sealants

Indications for Placing a Sealant

As sealants are usually placed in erupted (pre) molars, the level of caries experience of the child in their primary dentition is a good predictor of carious lesion development in pits and fissures of permanent molars (Disney et al. 1992). But being a high-caries risk child is not enough of a reason to place a sealant according to cost-effective principles. Also the caries risk at the tooth surface level should be established. Pits and fissure morphology (medium and deep) in combination with or without signs of carious lesion activity (presence of biofilm, roughness and/or whitish colour of the surface) are factors that determine the state of carious lesion in pits and fissures (**see Chaps. 9, 11, 16, 19**).

Sealing aims to modify patent pits and fissures into smooth surfaces that are protected from bacterial colonisation and exposure to fermentable substrates and that can be cleaned easily. The strategy is effective not only as a preventive measure but also in arresting non-cavitated enamel carious lesions in pits and fissures (Griffin et al. 2008). The superiority of pit and fissure sealants over fluoride varnish application in the prevention of occlusal carious lesions has been reported (Hiiri et al. 2010).

Glass-ionomers are more hydrophilic than are resin-based materials. It is therefore logical to assume that a glass-ionomer rather than a resin-based material should be used in sealing carious lesion-prone pits and fissures that cannot be kept absolutely moisture-free, such as in just erupting molars and in children with behaviour problems.

Resin-Based Sealants

Resin-based materials, auto- and light-cured, have a long tradition of use as a material for sealing pits and fissures. Controversy exists about whether a resin sealant needs to be applied under rubber dam or under cotton wool roll isolation. If the latter method is used, the dentist has to ensure that the tooth surface will not be contaminated with saliva and kept moisture-free after washing the etch gel away. Four-handed dentistry might then be a necessity. Etching and light-curing time differs from one product to the other and it is therefore important to read the manufacturers' instructions. When using light-cured resin sealant material, the dentist has to realise that the material can shrink by up to 4% and that unpolymerised sealant, containing Bisphenol A (BPA) and/or BPA-DM, is left at the surface layer. This layer can easily be removed when adjusting the bite or through wiping the surface with a cotton pellet.

One of the guiding principles of MID is that biomimetic dental material is used. As the toxic BPA and BPA derivates are released from dental resins (Fleisch et al. 2010; Kingman et al. 2012), this material needs to be adapted. These substances have been linked to a number of biological disorders (Eng et al. 2013; Jedeon et al. 2013; Yeo et al. 2013). This development has led the World Dental Federation (FDI 2013) to issue a policy statement on BPA, in which it discourages BPA use in the manufacturing of dental materials.

Atraumatic Restorative Treatment (ART) High-Viscosity Glass-Ionomers

ART sealants use a high-viscosity glass-ionomer, which is placed over carious lesion-prone pits and fissures under finger pressure. Hand instruments (such as an excavator and an applier/carver) are used for adjusting the bite and removing excess glass-ionomer material. In applying this approach, sealants can be placed in situations independent of the need for rotary instruments and thus electricity and running water.

Effectiveness of Fissure Sealants

In the literature, effectiveness is often expressed as the survival of fully and partially retained sealants and as the survival of cavitated dentine carious lesion-free tooth surface.

We know that sealants deteriorate over time. The rate of sealant deterioration varies from brand to brand but is on average higher among the group of glass-ionomer- than resin-based materials (Kühnisch et al. 2012). Among the glass-ionomers, retention of the high-viscosity type, particularly when applied under finger pressure as part of the ART approach, is on average higher than for the medium-viscosity type (van 't Hof MA et al. 2006). Encapsulated high-viscosity glass-ionomers (HVGIC) show higher mechanical strengths values than the hand-mix version (Dowling and Fleming 2009).

Despite the early exposure of parts of pits and fissures to the oral environment, the failure rate, expressed as the development of a cavitated dentine carious lesion, is not higher in glass-ionomer-based than in resin-based sealants (Beiruti et al. 2006a; Yengopal et al. 2009; Ahovuo-Saloranta et al. 2013). This phenomenon led Frencken and Holmgren (1999) to state that sealant retention should be considered only a surrogate endpoint of sealant effectiveness. The true endpoint is the absence of a cavitated dentine carious lesion in pits and fissures.

Comparison Between ART Sealants and Resin Sealants

As most long-term comparisons between the effectiveness of glass-ionomer-based materials and resin composite sealants over the last decade have used HVGIC applied according to the ART approach, it is of interest to analyse the outcomes of these comparisons. A total of five research articles could be retrieved. These covered studies of 2–5 years long carried out between 2006 and 2015 in Brazil, China and Syria, using the hand-mixed high-viscosity glass-ionomers Fuji IX (GC, Tokyo, Japan), Ketac Molar (3M ESPE, Seefeld, Germany) and Ketac Molar Easymix (3M ESPE, Seefeld, Germany) and the light-cured resin sealants Clinpro (3M ESPE, Seefeld, Germany), Delton (3M, St Pauls, USA), Fluoroshield (Dentsply, York, USA) and Helioseal (Ivoclar, Schaan, Liechtenstein).

Of the five studies, one showed a significantly higher cavitated dentine carious lesion-preventing effect in occlusal surfaces for ART/HVGIC than for resin composite sealants (Beiruti et al. 2006b), while no difference was obtained in the four remaining studies. Three studies used the same ART carious lesion assessment criteria (Beiruti et al. 2006b; Zhang et al. 2014; Hilgert et al. 2015) while four studies sealed only high-caries risk occlusal surfaces in first permanent molars (Beiruti et al. 2006b; Zhang et al. 2014; Liu et al. 2014; Hilgert et al. 2015) (Table 18.2). Given that, in addition to the methodological differences, different brands of materials and different operators were used, it is remarkable that sealants produced through the ART procedure using high-viscosity glass-ionomers show a similar or significantly higher performance than resin composite sealants, which were considered to be the reference sealant material (Deery 2013).

On the basis of extensive evidence, the use of dental sealants is strongly recommended for all at-risk surfaces. Both resin composite material and high-viscosity glass-ionomers, in combination with the ART approach, show good results (Table 18.3).

18.4 Managing Dentine Carious Lesions

18.4.1 How Does One Manage a Dentine Carious Lesion?

Providing a response to this question is not straightforward. The answer will depend on the stage of the carious lesion. Activities aimed at managing such a lesion should be directed at inactivation/control of the disease process, preservation of dental hard tissue, avoidance of initiating the cycle of re-restorations, and preservation of the tooth for as long as possible (Schwendicke et al. 2016).

Table 18.2 Comparison of the effectiveness of ART/HVGIC and resin composite sealants in preventing cavitated dentine carious lesion development in occlusal surfaces by year of study

		ART/HVGIC		Resin composite		Test outcome
Author	Year	*N*	%	*N*	%	*p*-value
Beiruti et al. (2006b)	5	139	94.1	115	78.8	0.003
Barja-Fidalgo et al. (2009)	5	21	87.0	28	80.0	0.27
Zhang et al. (2014)	4	239	97.3	297	96.4	0.31
Liu et al. (2014)	2	179	92.7	178	96.1	0.17
Hilgert et al. (2015)	3	69	90.2	169	91.4	0.59

N number of occlusal sealants, *ART/HVGIC* atraumatic restorative treatment/high-viscosity glass-ionomer cement

Inactivating the disease process is achieved by controlling the amount and frequency of free sugar intake daily and by removing the (cariogenic) biofilm from any tooth surface on a daily basis. Preservation of dental hard tissue is achieved by applying minimally invasive operative interventions and by removing only soft to firm tooth tissue from within a tooth cavity, allowing the remaining demineralised dentine to remineralise. The repeat restoration cycle can be avoided if the cleaned cavity is restored under optimal clinical conditions with an appropriate restorative material. An additional measure is the protection of the margins with a sealant material, which results in a so-called sealant-restoration (Simonson and Stallard 1977). Daily removal of the biofilm from all tooth surfaces will ensure that the tooth is preserved for a long time, provided that the periodontal tissues are kept healthy.

Table 18.3 Overview of the preventive agents and their evidence-based effectiveness

Non-fluoride agents	
CPP-ACP	Lack of evidence that it is superior to protection offered by fluoride agents
Ozone	Lack of evidence
Chlorhexidine	The evidence for the varnish is low. It may be a short-term option for carious lesion control in individuals at high-caries risk who have high microorganism counts. There is a lack of evidence for mouthwash and gel
Sealants	The evidence is high compared to no sealing. Particularly suitable for high-caries risk children

The MID philosophy seeks to preserve natural tooth tissue for as long as possible through not removing enamel and dentine tissue unnecessarily and by supporting remineralisation of demineralised enamel and dentine. Hence, non-restorative treatments have a place in managing dentine carious lesions within MID. For permanent teeth, such a treatment is suggested for non-cavitated dentine carious lesions, while in primary teeth this treatment is advocated for both non- and cavitated dentine carious lesions, as shown in Fig. 18.1.

18.4.2 Non-cavitated Dentine Carious Lesions

Non-cavitated enamel carious lesions can be managed through diet control, biofilm control with fluoride-containing toothpaste and, on indication of high caries activity in pits and fissures, through the application of a fissure sealant. These activities have been shown to be effective in reducing or stopping the activity of the caries process (Frencken et al. 2012a). But what would be the treatment for a

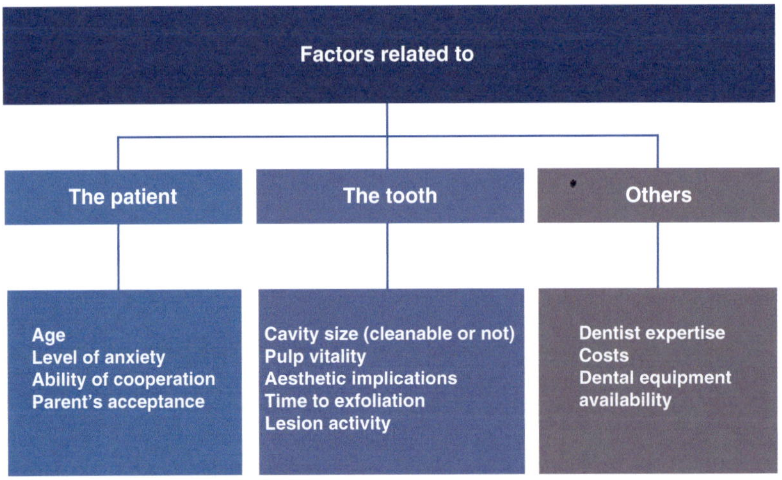

Fig. 18.1 Factors that should be considered when opting for non- or restorative treatment in the primary dentition

dentine carious lesion without an obvious cavitation? This condition is recorded when the ICDAS system and the CAST instrument (Code 4) are used. It is obvious that such lesions present a challenge to the dental practitioner. Can such a dentine carious lesion be sealed over in the same way as enamel carious lesions? Unfortunately, not many studies have investigated this condition; however, a few approaches have been proposed. It has been suggested that active lesions that are visible on radiographs can be either sealed or restored according to the MID principles (Ismail et al. 2013). Although not much evidence exists regarding the use of noninvasive procedures in this type of carious lesion, the application of pit and fissure sealants over non-cavitated dentinal occlusal carious lesions has been shown to be effective in arresting carious lesion progression after 36 months of follow-up in a group of high-caries risk patients (Borges et al. 2012).

It appears that insufficient evidence is available to guide the dental practitioner in the best way to treat such a condition. Strangely, more information, originating from decades ago, is available for treating small cavitated dentine carious lesions. A similar question as posed above can be formulated: Do small cavitated dentine carious lesions need to be treated restoratively or could a sealant be an effective treatment? This issue is dealt with in the section below.

18.4.3 Small Cavitated Dentine Carious Lesions

Evidence about sealing cavitated dentine carious lesions in permanent teeth comes from a clinical trial in which medium-sized cavities in occlusal surfaces were treated with a sealant restoration without removing soft 'infected' dentine. The study showed a success rate of 86% after 10 years (Mertz-Fairhurst et al. 1998). Since then, discussions have been held in the literature and in congresses about the need to remove all soft dentine tissue from tooth cavities in order to stop carious lesion progression. The slogan 'The Seal is the Deal' was born (Kidd 2004a). Would this slogan be applicable for treating small dentine carious lesions in pits and fissures? A few studies to this effect have been published.

Already in the mid-eighties, Mertz-Fairhurst et al. (1986) showed that sealing over small dentine lesions in pits and fissures stopped carious lesion progression. The authors based this finding on the assessment of lesion depth and bacterial counts and on radiographic and clinical examination. Years later, small dentine lesions (<0.9 mm orifice) in subjects that were on average 14-year-old were sealed with a medium-viscosity glass-ionomer according to the ART principles. These sealants had prevented dentine lesion progression in 87.4% of the cases after 3 years in this low-caries risk group, which was a significantly higher percentage than for small dentine lesions that were left untreated (Frencken et al. 1998). In a medium-caries risk group of 7-year old, dentine carious lesion progression was stopped in 68.2% of small dentine carious lesions (<0.9 mm orifice) that were sealed over with resin composite and high-viscosity glass-ionomers after 5 years (Beiruti et al. 2006b). These studies compared the therapeutic sealant to no sealant use but what might one expect if the effectiveness of the therapeutic sealant were compared to a restoration?

Such an investigation has been performed in primary teeth over 18 months (Hesse et al. 2014) and in permanent teeth over 2–3 years (Bakhshandeh et al. 2012). Compared to conventional restorative treatment, the survival of sealed over cavities with a resin fissure sealant material was significantly lower in both studies. The results of these studies show that not only should one attempt to stop carious progression in these cavities noninvasively but that this practice is limited by the strength of the sealing material used. According to an in vitro study, sealing small cavitated dentine carious lesions in pits and fissures showed a higher level of micro-leakage and insufficient penetration of resin sealant material into the cavity, compared to sound pits and fissures (Hevinga et al. 2008).

Evidence so far shows that sealing over obvious dentine cavities with a (resin) fissure material is not indicated but that sealing over small dentine carious cavities is worth pursuing. The reasoning for performing this treatment on small dentine carious lesions relates to the fact that an invasive intervention can still be performed should the sealant not function well anymore. More research regarding this noninvasive treatment is necessary before this treatment becomes commonly used.

18.4.4 Obvious Cavitated Dentine Carious Lesions in Primary Teeth

18.4.4.1 Cleansable Cavitated Dentine Carious Lesions

From a cariological point of view, removing the biofilm from within the cavity with a toothbrush and fluoride-containing toothpaste, sometimes supported by regular application of a fluoride varnish in the cavity or a glass-ionomer base, can inactivate open cavitated dentine carious lesions. But, for this strategy to be effective, the cavity should be cleansable or made cleansable by removing obstructing enamel structure and/or dentine tissue with rotary or hand instruments. G.V. Black (1908) wrote about this noninvasive, non-restorative cavity control treatment as follows: 'All buccal and labial cavities in which decay is burrowing should be fully opened by clipping away all the overhanging enamel and left as wide open as possible in order to admit free washing, both in artificial cleaning and in fresh clean saliva.' But, what evidence exists for recommending non-restorative procedures? Some techniques have been proposed and investigated for application in the primary dentition. These are discussed below.

Ultraconservative Treatment

Two retrospective studies carried out in the UK in which primary teeth remained unrestored but received preventive care showed that the majority of the teeth (82%) exfoliated naturally and symptomless (Tickle et al. 2002; Levine et al. 2002). Considering these results and the fact that primary teeth have a relatively short life span, a prospective study was performed that compared a mainly non-restorative procedure with two restorative procedures. The rationale behind the study design was that regular toothbrushing with fluoridated toothpaste (1 100 ppm) would be sufficient for preventing medium- to large-sized cavitated dentine carious lesions from progressing while the difficult-to-clean small cavities could be restored using the ART approach (Frencken et al. 2012b). Some medium and large cavities were opened further using hand instruments to allow proper removal of biofilm with a toothbrush. This protocol was termed 'ultraconservative treatment' (UCT). The UCT protocol was compared to the ART and to amalgam restorations in a group of high-caries risk children aged 6 to 7 years. Results showed no significant difference between the survival rates of teeth that were restored and those treated using the UCT protocol after 3.5 years (Mijan et al. 2014). There was also no significant difference in the exfoliation pattern of primary molars between the three treatment protocols after 3.5 years (Mijan et al. 2015). About 88% of teeth treated using UCT exfoliated without any pathology and/or toothache (Mijan et al. 2015).

Such results reinforce the idea postulated by Kidd (2004) that nonoperative treatments can lead cavitated deciduous teeth to exfoliate without pain. However, it is important that more studies in which similar approaches are tested are conducted. These are necessary not only to generate evidence about this treatment protocol but because nonoperative approaches based on diet and oral hygiene control may turn out to be the best strategy for overcoming the reality reported by Marcenes et al. (2013), that untreated cavitated dentine lesions in primary teeth affect more than 620 million children in the world. Treating these cavities restoratively is simply not possible and might not be needed.

Silver Diamine Fluoride

The effectiveness of removing the biofilm from within a cavity in controlling carious lesion progression was thought years ago to be increased by placing silver diamine fluoride (SDF) in the open cavity. SDF is a combination of silver nitrate and sodium fluoride ($Ag(NH_3)_2F$). When applied to carious tissues, it inhibits carious lesion progression by its interaction with bacteria (Knight et al. 2007). For that reason, open cavities have been treated using SDF, particularly in primary teeth. The main disadvantage of using SDF is that the lesions treated will be stained black and might displease some children and parents.

In terms of effectiveness, a series of clinical trials has shown that the application of 38% SDF was effective in arresting dentine cavitated carious lesions in upper anterior teeth of children aged 3 to 5 years (Lo et al. 2001; Chu et al. 2002) and in primary canines and molars of 6-year-old schoolchildren (Llodra et al. 2005). Different concentrations (12% and 38%) of SDF were tested in arresting dentine carious lesions in children aged 5, and the results showed that a single spot application of 38% SDF is more effective than the 12% concentration after 24 months but that the effectiveness decreases over time (Yee et al. 2009).

It is concluded that SDF can be considered an alternative treatment for primary teeth where other caries control strategies are not available. However, the optimum frequency of application needs to be investigated.

Hall Technique

The Hall Technique (HT) cannot be considered a nonoperative approach when compared to the UCT and to the use of SDF. However, this technique also differs from the conventional restorative approaches. It requires the placement of a preformed metal crown over a cavitated dentine carious lesion, without the use of local anaesthesia and the removal of carious tissue (Innes et al. 2006). Because of this description, HT has been classified as a conservative way of managing dentine carious lesions in primary molars (Leal 2014).

Results from a 5-year follow-up clinical trial in which the failure rates of the HT were compared with those from restorations placed by general dental practitioners in the UK showed that the HT crowns performed significantly better than the conventional restorations (Innes et al. 2011). Additionally, when the technique was compared to a nonoperative approach (no carious tissue removal, teaching brushing and fluoride application) and to the placement of compomer restorations, it was found that HT crowns were significantly more successful clinically than the other approaches after 1 year (Santamaria et al. 2014). When compared retrospectively to the traditional way of performing stainless steel crowns, it was found that the success rate of the two procedures was similar (Ludwig et al. 2014).

Although this strategy seems to be an effective way of managing carious lesions, barriers to its implementation were brought up by undergraduates. These included financial pressures and the ease of using glass-ionomer cement as an alternative treatment option (Gilchrist et al. 2013). However, in a study that assessed parents, children and dentists' perceptions of the HT in comparison to a nonoperative and to the conventional approaches, more than 77% of the dentists who performed the treatment reported that both HT and the nonoperative approach were very easy or easy to perform (Santamaria et al. 2015).

The HT seems to have potential for guiding cavitated dentine carious lesions to exfoliation in an atraumatic way but the evidence is still not abundant.

18.4.5 Restorative Management of Carious Lesions

According to Kidd (2004), the aims of restorative management are to aid biofilm control at the restored surface of the tooth instead of removing it from within the cavity; protect the pulp-dentine complex and arrest the carious lesion by sealing it; and restore the function, form and aesthetic appearance of the tooth.

Within the MID philosophy for dental caries, the principal guideline for managing a cavitated tooth is to remove the soft dentine, to leave the firm to hard demineralised dentine behind and to restore the cleaned cavity with a restorative material that has optimum biological and physical properties (Frencken et al. 2012a). Demineralised dentine has the ability to remineralise, as Fusayama (1993) showed decades ago.

Remineralisation of demineralised dentine occurs through (i) the function of the odontoblast process, providing calcium and phosphate from the vital pulp (Fusayama 1993); (ii) diffusion of ions (fluoride, calcium and phosphate) from materials placed on the floor of a restored cavity (Ngo et al. 2006; Peters et al. 2010); and (iii) contact of saliva with the carious lesion, providing calcium and phosphate, notably in root dentine in conjunction with oral hygiene measures (van Loveren and Duggal 2001)

Retention of decomposed dentine and remnants of cariogenic biofilm in a cavity skillfully restored with a well-manufactured restorative material that seals the cavity and restoration margin leads to the depletion of the cariogenic potential of those remnants of dental biofilm. Systematic reviews have reported that microorganisms left behind in cavities sealed over have no further ability to drive the caries process once they are disconnected from the oral cavity. The microorganisms are deprived of the source of metabolic nutrition required for their survival and for the production of acid, which demineralises tooth surfaces. This situation leads to a change in the environment of cariogenic microorganisms and inhibits their metabolic ability (Mertz-Fairhurst et al. 1986; Handelman et al. 1987; Oong et al. 2008). If the restoration margin is also sealed, this increases the chance not only of increased longevity of the restored tooth but also of a reduction in the development of secondary caries (Martin et al. 2013).

18.4.5.1 Principles for the Removal of Demineralised Carious Dentine

In February 2015, a group of 21 cariologists from 12 different countries met in Leuven, Belgium, and formed the International Caries Consensus Collaboration (ICCC). The ICCC agreed by consensus on the following guidelines for the removal of carious tissue (Schwendicke et al. 2016):

- Preserve non-demineralised and remineralisable tissue.
- Achieve an adequate seal by placing the peripheral restoration onto sound dentine and/or enamel, thus controlling the carious lesion and inactivating remaining bacteria.
- Avoid discomfort/pain and dental anxiety as both impact significantly on treatment/care planning and outcomes. Methods that are less likely to lead to dental anxiety are preferable.
- Maintain pulpal health by preserving residual dentine (avoiding unnecessary pulpal irritation/insult) and preventing pulp exposure, i.e. leave soft dentine in proximity to the pulp if required. Avoiding pulpal exposure has great impact both on the lifetime prognosis of the tooth and long-term treatment costs (Whitworth et al. 2005; Bjørndal et al. 2010). This preservation is more likely to occur even if the softer, bacterial-containing dentine is left over the floor of the cavity.
- Maximise longevity of the restoration by removing enough soft dentine to place a durable restoration of sufficient bulk and resilience.

The consensus meeting further agreed that:

> When dealing with teeth with sensible (vital) pulps, free from pathologic signs and symptoms, these last two aims, maintaining pulpal health and maximising restoration longevity, might need to be balanced against each other. In deep lesions (radiographically involving the inner pulpal third or quarter of dentine, or with clinically assessed risk of pulpal exposure), preservation of pulpal health should be prioritised. In shallow or moderately deep lesions (those not reaching the inner third or quarter of the dentine), restoration longevity is more important.

18.4.5.2 How Much Demineralised Carious Dentine Needs to be Removed?

The many studies that have investigated the state of demineralised dentine under well-sealed restorations have demonstrated that not all demineralised dentine needs to be removed (Frencken et al. 2012a). Removing all discoloured dentine prohibits the demineralised dentine from remineralising and weakens the tooth unnecessarily. The latter goes against the main aim of MID, which is keeping teeth for life.

The ICCC group proposed five strategies for the removal of carious tissue in teeth with vital pulps and no irreversible pulpitis. These strategies are based on the level of hardness of the remaining dentine. As, over the years, the literature has produced a number of different names for (almost) the same situation, researchers, dental professionals and the readers in general have become confused. The ICCC has suggested new names for the various methods of removing carious tissue to align these methods and avoid confusion. What is meant by the various (non) selective removals is presented below (Innes et al. 2016).

> *Nonselective removal to hard dentine* (formerly termed 'complete excavation' or 'complete caries removal') uses the same criterion in assessing the endpoint of carious tissue removal for all parts of the cavity, i.e. peripherally and pulpally. Only hard dentine is left so that demineralised dentine that is 'free' of bacteria is completely removed. This removal method is considered overtreatment and no longer advocated.
>
> *Selective removal to firm dentine* leaves 'leathery' dentine pulpally; a hand excavator encounters feeling of resistance while the cavity margins and peripheral dentine are left hard (scratchy) after removal. Selective removal to firm dentine is the treatment of choice for both dentitions, in shallow or moderately deep cavitated dentine lesions (i.e. lesions that extend radiographically less than the pulpal third or quarter of dentine). In deeper lesions, selective removal to firm dentine bears significant risks for the pulp, which is why other strategies should be considered.
>
> *Selective removal to soft dentine* is recommended in deep cavitated lesions (i.e. extending into the pulpal third or quarter of the dentine). Soft carious tissue is left over the pulp to prevent exposure and 'stress' of the pulp, promoting pulpal health, while peripheral enamel and dentine are prepared to hard dentine, to allow a tight seal and placement of a durable restoration. Selective removal to soft dentine significantly reduces the risk of pulpal exposure compared with nonselective removal to hard or selective removal to firm dentine.
>
> *Stepwise removal* is carious tissue-removal method performed in two stages (visits) (Bjørndal et al. 1997). Soft carious tissue is left over the pulp in the first step, while peripheral dentine is prepared to hard dentine to allow a complete and durable seal of the lesion. A provisional restoration is placed, which should be sufficiently durable to last up to 12 months to allow changes in the dentine and pulp to take place. The subsequent removal of this provisional restoration should then be followed by the selective removal to firm dentine pathway with the placement of a definitive restoration aiming for longevity. This technique has previously been known as 'two-step excavation'.

In summary, the amount of tissue that needs to be removed and how much carious tissue is left behind will depend on the clinical aspects of the lesion (depth and size) and the risk of pulp exposure. It should be the dentist's task to weigh up the advantages of pulp preservation against restoration longevity in order to provide the best treatment so that the tooth survives for as long as possible.

18.4.5.3 Which Dentine Carious Tissue Removal Method Is Preferable?

Most of the studies that have investigated the efficacy of the various carious tissue-removal methods have used different endpoints to delineate decomposed dentine. These endpoints cannot be related to the ICCC suggested strategies for the removal of dentine carious tissue. However, using results of available in vitro studies on this topic, it appears that rotating round metal burs have the tendency to over-prepare cavities and that laser and oscillation techniques underprepare cavities. Self-limiting burs made of polymer and ceramic material have also been found to underprepare cavities. The most appropriate dentine carious tissue-removal methods used either a chemo-mechanically applied gel or a metal hand excavator (Frencken et al. 2012a). In the philosophy of minimally invasive intervention, it may be more appropriate to consider pain, maintenance of pulpal health and retention of the tooth as relevant endpoints than the classical hardness, moisture, colour, fluorescence property and dye stainability (Schwendicke et al. 2016).

The ICCC purposely did not advise which carious tissue-removal method should be used. But following the group's guidelines, the patient-centred item (avoid discomfort/pain and anxiety) should be considered important. It is known that dental anxiety, developed at a young age, may lead to avoidance of self-care and seeking professional care and, eventually, to poor oral health. As hand instruments appear to cause less dental anxiety and discomfort/pain in children (Frencken et al. 2012b) and have been shown to be selective in removing carious tissues, a treatment using hand excavation should be preferred over rotary-driven excavation when removing carious tissues from dentine.

18.4.5.4 Disinfecting Excavated Tooth Cavities

Disinfecting the cavity before restoring it has been a common activity for a prolonged period of time. It was originally performed to ensure that as many microorganisms as possible were killed, which reduced the chance of the onset of a new carious lesion alongside the restoration margin. This action is associated with the erroneous thought that a carious lesion is solely caused by microorganisms, independent of the presence of fermentable substrate. We have argued and provided evidence that microorganisms, retained under a well-sealed restoration, are reduced in numbers over time and have no potential to demineralise the enamel and dentine further, provided that the seal remains secured.

The proof of the pudding should come from studies that have investigated the longevity of restorations in which the cavity was treated with and without a disinfectant. Common disinfection agents are 2% chlorhexidine solution and ozone gas. No significant difference was reported for restoration survival between cavities without disinfection and those disinfected with a 2% chlorhexidine solution using glass-ionomers after 2 years (Ersin et al. 2006) and 5 years (Farag et al. 2009). Long-term studies on cavity disinfection with ozone gas prior to restoration are lacking. In summary, no data is available to support the proposed need for cavity disinfection prior to restoration to increase the longevity of the restoration and the restored tooth.

18.4.5.5 Cavity Lining

Certain materials (predominantly calcium hydroxide-based and glass-ionomer-based) have been applied to the floor of the cavity for protective, therapeutic or structural reasons. The structural reason relates to the placement of amalgam and intra-coronal cast metal restorations. A therapeutic lining material may be placed in the base of very deep cavities in order to stimulate the odontoblasts to lay down reparative dentine, encourage remineralisation of the dentine and provide a hostile environment for any microorganism that may remain in the base. The protective action of a liner may prohibit chemical insults to the pulp (Kidd et al. 2004a).

We have presented evidence that microorganisms under a well-sealed restoration are inactive and reduced in number, becoming less threatening. Compared to placing no lining, a systematic review that included a limited number of cavities showed that, from the seven types of liners studied, only a mineral trioxide liner had a substantial antimicrobial effect (Schwendicke et al. 2015). That this additional antimicrobial effect is helpful in prolonging the life of a severely decayed tooth is not strongly supported by clinical studies.

Does a liner facilitate remineralisation of remaining dentine? This topic was studied and the authors concluded that remineralisation of the remaining dentine may not require a liner as it appears to be mediated by pulpal activities (Corralo and Maltz 2013). Further information comes from a systematic review (Schwendicke et al. 2015). Using failure, defined as the need to re-retreat after more than 1-year follow-up, as an inclusion criterion, three randomised clinical trials were included in a systematic review that investigated the effectiveness of cavity liners. The review concluded that strong recommendations for using cavity liners are unsubstantiated, but firm evidence for omitting calcium hydroxide lining is also unavailable. Placing a liner may be indicated for pulp protection from monomers released from resin composite materials (Galler et al. 2005; Modena et al. 2009).

The ICCC group agreed on a weak graded recommendation that reads as follows (Schwendicke et al. 2016):

> Placement of cavity lining materials is not necessary to control the sealed carious lesion but might be beneficial in impeding monomer penetration and avoidance of fracture of the remaining dentine when resin composite is the restorative material.

18.4.5.6 Restorative Materials

With the signing and ratification by governments of the 2013 'Minamata Treaty on Mercury', the future for amalgam in dentistry had been decided.

The Treaty has created the opportunity to develop a restorative material(s) that has (have) biomimetic characteristics. Restorative materials of the future should be biologically sound and physically strong enough to function in an oral environment for up to 80 years. Dental materials that contain toxic elements, such as resin composite, need to be changed (FDI 2013). These materials need to be adapted by removing/replacing the monomers. For this reason glass-based materials are currently the most biomimetic dental materials. A glass-ionomer cement contains biological features but has too low flexural strength, in general. The level of flexural strength differs according to the brand of glass-ionomer.

Minimally invasive interventions and adhesive materials and systems go hand in hand. Resin-based and glass-ionomer-based materials each have strengths and weaknesses. These days, the quality of resin-based restorations is high (Kopperud et al. 2012). However, it is important to highlight that one of the factors related to the longevity of posterior composite restorations is the patient caries risk at baseline (Demarco et al. 2012), which reinforces the need for assessing patients' behavioural profiles before deciding which material to use. Glass-ionomer restorative materials have improved in strength over the last few decades. A glass-ionomer restorative was recommended initially for cavities in non-stress-bearing tooth surfaces. However, the latest systematic review on restoration comparison concluded that the survival rates of high-viscosity glass-ionomer restorations placed in stress-bearing surfaces in both primary and permanent dentitions were equal to or higher than those of comparable amalgam restorations (Mickenautsch et al. 2010). A systematic review conducted in 2013 did not report a difference between high-viscosity glass-ionomers and composite resin restorations in primary teeth (Raggio et al. 2013).

Dental practitioners ought to know the chemistry, characteristics and handling features of the restorative material that they are using. For choosing the most appropriate material for a particular situation, they need to be lifelong trainees. Proper application of that knowledge in clinical practice is the basis for a long-lasting restoration.

18.4.5.7 Restoring a Cleaned Cavity

The manner in which a cavity is restored makes an important contribution to the life expectancy of the tooth. It is not the intention of this chapter to provide explanations about operational techniques. In order to get this information, the reader needs to turn to textbooks about operative procedures. However, all minimally invasive operative restorative procedures should ensure the presence of a tight seal of the restorative material in the cavity to the enamel and dentine. This implies that the coronal part of the cavity should be as free from soft dentine as possible in order to obtain a secure bond of the adhesive material used to the available tooth structure. A further increase in tooth life expectancy is obtained by sealing the margins of the restoration and the adjacent pits and fissures when available and indicated. The restoration margin is the weakest part of the restored tooth. It is the most common reason for replacement of the restoration (Kidd et al. 2004b) and is reinforced if sealed over. Sealing remaining pits and fissures may prevent the occurrence of dentine carious lesions.

Already in the mid-1970s, Simonson and Stallard (1977) showed the advantage of this sealant-restoration method in occlusal surfaces, which they called the preventive resin restoration. At that time a small cavity was prepared according to the selective removal to hard dentine approach, restored with a resin composite and sealed over, including the adjacent pits and fissures, with a resin sealant material. The 5- and 9-year survival rates of restorations produced in this way were 95% (Welbury et al. 1990) and 75% (Houpt et al. 1994), respectively. In a comparative study, Mertz-Fairhurst et al. (1998) showed that the 10-year survival rates of sealed restorations of modified amalgam (98%) and resin composite (87%) material over frank cavitation were clinically superior to unsealed amalgam restorations placed according to the 'extension for prevention' principle (83%).

A sealant restoration using high-viscosity glass-ionomer as the restorative and as the sealant material is called the atraumatic restorative treatment (Frencken et al. 1994). This caries lesion management concept is presented below.

18.4.5.8 The Atraumatic Restorative Treatment

ART was introduced almost 30 years ago, when researchers were challenged to manage cavitated dentine lesions in an environment in which the rotary-driven restorative care was not possible because of the lack of electricity and/or piped water. At that time, the dentists made use of what was available in dentistry for many years: hand instruments for enlarging small cavity openings and for selective removal of carious dentine to soft (deep cavities) or firm (medium cavities) stages in vital teeth. Today, in completing this process, local anaesthesia is seldom needed and used in children; the ART process causes less dental anxiety than the traditional approach of using the drill.

Another pillar of the ART procedure is the use of adhesive materials, with a preference for HVGIC, since the large majority of the studies in which the ART approach was tested used this dental material. A great advantage of using HVGIC over composite resin is that it allows the practitioner to use the press-finger technique to place the material into the cavity, which leads to what is called a sealant-restoration. This occurs because by using the finger to press the glass-ionomer cement (GIC), it will penetrate the cavity and some excess will spread along the cavity margins and over the pit and fissures, sealing both areas. This is considered an extra preventive effect provided by this approach.

The effectiveness of ART restorations comes from the most recent meta-analysis (de Amorim et al. 2012). The meta-analysis concludes that:

- ART using high-viscosity glass-ionomer can be used safely in single-surface cavities in both primary and permanent posterior teeth.
- ART using high-viscosity glass-ionomer cannot be used routinely in multiple-surface cavities in primary posterior teeth.
- Insufficient information is available for conclusions to be drawn about ART restorations in multiple surfaces in permanent posterior teeth and in anterior teeth in both dentitions.

How Do ART Restorations Compare with Traditional Restorations? Systematic reviews and meta-analyses show that the longevity of ART restorations in primary teeth is no different from that produced using traditional methods with either amalgam (Mickenautsch et al. 2010; Mickenautsch and Yengopal 2012) or resin composite (Raggio et al. 2013). Similarly, in comparing ART and conventional restorations in primary teeth, there appears to be no difference in the longevity of single-surfaces restorations in the permanent dentition (Frencken et al. 2004; Mickenautsch et al. 2010). Dentine carious lesion development at the margin of ART glass-ionomer restorations was reported to be low (Lo et al. 2007; Zanata et al. 2011). This finding is supported by the results of another systematic review, which showed that glass-ionomer had a higher caries-preventive effect than amalgam restorations in permanent teeth, with no difference in primary teeth (Mickenautsch and Yengopal 2011).

It is concluded therefore that, for the moment, current evidence restricts the unconditional use of ART to the treatment of cavitated dentine carious lesions that affect single surfaces in both primary and permanent teeth.

18.5 How to Manage a Defective Restoration

Restorations deteriorate over time and some become defective to various degrees. Deciding when and in which way to intervene appears to be inconsistent among dentists as they do not always use objective criteria (Bader and Shugars 1993; Gordan et al. 2015). If in doubt, they tend to replace rather than repair a defective restoration (Mjör et al. 2000; Mjör et al. 2002). Repairing includes removing the defect only and re-restoring it or sealing the defect with a sealant material. Replacement of restorations constitutes over 50% of the work performed by general dental practitioners in their practices

(Mjör et al. 2000; Mjör et al. 2002). The most common reasons for restoration replacement in permanent and primary teeth are secondary carious lesions and staining of the margins of existing restorations (Pink et al. 1994; Deligeorgi et al. 2000). Certainly, positively assessed secondary carious lesions need to be treated restoratively. But whether the lesion is treated through a repair process or through a total replacement of the restoration is dependent on the size of the carious lesion. Staining of margins is frequently related to loss of bonding of composite resin material. The treatment of this defect may consist of sealing the defect, repolishing or refurbishing it or doing nothing and monitoring it, depending on the position of the defect.

Knowing that a replacement will enlarge the cavity unnecessarily and inevitably weaken the tooth, repairing, sealing, polishing and refurbishing the defected restoration comply more with the principles of the MID concept. But are these alternative options as good as the one that replaces the defective restoration totally? So far, prospective studies have shown that repaired restorations through removal of tissue in the defected area in permanent teeth have the same or increased longevity as restorations that were replaced completely over a period of 10 years for amalgam restorations (Moncada et al. 2015).

A recently published study followed a 'Bravo' score (the surface of the restoration has minimal surface defects) over a period of 10 years. A defect with a Bravo score was treated either through full replacement of the restoration or sealing the defect, or it received no treatment. The study showed no significant differences between the three treatments types after 10 years. Unfortunately, the number of treated teeth was low (Moncada et al. 2015).

An overview regarding restoration margins concludes that margin defects without visible evidence of soft dentine on the wall or base of the defect should be monitored, repaired or resealed, instead of total restoration replacement (Dennison and Sarrett 2012). This conclusion is in line with the strong graded recommendation of the ICCC group that reads: 'Re-treatment of restorations should aim to repair by resealing, refurbishing or repolishing where possible and replacement should be the last resort' (Schwendicke et al. 2016).

18.6 Concluding Remarks

The way the dental profession manages dental caries ought to be changed. Dental caries is preventable and it is, therefore, unacceptable that untreated cavitated dentine carious lesions in permanent and primary teeth are number one and ten, respectively, on the list of most prevalent medical conditions over the period 1990-2010. This outcome calls for a greater emphasis on keeping healthy teeth healthy, right from birth into old age. People need to be convinced that a diet low in sugar consumption and twice daily toothbrushing with a fluoridated toothpaste are an absolute necessity if they wish to keep on enjoying the advantages of a good set of teeth. Exercising these two fundamental measures for keeping tooth cavities away is possible for a large part of the world population. However, societies exist in which maintaining oral health does not have a high priority for a number of reasons and in some societies toothbrush and (fluoride) toothpaste are not always available. The major task of the dental profession is to guide the public in creating an environment at home, school, the work place and institutions, in which these two carious lesion-preventive actions can be exercised. This requires, among other things, that dental training institutions shift the emphasis in the curriculum from teaching young students cavity-curing topics to teaching them cavity-preventive topics.

This chapter outlines some additional carious lesion-preventive measures and assesses evidence for their level of usefulness. It further provides information on how to keep cavitated teeth functional for many decades to come, using the latest state-of-the-art knowledge about cariology and restorative dentistry, all encompassed in the

MID philosophy. The dental profession has to act now and has to act on a broad scale. It knows how to prevent dental caries and it has to support the public in achieving this.

Acknowledgement We thank Mrs. S. van Tonder for having edited the chapter skillfully.

References

Ahovuo-Saloranta A, Forss H, Walsh T, Hiiri A, Nordblad A, Mäkelä M, Worthington HV. Sealants for preventing dental decay in the permanent teeth. Cochrane Database Syst Rev. 2013;3, CD001830.

Almaz ME, Sönmez IS. Ozone therapy in the management and prevention of caries. J Formos Med Assoc. 2015;114:3–11.

Alves LS, Fontanella V, Damo AC, Ferreira de Oliveira E, Maltz M. Qualitative and quantitative radiographic assessment of sealed carious dentin: a 10-year prospective study. Oral Surg Oral Med Oral Pathol Oral Radiol Endod. 2010;109:135–41.

Andersson A, Sköld-Larsson K, Hallgren A, Petersson LG, Twetman A. Effect of a dental cream containing amorphous cream phosphate complexes on white spot lesion regression assessed by laser fluorescence. Oral Health Prev Dent. 2007;5:229–33.

Azarpazhooh A, Limeback H. Clinical efficacy of casein phosphopeptide-amorphous calcium phosphate (CPP-ACP): a meta-analysis. J Am Dent Assoc. 2008;139:915–24.

Backer-Dirks O, Houwink B, Kwant GW. The results of 6 1/2 years of artificial fluoridation of drinking water in the Netherlands. The Tiel-Culemborg experiment. Arch Oral Biol. 1961;5:284–300.

Bader JD, Shugars DA. Agreement among dentists' recommendations for restorative treatment. J Dent Res. 1993;72:891–6.

Bakhshandeh A, Qvist V, Ekstrand KR. Sealing occlusal caries lesions in adults referred for restorative treatment: 2–3 years of follow-up. Clin Oral Investig. 2012;16:521–9.

Barja-Fidalgo F, Maroun S, de Oliveira BH. Effectiveness of a glass ionomer cement used as a pit and fissure sealant in recently erupted permanent first molars. J Dent Child (Chic). 2009;76:34–40.

Baysan A, Beighton D. Assessment of ozone-mediated killing of bacteria in infected dentine associated with non-cavitated occlusal carious lesions. Caries Res. 2007;41:337–41.

Beiruti N, Frencken JE, van 't Hof MA, van Palenstein Helderman WH. Caries-preventive effect of resin-based and glass ionomer sealants over time: a systematic review. Community Dent Oral Epidemiol. 2006a; 34:403–9.

Beiruti N, Frencken JE, van't Hof MA, Taifour D, van Palenstein Helderman WH. Caries-preventive effect of a one-time application of composite resin and glass ionomer sealants after 5 years. Caries Res. 2006b; 40:52–9.

Bjørndal L, Larsen T, Thylstrup A. A clinical and microbiological study of deep carious lesions during stepwise excavation using long treatment intervals. Caries Res. 1997;31:411–7.

Bjørndal L, Reit C, Bruun G, Markvart M, Kjaeldgaard M, Nasman P, Thordrup M, Dige I, Nyvad B, Fransson H, Lager A, Ericson D, Petersson K, Olsson J, Santimano EM, Wennstrom A, Winkel P, Gluud C. Treatment of deep caries lesions in adults: randomized clinical trials comparing stepwise vs. direct complete excavation, and direct pulp capping vs. partial pulpotomy. Eur J Oral Sci. 2010;118:290–7.

Black GV. Operative dentistry, vol 1. Pathology of hard tissues of the teeth. Chicago: Medico-Publishing Co.; 1908.

Borges BC, de Souza BJ, Braz R, Montes MA, de Assunção Pinheiro IV. Arrest of non-cavitated dentinal occlusal caries by sealing pit and fissures: a 36-month, randomised controlled clinical trial. Int Dent J. 2012;62:251–5.

Buonocore MG. A simple method of increasing the adhesion of acrylic filling materials to enamel surfaces. J Dent Res. 1955;34:849–53.

Burke FJT. Minimal intervention isn't just small cavities! Dent Update. 2008;35:509.

Burke FJ. Ozone and caries: a review of the literature. Dent Update. 2012;39:271–2, 275–278.

Chu CH, Lo EMC, Lin HC. Effectiveness of silver diamine fluoride and sodium fluoride varnish in arresting dentin caries in Chinese pre-school children. J Dent Res. 2002;81:767–70.

Corralo DJ, Maltz M. Clinical and ultrastructural effects of different liners/restorative materials on deep carious dentin: a randomized clinical trial. Caries Res. 2013;47:243–50.

de Amorim RG, Leal SC, Bezerra AC, de Amorim FP, de Toledo OA. Association of chlorhexidine and fluoride for plaque control and white spot lesion remineralization in primary dentition. Int J Paediatr Dent. 2008;18:446–51.

de Amorim RG, Leal SC, Frencken JE. Survival of atraumatic restorative treatment (ART) sealants and restorations: a meta-analysis. Clin Oral Investig. 2012;16:429–41.

Deery C. Strong evidence for the effectiveness of resin based sealants. Evid Based Dent. 2013;14:69–70.

Deligeorgi V, Wilson NH, Fouzas D, Kouklaki E, Burke FJ, Mjör IA. Reasons for placement and replacement of restorations in student clinics in Manchester and Athens. Eur J Dent Educ. 2000;4:153–9.

Demarco FF, Corrêa MB, Cenci MS, Moraes RR, Opdam NJ. Longevity of posterior composite restorations: not only a matter of materials. Dent Mater. 2012;28:87–101.

Dennison JB, Sarrett DC. Prediction and diagnosis of clinical outcomes affecting restoration margins. J Oral Rehabil. 2012;39:301–18.

Derks A, Katsaros C, Frencken JE, van't Hof MA, Kuijpers-Jagtman AM. Caries-inhibiting effect of preventive measures during orthodontic treatment with fixed appliances. A systematic review. Caries Res. 2004;38:413–20.

Disney JA, Graves RC, Stamm JW, Bohannan HM, Abernathy JR, Zack DD. The University of North Carolina Caries Risk Assessment study: further developments in caries risk prediction. Community Dent Oral Epidemiol. 1992;20:64–75.

Dowling AH, Fleming GJ. Are encapsulated anterior glass-ionomer restoratives better than their hand-mixed equivalents? J Dent. 2009;37:133–40.

Du MQ, Tai BJ, Jiang H, Lo EC, Fan MW, Bian Z. A two-year randomized clinical trial of chlorhexidine varnish on dental caries in Chinese preschool children. J Dent Res. 2006;85:557–9.

Elderton R. Principles in the management and treatment of dental caries. In: Elderton R, editor. The dentition and dental care. Oxford: Heinemann Medical Books; 1990. p. 237–62.

Eng DS, Lee JM, Gebremariam A, Meeker JD, Peterson K, Padmanabhan V. Bisphenol A and chronic disease risk factors in US children. Pediatrics. 2013;132:e637–45.

Ersin NK, Uzel A, Aykut A, Candan U, Eronat C. Inhibition of cultivable bacteria by chlorhexidine treatment of dentin lesions treated with the ART technique. Caries Res. 2006;40:172–7.

Farag A, van der Sanden WJ, Abdelwahab H, Mulder J, Frencken JE. 5-Year survival of ART restorations with and without cavity disinfection. J Dent. 2009;37:468–74.

FDI World Dental Federation. FDI policy statement on bisphenol-A in dental restorative and preventive materials. Adopted by the FDI General Assembly: 30 August 2013 – Istanbul, Turkey. Int Dent J. 2013;63:284.

Fleisch AF, Sheffield PE, Chinn C, Edelstein BL, Landrigan PJ. Bisphenol A and related compounds in dental materials. Pediatrics. 2010;126:760–8.

Frencken JE, Holmgren CJ. Atraumatic restorative treatment for dental caries. Nijmegen: STI book b.v.; 1999.

Frencken JE, Songpaisan Y, Phantumvanit P, Pilot T. An atraumatic restorative treatment (ART) technique: evaluation after one year. Int Dent J. 1994;44:460–4.

Frencken JE, Makoni F, Sithole WD, Hackenitz E. Three-year survival of one-surface ART restorations and glass-ionomer sealants in a school oral health programme in Zimbabwe. Caries Res. 1998;32:119–26.

Frencken JE, Holmgren CJ, van Palenstein Helderman WH. Basic package of oral care. Nijmegen: WHO Collaborating Centre for Oral Health Care Planning and Future Scenarios; 2002.

Frencken JE, van't Hof MA, van Amerongen WE, Holmgren CJ. Effectiveness of single-surface ART restorations in the permanent dentition: a meta-analysis. J Dent Res. 2004;83:120–3.

Frencken JE, de Amorim RG, Faber J, Leal SC. The Caries Assessment Spectrum and Treatment (CAST) index: rational and development. Int Dent J. 2011;61:117–23.

Frencken JE, Peters MC, Manton DJ, Leal SC, Gordan VV, Eden E. Minimal intervention dentistry for managing dental caries – a review: report of a FDI task group. Int Dent J. 2012a;62:223–43.

Frencken JE, Leal SC, Navarro MF. Twenty-five-year atraumatic restorative treatment (ART) approach: a comprehensive overview. Clin Oral Investig. 2012b;16:1337–46.

Fusayama T. A simple pain-free adhesive restorative system by minimal reduction and total etching. Tokyo: Ishiyaku EuroAmerica Inc Tokyo; 1993. p. 1–21.

Fusayama T. The process and results of revolution in dental caries treatment. Int Dent J. 1997;47:157–66.

Galler K, Hiller KA, Ettl T, Schmalz G. Selective influence of dentin thickness upon cytotoxicity of dentin contacting materials. J Endod. 2005;31:396–9.

Gilchrist F, Morgan AG, Farman M, Rodd HD. Impact of the Hall technique for preformed metal crown placement on undergraduate paediatric dentistry experience. Eur J Dent Educ. 2013;17:e10–5.

Gordan VV, Riley 3rd J, Geraldeli S, Williams OD, Spoto 3rd JC, Gilbert GH, National Dental PBRN Collaborative Group. The decision to repair or replace a defective restoration is affected by who placed the original restoration: Findings from the National Dental PBRN. Tex Dent J. 2015;132:448–58.

Griffin SO, Oong E, Kohn W, Vidakovic B, Gooch BF; CDC Dental Sealant Systematic Review Work Group, Bader J, Clarkson J, Fontana MR, Meyer DM, Rozier RG, Weintraub JA, Zero DT. The effectiveness of sealants in managing caries lesions. J Dent Res. 2008;87:169–74.

Handelman SL, Leverett DH, Espeland M, Curzon J. Retention of sealants over carious and sound tooth surfaces. Community Dent Oral Epidemiol. 1987;15:1–5.

Hesse D, Bonifácio CC, Mendes FM, Braga MM, Imparato JC, Raggio DP. Sealing versus partial caries removal in primary molars: a randomized clinical trial. BMC Oral Health. 2014;14:58.

Hevinga MA, Opdam NJ, Frencken JE, Bronkhorst EM, Truin GJ. Can caries fissures be sealed as adequately as sound fissures? J Dent Res. 2008;87:495–8.

Hiiri A, Ahovuo-Saloranta A, Nordblad A, Mäkelä M. Pit and fissure sealants versus fluoride varnishes for preventing dental decay in children and adolescents. Cochrane Database Syst Rev. 2010;17, CD003067.

Hilgert LA, Leal SC, Mulder J, Creugers NH, Frencken JE. Caries-preventive effect of supervised toothbrushing and sealants. J Dent Res. 2015;94:1218–24.

Houpt M, Fuks A, Eidelman E. The preventive resin (composite resin/sealant) restoration: nine-year results. Quintessence Int. 1994;25:155–9.

Hugoson A, Koch G, Göthberg C, Helkimo AN, Lundin SA, Norderyd O, Sjödin B, Sondell K. Oral health of individuals aged 3–80 years in Jönköping, Sweden during 30 years (1973–2003). II. Review of clinical and radiographic findings. Swed Dent J. 2005;29:139–55.

Innes NPT, Stirrups DR, Evans DJ, Hall N, Leggate M. A novel technique using preformed metal crowns for managing carious molars in general practice – a retrospective analysis. Clin Oral Investig. 2006;200:451–4.

Innes NP, Evans DJ, Stirrups DR. Sealing caries in primary molars: randomized control trial, 5-year results. J Dent Res. 2011;90:1405–10.

Innes NPT, Frencken JE, Bjørndal L, Maltz M, Manton DJ, Ricketts D, Van Landuyt K, Banderjee A, Campus G, Doméjean S, Fontana M, Leal S, Lo E, Machiulskiene V, Schulte A, Splieth C, Zandona AF, Schwendicke F. Managing carious lesions: Consensus recommendations on terminology. Adv Dent Res. 2016; in print

Ismail AI, Telles M, Pitts NB, Ekstrand KR, Ricketts D, Longbottom C, Eggertsson H, Deery C, Fisher J, Young DA, Featherstone JD, Evans W, Zeller GG, Zero D, Martignon S, Fontana M, Zandona A. Caries management pathways preserve dental tissue and promote oral health. Community Dent Oral Epidemiol. 2013;41:e12–40.

James P, Parnell C, Whelton H. The caries-preventive effect of chlorhexidine varnish in children and adolescents: a systematic review. Caries Res. 2010;44:333–40.

Jedeon K, De la Dure-Molla M, Brookes SJ, Loiodice S, Marciano C, Kirkham J, Canivenc-Lavier MC, Boudalia S, Bergès R, Harada H, Berdal A, Babajko S. Enamel defects reflect perinatal exposure to bisphenol A. Am J Pathol. 2013;183:108–18.

Johansson E, Claesson R, van Dijken JWV. Antibacterial effect of ozone on cariogenic bacterial species. J Dent. 2009;37:449–53.

Kidd EA. How 'clean' must a cavity be before restoration? Caries Res. 2004;38:305–13.

Kidd EAM, Smith BGN, Watson TF. Pickard's manual of operative dentistry. 8th ed. Oxford: Oxford University Press; 2004a. p. 68.

Kidd EAM, Smith BGN, Watson TF. Pickard's manual of operative dentistry. 8th ed. Oxford: Oxford University Press; 2004b. p. 194.

Kingman A, Hyman J, Masten SA, Jayaram B, Smith C, Eichmiller F, Arnold MC, Wong PA, Schaeffer JM, Solanki S, Dunn WJ. Bisphenol A and other compounds in human saliva and urine associated with the placement of composite restorations. J Am Dent Assoc. 2012;143:1292–302.

Knight GM, McIntyre JM, Craig GG, Mulyani ZPS, Gully NJ. Differences between normal and demineralized dentine pretreated with silver fluoride and potassium iodide after an in vitro challenge by Streptococcus mutans. Aust Dent J. 2007;52:16–21.

Kopperud SE, Tveit AB, Gaarden T, Sandvik L, Espelid I. Longevity of posterior dental restorations and reasons for failure. Eur J Oral Sci. 2012;120:539–48.

Kühnisch J, Mansmann U, Heinrich-Weltzien R, Hickel R. Longevity of materials for pit and fissure sealing – results from a meta-analysis. Dent Mater. 2012;28:298–303.

Leal SC. Minimal intervention dentistry in the management of the paediatric patient. Br Dent J. 2014;216:623–7.

Levine RS, Pitts NB, Nugent ZJ. The fate of 1,587 unrestored carious deciduous teeth: a retrospective general dental practice based study from northern England. Br Dent J. 2002;193:99–103.

Listl S, Galloway J, Mossey PA, Marcenes W. Global economic Impact of dental diseases. J Dent Res. 2015;94:1355–61.

Liu BY, Xiao Y, Chu CH, Lo EC. Glass ionomer ART sealant and fluoride-releasing resin sealant in fissure caries prevention – results from a randomized clinical trial. BMC Oral Health. 2014;14:54.

Llodra JC, Rodriguez A, Ferrer B, Menardia V, Ramos T, Morato M. Efficacy of silver diamine fluoride for caries reduction in primary teeth and first permanent molars of schoolchildren: 36-month clinical trial. J Dent Res. 2005;84:721–4.

Lo EMC, Chu CH, Lin HC. A community-based caries control program for pre-school children using topical fluorides: 18-month results. J Dent Res. 2001;80:2071–4.

Lo ECM, Holmgren CJ, Hu D, Wan H, van Palenstein Helderman W. Six-year follow-up of atraumatic restorative treatment restorations placed in Chinese school children. Community Dent Oral Epidemiol. 2007;35:387–92.

Ludwig KH, Fontana M, Vinson LA, Platt JA, Dean JA. The success of stainless steel crowns placed with the Hall Technique: a retrospective study. J Am Dent Assoc. 2014;145:1248–53.

Marcenes W, Kassebaum NJ, Bernabé E, Flaxman A, Naghavi M, Lopez A, Murray CJ. Global burden of oral conditions in 1990–2010: a systematic analysis. J Dent Res. 2013;92:592–7.

Marthaler TM. A standardized system of recording dental conditions. Helv Odontol Acta. 1966;10:1–18.

Martin J, Fernandez E, Estay J, Gordan VV, Mjor IA, Moncada G. Minimal invasive treatment for defective restorations: five-year results using sealants. Oper Dent. 2013;38:125–33.

Massler M. Pulpal reactions to dental caries. Int Dent J. 1967;17:441–60.

McIntyre J. Minimal intervention dentistry. Ann R Australas Coll Dent Surg. 1994;12:72–9.

Mertz-Fairhurst EJ, Schuster GS, Fairhurst CW. Arresting caries by sealants: results of a clinical study. J Am Dent Assoc. 1986;112:194–7.

Mertz-Fairhurst EJ, Curtis JW, Ergle JW, Rueggeberg FA, Adair SM. Ultraconservative and cariostatic sealed restorations: results at year 10. J Am Dent Assoc. 1998;129:55–66.

Mickenautsch S, Yengopal V. Absence of carious lesions at margins of glass-ionomer cement and amalgam restorations: an update of systematic review evidence. BMC Res Notes. 2011;4:58.

Mickenautsch S, Yengopal V. Failure rate of atraumatic restorative treatment using high-viscosity glass-ionomer cement compared to that of conventional amalgam restorative treatment in primary and permanent teeth: a systematic review update. J Minim Interv Dent. 2012;5:63–124. Erratum in: J Minin Interv Dent 2012: 5: 209–210.

Mickenautsch S, Yengopal V, Banerjee A. Atraumatic restorative treatment versus amalgam restoration longevity: a systematic review. Clin Oral Investig. 2010;14:233–40.

Mijan M, de Amorim RG, Leal SC, Mulder J, Oliveira L, Creugers NHJ, Frencken JE. The 3.5-year survival rates of primary molars treated according to three

treatment protocols: a controlled clinical trial. Clin Oral Investig. 2014;18:1061–9.
Mijan MC, de Amorim RG, Mulder J, Frencken JE, Leal SC. Exfoliation rates of primary molars submitted to three treatment protocols after 3.5 years. Community Dent Oral Epidemiol. 2015;43:232–9.
Mjör IA, Moorhead JE, Dahl JE. Reasons for replacement of restorations in permanent teeth in general dental practice. Int Dent J. 2000;50:360–6.
Mjör IA, Shen C, Eliasson ST, Richter S. Placement and replacement of restorations in general dental practice in Iceland. Oper Dent. 2002;27:117–23.
Modena KC, Casas-Apayco LC, Atta MT, Costa CA, Hebling J, Sipert CR, Navarro MF, Santos CF. Cytotoxicity and biocompatibility of direct and indirect pulp capping materials. J Appl Oral Sci. 2009;17:544–54.
Moncada G, Fernández E, Mena K, Martin J, Vildósola P, De Oliveira Junior OB, Estay J, Mjör IA, Gordan VV. Seal, replacement or monitoring amalgam restorations with occlusal marginal defects? Results of a 10-year clinical trial. J Dent. 2015;43:1371–8.
Müller F, Naharro M, Carlsson GE. What are the prevalence and incidence of tooth loss in the adult and elderly population in Europe? Clin Oral Implants Res. 2007a;18:2–14.
Müller P, Guggenheim B, Schmidlin P. Efficacy of gasiform ozone and photodynamic therapy on a multispecies oral biofilm in vitro. Eur J Oral Sci. 2007b;115:77–80.
Ngo HC, Mount G, Mc Intyre J, Tuisuva J, Von Doussa RJ. Chemical exchange between glass-ionomer restorations and residual carious dentine in permanent molars: an in vivo study. J Dent. 2006;34:608–13.
Nyvad B, Machiulskiene V, Baelum V. Reliability of a new caries diagnostic system differentiating between active and inactive caries lesions. Caries Res. 1999;33:252–60.
Oong EM, Griffin SO, Kohn WG, Gooch BF, Caufield PW. The effect of dental sealants on bacteria levels in caries lesions: a review of the evidence. J Am Dent Assoc. 2008;139:271–8.
Organisation for Economic Co-operation and Development (OECD). Health at a glance 2015: OECD indicators. OECD Publishing; 2015. doi:10.1787/health_glance-2015-en.
Paris S, Meyer-Lueckel H. Inhibition of caries progression by resin infiltration in situ. Caries Res. 2010;44:47–54.
Peters MC, Bresciani E, Barata TJ, Fagundes TC, Navarro RL, Navarro MF, Dickens SH. In vivo dentin remineralization by calcium-phosphate cement. J Dent Res. 2010;89:286–91.
Pink FE, Minden NJ, Simmonds S. Decisions of practitioners regarding placement of amalgam and composite restorations in general practice settings. Oper Dent. 1994;19:127–32.
Pitts N. "ICDAS"— an international system for caries detection and assessment being developed to facilitate caries epidemiology, research and appropriate clinical management. Community Dent Health. 2004;21:193–8.
Raggio DP, Hesse D, Lenzi TL, Guglielmi CA, Braga MM. Is Atraumatic restorative treatment an option for restoring occlusoproximal caries lesions in primary teeth? A systematic review and meta-analysis. Int J Paediatr Dent. 2013;23:435–43.
Raphael S, Blinkhorn A. Is there a place for Tooth Mousse® in the prevention and treatment of early dental caries? A systematic review. BMC Oral Health. 2015;15:113.
Reynolds EC. Anticariogenic complexes of amorphous calcium phosphate stabilized by casein phosphopeptides: a review. Spec Care Dentist. 1998;18:8–16.
Santamaria RM, Innes NP, Machiulskiene V, Evans DJ, Splieth CH. Caries management strategies for primary molars: 1-yr randomized control trial results. J Dent Res. 2014;93:1062–9.
Santamaria RM, Innes NP, Machiulskiene V, Evans DJ, Alkilzy M, Splieth CH. Acceptability of different caries management methods for primary molars in a RCT. Int J Paediatr Dent. 2015;25:9–17.
Schwendicke F, Tu YK, Hsu LY, Gostemeyer G. Antibacterial effects of cavity lining: a systematic review and network meta-analysis. J Dent. 2015;43:1298–307.
Schwendicke F, Frencken JE, Bjørndal L, Maltz M, Manton DJ, Ricketts D, Van Landuyt K, Banderjee A, Campus G, Doméjean S, Fontana M, Leal S, Lo E, Machiulskiene V, Schulte A, Splieth C, Zandona AF, Innes NPT. Managing carious lesions: consensus recommendations on carious tissue removal. Adv Dent Res. 2016; in print
Simonson RJ, Stallard RE. Sealant restorations utilizing a diluted filled resin: one year results. Quintessence Int Dent Dig. 1977;8:77–84.
Slot DE, Vaandrager NC, Van Loveren C, Van Palenstein Helderman WH, Van der Weijden GA. The effect of chlorhexidine varnish on root caries: a systematic review. Caries Res. 2011;45:162–73.
Tickle M, Milsom K, King D, Kearny-Mitchell BA. The fate of the carious primary teeth of children who regularly attend the general dental service. Br Dent J. 2002;192:219–23.
Tyas MJ, Anusavice KJ, Frencken JE, Mount GJ. Minimal intervention dentistry – a review. FDI commission project 1–97. Int Dent J. 2000;50:1–12.
van 't Hof MA, Frencken JE, van Palenstein Helderman WH, Holmgren CJ. The atraumatic restorative treatment (ART) approach for managing dental caries: a meta-analysis. Int Dent J. 2006;56:345–51.
van Loveren C, Duggal MS. The role of diet in caries prevention. Int Dent J. 2001;51:399–406.
van Rijkom HM, Truin GJ, van't Hof MA. A meta-analysis of clinical studies on the caries-inhibiting effect of chlorhexidine treatment. J Dent Res. 1996;75:790–5.
Walsh T, Oliveira-Neto JM, Moore D. Chlorhexidine treatment for the prevention of dental caries in children and adolescents. Cochrane Database Syst Rev. 2015;4, CD008457.
Welbury RR, Walls AWG, Murray JJ, McCabe JF. The management of occlusal caries in permanent molars. A 5-year

clinical trial comparing a minimal composite with an amalgam restoration. Br Dent J. 1990;169:361–6.
Whelton H, O'Mullane D. The use of combinations of caries preventive procedures. J Dent Educ. 2001;65:1110–3.
Whitworth JM, Myers PM, Smith J, Walls AW, McCabe JF. Endodontic complications after plastic restorations in general practice. Int Endod J. 2005;38:409–16.
Wilson AD, Kent BE. A new translucent cement for dentistry. The glass ionomer cement. Br Dent J. 1972;132:133–5.
World Health Organization. WHO's oral health country/area profile programme (CAPP) databse. 2013. http://www.mah.se/CAPP/Country-Oral-Health-Profiles. Caries distribution world-wide and in relation to socio-economic inequalities within and between countries.
Yamayoshi T, Tatsumi N. Microbicidal effects of ozone solution on methicillin-resistant Staphylococcus aureus. Drugs Exp Clin Res. 1993;19:59–64.
Yee R, Holmgren C, Mulder J, Lama D, Walker D, van Palenstein HW. Efficacy of silver diamine fluoride for arresting caries treatment. J Dent Res. 2009;88:644–7.
Yengopal V, Mickenautsch S. Caries preventive effect of casein phosphopeptide-amorphous calcium phosphate (CPP-ACP): a meta-analysis. Acta Odontol Scand. 2009;67:1–12.
Yengopal V, Mickenautsch S, Bezerra AC, Leal SC. Caries-preventive effect of glass ionomer and resin-based fissure sealants on permanent teeth: a meta analysis. J Oral Sci. 2009;51:373–82.
Yeo M, Berglund K, Hanna M, Guo JU, Kittur J, Torres MD, Abramowitz J, Busciglio J, Gao Y, Birnbaumer L, Liedtke WB. Bisphenol A delays the perinatal chloride shift in cortical neurons by epigenetic effects on the Kcc2 promoter. Proc Natl Acad Sci U S A. 2013;110:4315–20.
Zanata RL, Fagundes TC, Freitas MC, Lauris JR, Navarro MF. Ten-year survival of ART restorations in permanent posterior teeth. Clin Oral Investig. 2011;15:265–71.
Zhang Q, van Palenstein Helderman WH, van't Hof MA, Truin GJ. Chlorhexidine varnish for preventing dental caries in children, adolescents and young adults: a systematic review. Eur J Oral Sci. 2006;114:449–55.
Zhang W, Chen X, Fan MW, Mulder J, Huysmans MC, Frencken JE. Do light cured ART conventional high-viscosity glass-ionomer sealants perform better than resin-composite sealants: a 4-year randomized clinical trial. Dent Mater. 2014;30:487–92.

Invasive and Noninvasive Therapies

19

Sophie Doméjean, Michèle Muller-Bolla, and John D.B. Featherstone

19.1 Prevention in Dental Practice

19.1.1 What Is Prevention?

Prevention is the cornerstone of the concept of minimal intervention (MI) in dentistry in general and in cariology in particular. MI aims to prevent and intercept caries disease and to avoid relapses by acting on the modifiable pathological and protective risk factors mentioned above (Sheiham 2002).

S. Doméjean
Département d'Odontologie Conservatrice, CHU Clermont Ferrand, Service d'Odontologie, Hôtel Dieu, F-63001 Clermont Ferrand, France

Université Clermont 1, UFR d'Odontologie, Centre de Recherche en Odontologie Clinique EA 4847, F-63000 Clermont Ferrand, France

M. Muller-Bolla
Département d'Odontologie Pédiatrique, UFR d'Odontologie, UNS, Pôle Odontologie, CHU Nice URB2i- EA 4462, Paris Descartes, France

J.D.B. Featherstone (✉)
Department of Preventive and Restorative Dental Sciences, School of Dentistry, University of California San Francisco, UCSF, Room S630, 513 Parnassus Avenue, Box 0430, San Francisco, CA 94143-0430, USA
e-mail: jdbf@itsa.ucsf.edu

Thus MI needs to include all three domains of prevention: primary, secondary, and tertiary without forgetting quaternary prevention (Featherstone and Domejean 2012; Fédération Dentaire Internationale 2002; Jamoulle 2015).

- *Primary prevention* before the onset of the disease can be considered both at a population and at a family or individual level. The population level aims to target populations or groups that have been shown to be at high risk to develop the caries disease, for example, low-income populations, migrants or refugees, people with low health literacy, or institutionalized people. Prevention may be done by public health programs such as information/education campaigns or delivery fluoride therapy to all involved. Examples are fluoridated water at a population level and school-based interventions (education, fluoride rinses, or dental sealants) in socially deprived areas/communities. The individual level deals with early intervention and personalized education in reference to the identified risk factors. Prevention messages may concern the whole family (e.g., dietary habits and oral hygiene recommendations) with the aim of preventing caries in younger children.
- *Secondary prevention* can also be considered at both population and individual levels. For example, at a population level, school-based programs may aim at the detection of patients who need

M. Goldberg (ed.), *Understanding Dental Caries*, DOI 10.1007/978-3-319-30552-3_19

dental care. At the individual level, secondary prevention includes the detection of asymptomatic carious lesions to identify those in need of therapy. The objective of the secondary prevention is to intercept detected lesions using different noninvasive chemical therapy and/or microinvasive and minimally invasive restorative techniques. Primary and secondary preventions have to be considered together; indeed, if a patient is already affected by the caries disease, it is recommended to combine the traditional treatment plan and primary prevention techniques by considering, for example, preventive dental sealants on the caries-free permanent molars. Furthermore some products or techniques are used for both primary and secondary preventions with the same (e.g., dental sealants) or different (fluoridated topic agents) clinical protocols/procedures.

- *Tertiary prevention* deals with symptomatic lesions and aims to prevent further complications of the disease and also integrates the prevention of treatment failures. It thus includes both restorative techniques and patient follow-up.
- *Quaternary prevention*: a fourth dimension has been recently considered in medicine. Quaternary prevention (Jamoulle 2015) is the process that protects a patient from unnecessary medical procedures. This approach will help to control the economic and human costs of healthcare. In simple terms identification of patients at risk for a particular disease can suggest interventions, which are ethically acceptable, and avoid excessive treatment. The newly implemented dimension may have a huge impact in dentistry in the upcoming years. In the present context, the concept of caries management by risk assessment coupled with minimal intervention dentistry fits this model.

Historically, approaches to oral care have focused on individual restorative care rather than on population-based preventive interventions. However, the financial and human resource costs of this approach are unaffordable for many countries and unsustainable on a global scale. Most oral diseases can largely be prevented through simple, cost-effective measures that involve reducing exposure to recognized risks and strengthening healthy behaviors. Prevention and oral health promotion are highly cost-effective strategies to address the global burden of oral diseases (Fédération Dentaire Internationale 2015). For instance, the Fédération Dentaire Internationale (FDI) stated that estimates from the USA show that every dollar spent on preventive dental care could save between US$8 and US$50 in restorative and emergency treatment, emphasizing the importance of increasing the focus on the prevention of oral disease (Fédération Dentaire Internationale 2015).

19.1.2 Individual Caries Risk Assessment

The establishment of an individualized prevention plan requires an evaluation of the factors related to the disease process itself. This phase is called “caries risk assessment” (CRA). The process should identify disease indicators (clinical signs of caries), biological risk factors (or pathological factors), and protective factors. CRA can be done with a small number of factors and allows subsequent modification of the pathological factors and enhancement of the protective factors. The aim is to alter the so-called caries balance toward protection rather than progress of the disease (Featherstone 2003).

Many CRA methods have been developed and described in the literature: e.g., the system “Caries Management by Risk Assessment” (CAMBRA) (Featherstone et al. 2007), the “Cariogram” (Bratthall and Hansel Petersson 2005), the “Caries Risk Pyramid” (Morou-Bermudez et al. 2011), the “Caries-Risk Assessment Tool” (CAT) of the American Academy of Pediatric Dentistry (AAPD) (American Association of Pediatric Dentistry 2013), the form of the Collège des Enseignants en Odontologie Pédiatrique (CEOP) (Collège des Enseignants en Odontologie Pédiatrique 2014), or the “Dundee Caries Risk Assessment Model” (DCRAM) (Macritchie et al. 2012). All are based on the identification of variables that can be grouped in various ways, such as non-modifiable factors represented by high-risk groups (elderly, disabled, low socioeconomic status) versus modifiable factors by the patient and/or the practitioner and environmental factors versus behavioral versus biological factors.

Fontana et al. consider that even if critics of CRA argue that it is difficult to identify with certainty patients at risk and that the evidence of the effectiveness of preventive measures for individuals at high risk is not always very strong, CRA still has the potential to enhance patient care by allowing the practitioner and the patient to understand the specific reasons for the caries activity and to tailor the treatment plan and recall interval accordingly (Fontana and Gonzalez-Cabezas 2012; Twetman et al. 2013). In the absence of clear-cut consensus (Tellez et al. 2013; Twetman 2015a; Mejare et al. 2014), the choice was made in the present chapter to describe the CRA based on "disease indicators," "pathological factors," and "protective factors" as used in the CAMBRA system (Table 19.1).

- *Disease indicators* include the variables directly related to caries experience that, regardless of age, is a reflection of caries activity, past or present. These are primarily clinical observations that indicate the presence

Table 19.1 Caries risk assessment checklist

Factors	Description	Is the factor modifiable?
Disease indicators Having a high predictive value for further lesion development	*Caries experience* (Previous restorations, carious lesions from early demineralization to deep lesion that may have a pulpal involvement)	*No* Neither by the dental practitioner nor by the patient
Pathological factors Directly linked to the onset of the disease	*Bad oral hygiene* (Low frequency, absence of regular use of fluoridated agent)	*Yes* By the patient after professional advice and recommendations Toothbrushing at least twice a day with a fluoridated toothpaste at a concentration and amount adapted to age and caries risk status
	Frequent consumption of carbohydrates	*Yes* By the patient after professional advice and recommendations, coupled with substitution with non-cariogenic sweeteners such as xylitol
	Decreased saliva flow (Temporary due to medication or permanent due to head and neck irradiation)	*No* Neither by the dental practitioner nor by the patient. Additional aggressive antibacterial therapy and pH control (sodium bicarbonate) are essential for these patients
	Deep pits and fissures	*Yes* Sealant placement by a dental professional
	High cariogenic bacteria count	*Yes* By the patient after professional advice and recommendations using proven antibacterial therapy
	Exposed roots (Factors of plaque retention and stagnation)	*No, but…* The patient should follow professional advice and recommendations in terms of oral hygiene
	Appliances (orthodontic and prosthodontic) (Factors of plaque retention and stagnation)	*No, but…* The patient should follow professional advices and recommendations in terms of oral hygiene and high-concentration fluoride therapy
Protective factors Stopping or even counterbalancing the pathological factors	*Good saliva function*	No need for change
	Remineralizing and antibacterial agents	No need for change except for high and extreme risk when aggressive fluoride therapy and antibacterial therapy are needed

of disease, rather than the factors that caused it. Caries experience is determined by the presence of existing lesions (from early non-cavitated lesions to deep dentin carious lesion close to the pulp), restorations, and missing teeth due to caries. Active carious lesions have a strong predictive value and are a very strong indicator of future carious lesions, even without considering other factors. In preschool children, we need to consider not only the child's caries experience but also the presence of cavitated active lesions among the parents, the caregivers, and the siblings.

- *Pathological factors* are directly linked to the onset of the disease; they include inadequate oral hygiene (low frequency of toothbrushing, absence of regular use of fluoridated agent), inadequate oral environment (decreased saliva flow, high count of cariogenic bacteria), and frequent consumption of carbohydrates. More recently, a genetic component has been identified but is so far impossible to assess clinically in adults (Vieira et al. 2014). In young children some additional factors have to be noted, such as unfavorable eating habits linked to prolonged breastfeeding; prolonged use of a "sippy cup" containing milk, juice, or a sweetened beverage; or sleeping with a bottle that contains liquids other than water. During the first year, the predictive value of salivary counts of mutans streptococci and lactobacilli is higher than at later ages.
- *Protective factors* include the biological and therapeutic components involved in stopping or even counterbalancing the pathological factors. These include remineralizing and antibacterial agents such as fluoride, calcium phosphate, chlorhexidine, hypochlorite, silver diamine fluoride, and agents currently in development or that will be developed in the future. Unfortunately, some pathological factors cannot be easily corrected by the dental professional, such as decreased saliva flow due to some antihypertensive drugs, mood-altering medications, and numerous other medications that have hyposalivatory side effects in some people. Increased efforts by the patient himself/herself and the use of aggressive fluoride therapy and antibacterial therapy are needed to overcome the high caries challenge in these cases.

More important than the risk level determination (low/high in the French Haute Autorité de Santé (Haute Autorité de Santé 2005) recommendations or low/moderate/high/extreme in CAMBRA (Featherstone et al. 2007)) is the specific identification of the pathological and protective factors in order to plan customized preventive strategies adapted to individual needs and ability of compliance; a customized preventive plan aims to counterbalance individual pathological factors by strengthening individual protective factors. These procedures have been validated by outcomes assessments in thousands of patients demonstrating the ability of CAMBRA CRA to identify high- and extreme-risk patients with between 70 and 90 % success (Doméjean et al. 2011; Chaffee et al. 2015a, b).

Omitting to consider the CRA is nowadays unethical; indeed, despite the lack of consensus (Tellez et al. 2013), it has been shown that traditional restorative strategies have no effect of the bacterial count and the carious process itself (Featherstone et al. 2012; Elderton 1992, 1996). Moreover, baseline CRA helps both the practitioner and the patient to objectively understand the evolution of the carious process through follow-up and regular CRA (Lapidos et al. 2016).

19.1.3 Strategies for Prevention

Numerous strategies are available and can be used alone or in combination according to the individual need and individual CRA of each patient. As seen in the previous chapter, dental caries is characterized by demineralization of tooth tissues at lowered pH following bacterial fermentation of dietary carbohydrates. Thus essential components of the caries prevention and management are related to preventing the early colonization of infants by cariogenic bacteria as well as the control of the diet in terms of frequency of ingestion of fermentable carbohydrates (such as glucose, sucrose, fructose, or cooked starch), the inhibition of bacterial metabolism, and other strategies preventing demineralization and/or enhancing the remineralization to counterbalance the drop of pH following carbohydrates intake.

The following paragraphs discuss prevention strategies including education (prevention of the early contamination and dietary counseling), dental sealants, fluoridated agent, and non-fluoridated agents.

19.1.3.1 Education

Preventing Early Colonization

It is critical to consider an infant oral care program in the context of a participating pair or mother-and-child dyad, which includes comprehensive maternal perinatal oral healthcare, counseling, and treatment (Ramos-Gomez et al. 2012). Indeed, caries is a transmissible, infectious disease and generally, colonization of mutans streptococci (MS) in the oral cavity of children is the result of transmission of these organisms from the child's primary caregiver; numerous studies showed that a direct relationship exists between MS levels in adult caregivers and that of caries prevalence in their children. Factors influencing colonization include frequent sugar exposure in the infants and habits that allow salivary transfer from mother/caregiver to infants. Maternal factors, such as high levels of MS, poor oral hygiene, low socioeconomic status, low education level, and frequent snacking, increase the risk of bacterial transmission to her infant (Tinanoff et al. 2002; Seki et al. 2006; Douglass et al. 2008; da Silva Bastos Vde et al. 2015).

In the light of these facts, dental professionals must recognize the essential role a mother/caregiver plays in ensuring her child's oral health (Albino and Tiwari 2016). Improving expectant mothers' and caregiver's oral health by reducing pathogenic bacteria levels in their own mouths will delay the acquisition of oral bacteria and the development of early childhood caries in their children, and an effective perinatal program should institute practices such as therapeutic interventions and lifestyle modification counseling both during pre- and postpartum to reduce maternal MS and lactobacilli levels (Ramos-Gomez et al. 2012). Education aims also to inform the mother/caregiver of simple items such as using the same spoon may lead into early contamination.

Toothbrushing

Although the relationship between the presence of plaque and caries is not as clear as with gingivitis, there is clear evidence that the presence of plaque makes teeth more at risk of caries (Zenkner et al. 2013). It is illusionary to think that toothbrushing even combined with flossing results in a perfect plaque removal; nevertheless regular disruption of biofilm has been shown to play a key role in maintaining oral health in general and in caries prevention in particular. Effective toothbrushing depends on a number of factors including motivation, knowledge, and manual dexterity. Classically, toothbrushing is recommended at least twice a day (after breakfast and at bedtime); frequency can be increased according to the patient need (in case of orthodontic appliances favoring plaque stagnation and retention) and compliance. Emphasis has to be on frequency of the toothbrushing more than on the technique, as there is no consensus yet on the effectiveness of different methods/techniques; nevertheless, the Bass method is the most popular (Muller-Bolla and Courson 2013). For young patients, toothbrushing has to be supervised by an adult (for better plaque removal and to avoid ingestion of fluoride toothpaste). Manual toothbrushing is the method with the better cost-effectiveness ratio; nevertheless, powered (or "electric") toothbrushes were shown to provide a significantly better plaque removal in both short and long terms. Dental floss must be used once a day (Yaacob et al. 2014; Re et al. 2015). Other tooth-cleaning tools, like waxed dental floss, dental picks, sticks, mini-brushes, oral irrigator (with low water pressure), may be useful to optimize plaque removal in proximal areas (Berchier et al. 2008; Slot et al. 2008). Toothpaste and toothbrushing cannot be considered separately; even though toothbrushing without fluoride toothpaste helps improve oral hygiene and gingival health, it has no caries-preventive effect.

Dietary Counseling

Frequent snacking is not only strongly associated with increased risk of dental caries progression, but also with type 2 diabetes and obesity. Snacking has gained an increasing role as a risk indicator for caries development (Lingström et al. 1994). Energy-dense, low-nutrient-dense foods are often characterized by a high content of added sugar, but several modern snack products such as chips (crisps), popcorn, and shrimp crackers, while not sweet, are still potentially cariogenic due to their content of extensively hydrolyzed starch (Lingström et al. 2000, 2003). Moreover, sweetened and flavored beverage consumption has increased dramatically over the past decades in most of the industrialized countries and particularly in the USA with carbonated soft drinks being consumed the most frequently and most often by children, teens, and young adults (Reddy et al. 2015). It is interesting to notice that different snacking patterns have been reported based on household income: individuals with income at or below the poverty line in the USA more frequently consumed potato chips, fried potatoes, whole milk, and fruit drinks, whereas those with higher incomes consumed more grain-based salty snacks, fruits, skim milk, soft drinks, coffee, and tea (Johansson et al. 2010).

The type and frequency of carbohydrates consumed is of major importance when dealing with caries prevention (Peres et al. 2016); but other important dietary factors are consistency and degree of retention.

Dietary counseling should aim at reducing both the amount and the frequency of carbohydrate intake (Table 19.2).

Table 19.2 Dietary advice for patients

Identify the fermentable carbohydrates	Fermentable carbohydrates can be found in various forms in food. Some foods can be rich in sugar without having a sweet taste. The sugar content may be verified on the nutrition facts label. Many foods (chips, cereals, etc.) contain cooked starch, which has a high cariogenic potential
Meal frequency	Have 3 or 4 meals per day Avoid snacking between meals Take time for a real breakfast which may be the most important meal (25 % of the total calorie intake per day) If snacking is necessary or cannot be stopped, choose some sugar-free food Avoid drinking or eating sweetened foods all day long (better to consume them during the meals)

19.1.3.2 Dental Sealants

Dental sealants were introduced in the 1960s. Their caries-preventive effect in the pits and fissures of mainly the occlusal tooth surfaces has been well described for high caries risk (Ahovuo-Saloranta et al. 2013). Although studies have utilized first permanent molars, by extension, the results indicate that sealants are effective and should also be recommended for second permanent molars and premolars. While most of the studies and recommendations target children and adolescents, dental sealants also represent an effective preventive measure in adult patients on lifelong therapies capable of producing a number of systemic and oral complications, including xerostomia, which may increase caries susceptibility (Gore 2010).

Comparison of dental sealants to fluoride varnish showed contradictory results; a 2010 literature review presented some evidence toward the superiority of sealants in the prevention of occlusal carious lesions (Hiiri et al. 2010), when the results of a randomized controlled trial with parallel groups concluded that they are all effective in preventing pit and fissure carious lesions in permanent molars (Liu et al. 2012).

Deep pits and fissures have been clearly related to caries risk in occlusal surfaces, and in this case sealants are strongly recommended.

Dental sealants have also been proposed for proximal lesions; it seems that they are rarely used due to the difficulties to access the lesion (need for orthodontic separator); resin infiltration, with a simplified clinical protocol, may be as effective as dental sealant for such lesions (Martignon et al. 2012).

Apart from the indication for primary prevention, dental sealants have also been shown to be an effective noninvasive management strategy for non-cavitated carious lesions and defective restorations (Holmgren et al. 2014).

19.1.3.3 Fluoridated Agents

Fluoride has been used for over 70 years in caries prevention and remains the cornerstone of modern noninvasive dental caries prevention and management based upon a large body of scientific evidence demonstrating its effectiveness. However, the evidence is still evolving and varies for different modes of delivery. Even though systemic fluoride methods were originally designed to promote caries protection by ingestion, anticaries benefits are delivered primarily through topical effects due to the direct contact of fluoride with the tooth surface and penetration of the plaque and enamel of dentin, especially into carious lesions. Obviously fluoride topical effects occur prior to ingestion, but also the beneficial effects can be partly explained by the ingested fluoride that returns to the oral cavity via the saliva (Sampaio and Levy 2011). Thus, the effect of fluoride is local – topical – on the tooth surface and inside precavitated or cavitated lesions: inhibiting bacterial acid production, stopping enamel demineralization, enhancing remineralization (repair), and improving enamel resistance to future acid attacks. The evidence for these fluoridation methods and corresponding products varies from very strong to weak, so that the choice of the most suitable fluoride strategy depends on many factors, including the evidence of effectiveness, the setting, and the resources available in each country or community. Effective fluoride products are available in some countries but not others, and high-concentration fluoride products are not available in numerous countries, making fluoride therapy for high-risk individuals very difficult. Fluorides are safe and effective if applied at recommended levels. However, exposure to higher-than-recommended levels of fluoride during tooth development (between birth and four years of age) may cause dental fluorosis (Fédération Dentaire Internationale 2015)

Fluoride Toothpaste

Fluoride toothpaste sold without restriction over the counter is currently the most widespread fluoride delivery method for individuals and the evidence for its caries-preventive effect in both primary and permanent dentitions is strong (Fédération Dentaire Internationale 2015; Marinho et al. 2003a, b, 2004a, b; Marthaler 2003). Recommendations concern all patients whatever the age and the WHO states that, for public health, based on scientific evidence, every effort must be made to develop affordable fluoridated toothpastes for use in developing countries (Petersen and Lennon 2004). Moreover, its use in combination with water or salt fluoridation is safe.

Recommendations have to be adjusted according to age and risk level. Thus most of the current recommendations consider concentration of fluoride as well as the amount must be adjusted to age (a smear of toothpaste for children up to 3 years old and a pea-size amount after 3 years of age, for example, for the recent recommendations edited by the Scottish Intercollegiate Guidelines Network), particularly for young children to prevent from fluorosis (from fluoride swallowing and ingestion) whom require supervised toothbrushing by an adult (parents, caregivers) (Scottish Intercollegiate Guidelines Network 2014). Moreover, in order to maximize the topical effect of the fluoride toothpastes, patients should be encouraged to spit out excess toothpaste and not rinse with water after brushing. It has to be noted that fluoride toothpaste at a concentration below 1,000 ppm has not been demonstrated to be effective in caries control. In Europe, toothpaste now commonly contains 1,450 ppm fluoride in some form, whereas in other countries they tend to be at 1,000 ppm F.

More recently, toothpaste combining fluoride (1,450 ppm) and arginine (1.5 %) has been developed and studied toward its potential caries-preventive effect, assuming that arginine as an alkali-generating substrate could further counter the acid accumulation within the oral biofilm and thus serves as a promising approach to caries prevention and management. In vitro results showed that the combinatory application of fluoride and arginine has a potential synergistic effect in maintaining a healthy oral microbial equilibrium and thus represents a promising ecological approach to caries management (Zheng et al. 2015). In vivo results support the conclusion that dentifrices containing 1.5 % arginine, an insoluble calcium compound, and 1,450 ppm fluoride may provide significantly greater protection against caries lesion cavitation, in a low to moderate caries risk population, than dentifrices containing 1,450 ppm fluoride alone (Kraivaphan et al. 2013; Li et al. 2015) (Table 19.3).

The evidence indicates that, for preventing caries in children and adolescents, toothpastes of at least 1,000 ppm fluoride should be used. From 1,000 ppm fluoride, there is a dose-response relationship for caries prevention that should be taken into account when advising children from 3 to 6 years old at high risk for caries. For younger children, consideration should be given, when brushing with concentrations greater than 1,000 ppm fluoride, to their risk of developing mild fluorosis; a risk-benefit decision needs to be discussed with parents/guardians.

For high-risk patients presenting with non-cavitated carious lesions (aged over 6 years) or high-risk patients having root caries lesions (when roots are exposed), toothpaste with 5,000 ppm fluoride has been shown to be superior for caries control compared to 1,450 ppm F toothpaste (Nordstrom and Birkhed 2010; Ekstrand et al. 2013; Srinivasan et al. 2014).

Table 19.3 Toothbrushing recommendations

Tools	Manual or powered toothbrush[a] Dental floss Fluoride toothpaste (see below)
Toothbrushing frequency	At least twice a day: After breakfast At bedtime (no eating no drinking (except water) after bedtime brushing)
Toothbrush lifespan	Approximately every 2 months maximum

[a]Powered toothbrushes may enhance the compliance of young patients and may result in better plaque control for elderly patients or those with problem of dexterity

Fluoride Varnish

The most commonly used and evaluated concentration of fluoride in varnish vehicles is 22,600 ppm (Marinho et al. 2002a, 2003a, 2004a, b, 2013; Twetman 2015b). Its use for high-caries-risk patient is recommended at least 2 times per year (maximum 4 times per year). Fluoride varnish is a delivery system easily used by a dental practitioner or another trained professional (e.g., dental hygienists, dental therapists, pediatricians) whatever the age of the patient (even for infants) by bypassing the risk of ingestion and thus the risk of fluorosis. Several systematic reviews and meta-analysis on the topics have been published describing the effectiveness of fluoride varnishes (Marinho et al. 2002a, 2003a, 2004a, b, 2013; Twetman 2015b).

Fluoride varnishes have also their indications in the field of secondary prevention for non-cavitated carious lesion (one application per week during 6 to 8 weeks up to remineralization).

Fluoride Mouthwashes

They are indicated for moderate or high-caries-risk patients older than 6 years, as the young patient is not able to spit out the fluoride solution; when prescribed for children, an adult must supervise their use (Scottish Intercollegiate Guidelines Network 2014). Fluoride mouthwashes have been shown to have a clear caries prevention effect in the absence of daily fluoride toothpaste use; nevertheless, there were inconsistent results when viewed against the background of fluoride toothpaste use (Marinho et al. 2003a, c, 2004a, b; Twetman 2015b).

Fluoride Gels

The effectiveness of fluoride gels as caries-preventive agents has been reported in both deciduous and permanent teeth (Marinho et al. 2002b, 2003a, 2004a, b, 2015). They are indicated for high-caries-risk patients aged 6 years. High-concentration fluoride gels (≥12,300 ppm)

may be applied in disposable trays, which fit loosely over the teeth. Several guidelines recommend the alternative use of fluoride gels to fluoride varnish, but there is no clinical evidence in favor of one or the other. Some other recommendations, such as in Scotland (Scottish Intercollegiate Guidelines Network 2014) or Australia (Australian Dental Association 2012), recommend their use only in the absence of fluoride toothpaste. The European Association of Paediatric Dentistry (EADP) (European Association of Paediatric Dentistry 2009) or the New Zealand Guidelines Group (Ministry of Health New Zealand 2009) recommend that the patient should sit in upright position, should not swallow, and must be allowed to expectorate freely after application (teeth should be wiped at the end of the session with gauze; refrain from eating or drinking for 20–30 min after application). In general, fluoride gels are less recommended than fluoride varnishes; this may be explained by the limitation due to age but also by the limited distribution at professional concentrations (≥12,300 ppm) in some countries like in France, for example, and the additional cost represented by the individualized tray.

Comparison of the Caries-Preventive Effectiveness of One Form of Topical Fluoride Intervention with Another

A literature review published in 2004 proposed to assess the caries-preventive effect of one fluoridated topical agent to another. It concluded that fluoride toothpastes in comparison to mouthrinses or gels appear to have a similar degree of effectiveness for the prevention of dental caries in children in permanent teeth. It also reported that there was no clear suggestion that fluoride varnish is more effective than mouthrinses; moreover, the evidence for the comparative effectiveness, on temporary teeth, of fluoride varnishes and gels and mouthrinses and gels is inconclusive; nevertheless, a tendency of a superior effect of fluoride varnish is suggested (Marinho et al. 2004a).

Another literature review from the same team compared the caries prevention effectiveness of two topical fluoride agents combined with one of them alone, and it appears that mouthrinses, gels, or varnishes used in addition to fluoride toothpaste achieve a modest reduction in caries compared to toothpaste used alone (the prevented fraction was increased about 10%) (Marinho et al. 2004b).

Slow-Release Fluoride Devices

Slow-release fluoride devices (e.g., slow-dissolving fluoride-releasing glass beads) have been more recently proposed for the prevention, the arrest, or the reversal of the progression in both temporary and permanent teeth carious lesions. So far, there is insufficient evidence to determine whether slow-release fluoride devices (such as glass beads) help reduce dental decay (retention of the beads is a problem) (Chong et al. 2014).

Fluoride Tablets, Drops, Chewing Gums, and Lozenges

The prescription of fluoride supplements like tablets, drops, chewing gums, and lozenges is subordinated by several factors: the patient age, his/her individual caries risk level, the level of fluoride in drinking water, and the determination of dietary fluoride (in order to prevent intake of excess fluoride) (European Association of Paediatric Dentistry 2009). A 2011 literature review and meta-analysis showed that fluoride supplements are associated with a caries increment reduction when used in permanent teeth versus no other preventive fluoride treatment. The preventive effect was not significantly different when fluoride supplements were compared to other fluoridated topic agents. Unfortunately, many of the studies included in the cited review had been conducted at a time when topical fluorides were not widely used suggesting that there is a lack of evidence from the review to make actual good recommendations because, at the present time, the effect of fluoride supplements in children using fluoride toothpastes on a regular basis would probably be limited (Tubert-Jeannin et al. 2011).

Furthermore, when the fluoride supplements were compared with the use of topical fluorides (toothpastes, varnishes, rinses) or with the use of other preventive measures (xylitol lozenges), there was no differential effect (Table 19.4).

Table 19.4 The different fluoridated topic agents and their effectiveness (when compared to a placebo or the absence of treatment) – prevented fraction recorded in randomized clinical trials (based on D(M)FS and d(m)fs increment during follow-up)

	Concentration	Frequency of use	Prevented fraction[b] (CI 95 %)
Toothpastes (Walsh et al. 2010)	<1,000 ppm	Daily use (at least two times)	No evidence of effectiveness
	1,000–1,250 ppm		Permanent teeth: 23 % (19–27 %)
	2,400–2,280 ppm		Permanent teeth: 36 % (27–44 %)
Varnishes (Marinho et al. 2013)	≥22,600 ppm	Biannual (Professional application)	Permanent teeth: 43 % (30–57 %) Deciduous teeth: 37 % (24–51 %)
Gels[a] (Marinho et al. 2015)	<13,500 ppm	Biannual (Professional application during a minimum of 4 min)	Deciduous teeth: 20 % (1–51 %)
	≥13,500 ppm		Permanent teeth: 38 % (24–52 %)
Mouthwashes (Marinho et al. 2003c)	0.2 (1,000 ppm) at 0.1 %	Weekly use	Permanent teeth: 26 % (23–30 %)
	0.05 at 0.02 %	Daily use	

The prevented fraction gives the percentage of cases that can be prevented if a population is exposed to an intervention, compared to an unexposed population

CI 95 %: range of values that you can be 95 % certain contains the true mean of the population

[a]Some, at 1,500 ppm, are for use at home

[b]Prevented fraction when compared to a placebo or the absence of treatment

19.1.3.4 Non-fluoridated Agents

Various non-fluoridated agents and molecules like xylitol, chlorhexidine, and casein phosphopeptide-amorphous calcium phosphate (CPP-ACP) have been tested toward their potential caries-protective effect. In light of the results of the clinical surveys investigating their effectiveness, they cannot be considered to be effective alternatives to fluoride, which is nowadays the key molecule for caries prevention (best ratio cost-effectiveness). However, when considering caries management by risk assessment and the management of high- and extreme-risk individuals, fluoride alone is not enough to be effective. An antibacterial agent and potentially pH control must be added to swing the cries balance from caries progression to arrest or reversal. Likewise, the antibacterial agents alone are not effective in high- or extreme-caries-risk individuals.

Xylitol-Containing Products

Xylitol is a non-cariogenic natural sugar alcohol with antibacterial properties that has shown to have potential in caries prevention in children by interfering with MS colonization. Indeed, xylitol gum consumption by mothers with high MS levels is associated with a significant reduction in the mother-to-child transmission of salivary MS (Lin et al. 2016). After the eruption of the first teeth, xylitol has been added to tooth wipes considered by the AAPD as an important tool for oral hygiene care in infants and toddlers (American Association of Pediatric Dentistry 2008); the results of a clinical study clearly showed that daily xylitol-wipe application markedly reduced the caries incidence in young children as compared with wipes without xylitol, suggesting that the use of xylitol wipes may be a useful adjunct for caries control in infants (Zhan et al. 2012). There is also some evidence to suggest that using a fluoride toothpaste containing xylitol may reduce tooth decay in the permanent teeth of children by 13 % over a 3-year period when compared to a fluoride-only toothpaste. Nevertheless, there is nowadays no evidence toward the effectiveness of xylitol used as a natural sweetener used in products such as sweets, lozenges, and candy in children and adults (Bader et al. 2013; Riley et al. 2015).

Xylitol chewing gums (5 times per day) have been shown to have a caries-preventive effect, but this conclusion might be due to the stimulation of the saliva flow (Twetman 2009; Campus et al. 2013); thus, they might be recommended in high-caries-risk patients presenting a decreased saliva flow. A further advantage of xylitol is that the cariogenic bacteria cannot ferment it, so if xylitol products (gum or lozenges) are substituted for sugar-containing snacks, the frequency of fermentable carbohydrate consumption is immediately reduced and one of the significant caries risk factors is essentially eliminated.

Chlorhexidine

Chlorhexidine is an antibacterial agent; a number of over-the-counter and professionally administered chlorhexidine-based preparations are available in a variety of formulations and in a range of strengths depending on the country, the marketing, and government regulations. Chlorhexidine/thymol varnish has been shown to have a preventive effect on root caries lesions and is currently recommended by the American Dental Association (American Dental Association 2011). It has been demonstrated in a controlled clinical trial in high-caries-risk adults that 0.12 % chlorhexidine gluconate mouthrinse used once a day for one week every month, in conjunction with fluoride toothpaste, was effective in reducing mutans streptococci levels and reducing dental decay by 24 % over a 2-year period by altering the balance between pathological and protective caries risk factors (Featherstone et al. 2012). However, a recent literature review reported that there is little evidence on chlorhexidine varnishes and gels to either support or refute the assertion that chlorhexidine is more effective than placebo or no treatment in the prevention of caries or the reduction of mutans streptococci levels in children and adolescents (Walsh et al. 2015); moreover, there were no trials on other products containing chlorhexidine such as sprays, toothpastes, chewing gums, or mouthrinses.

A recent outcomes study, involving approximately 12,000 high-risk adult patients, showed a reduction in new decayed teeth of 20 to 40 % in those patients who used combined fluoride and chlorhexidine therapy compared to those who did not. The combined therapy used high-concentration fluoride toothpaste (5,000 ppm F) daily and 0.12 % chlorhexidine mouthrinse once daily for one week each month (Chaffee et al. 2015b).

CPP-ACP

Based on the pioneering work of Reynolds, who developed Recaldent® (casein phosphopeptide-amorphous calcium phosphate (CPP-ACP) technology) (Reynolds et al. 2008), some products containing the active ingredient CPP-ACP have been developed. Calcium and phosphate ion releasing in the saliva and dental plaque are supposed to decrease demineralization and enhance remineralization (Nongonierma and Fitzgerald 2012). If there is some evidence toward the effect of CPP-ACP chewing gums to slow down and enhance the regression of proximal carious lesions (secondary prevention) (Morgan et al. 2008), the overall findings did not show so far any significant benefits of CPP-ACP paste over brushing with fluoride toothpaste for the caries prevention (Sitthisettapong et al. 2012; Raphael and Blinkhorn 2015). Moreover, there are contradictory findings toward the caries-preventive effects of toothpaste combining CPP-ACP and fluoride, and varnishes combining both CPP-ACP and fluoride have not been evaluated yet (Li et al. 2014).

CPP-ACP pastes are not an alternative to fluoride toothpaste but may be considered for high-caries-risk patients with decreased saliva flow as extra regimen (fluoride toothpaste being the principal preventive strategy) especially to enhance remineralization or prevention of smooth surface white spot lesions.

Other Molecules

Numerous other approaches, as alternative to fluoride, are currently under study for their potential caries-preventive or caries therapeutic effects.

For example, recent insights in medical science indicate that probiotics play an important role in health and well-being. The conceptual thinking is that a harmless effector strain is implanted into the host's microflora to maintain or restore a natural microbiome by interference and/or inhibition of other microorganisms and especially pathogens (Twetman 2012). Furthermore, a systemic modulation of immunological parameters is thought to be a part of the interaction. Whether bacterial interference or bacteriotherapy applies to dental caries is still an open question. In dentistry, bacterial interference with probiotic bacteria to support the stability and diversity of oral biofilms has gained similar interest (Twetman and Keller 2012). First investigations into metabolic activity, co-aggregation, growth inhibition, bacteriocin production, and adhesion have collectively suggested a potential role for probiotic lactobacilli and bifidobacteria to modulate the oral microbial ecology (Twetman and Keller 2012). Moreover, a recent placebo-controlled randomized trial demonstrated that the regular long-term intake of probiotic-supplemented milk may reduce caries development in high-caries preschool children (Rodríguez et al. 2016). However, further large-scale trials with orally derived anticaries candidates are needed before it can be recommended to adopt bacteriotherapy for preventing and controlling caries in clinical practice.

In the same manner, results from in vitro and preliminary in vivo studies have shown polyphenols, plant (e.g., green tea, cocoa, etc.), and fungal extracts show promise as caries-preventive agents (inhibition of biofilm formation, disruption of biofilms) (Ferrazzano et al. 2009, 2011; Spratt et al. 2012; Thomas et al. 2015).

19.1.4 Follow-Up

Follow-up is a key phase of a prevention-oriented treatment plan; it concerns the reinforcement of patient education, monitoring the effectiveness of all preventive and control measures implemented and therapeutic measures (e.g., the integrity of therapeutic sealants and restorations) (Featherstone and Domejean 2012). During follow-up visits, potential failures can be intercepted, and the recall interval adjusted based on new clinical findings and the behavior of the patient (Lapidos et al. 2016).

Nowadays, the evidence for using a one-recall-interval-fits-all protocol to reduce caries incidence is weak; there is also little evidence to either support or refute the practice of encouraging 6 monthly dental checks in adults or children. There is not clear-cut consensus about the best recall interval for a given caries risk level (Patel et al. 2010; Beirne et al. 2007).

The determination of the recall interval must be a joint decision between both the patient and the dental practitioner. The National Institute for Clinical Excellence (NICE) guidelines (National Institute for Clinical Excellence 2004) stated that:

- Recall interval must be influenced by the risk factors that may influence the patient's oral health, the outcome of previous care episodes, the suitability of previously recommended intervals, and the patient's ability or desire to visit the dentist at the recommended interval.
- The dentist should discuss the recommended recall interval with the patient and record this interval, and the patient's agreement or disagreement with it, in the current record-keeping system.
- The recall interval should be reviewed again at the next oral health review, to learn from the patient's responses to the oral care provided and the health outcomes achieved. This feedback and the findings of the oral health review should be used to adjust the next recall interval chosen.
- Patients should be informed that their recommended recall interval may vary over time.

Moreover, the optimum recall interval varies with the level of caries risk assessed by the CRA procedure (Jenson et al. 2007) (Table 19.5).

Table 19.5 Recall intervals for caries management

Recall intervals and NICE recommendations	
The shortest interval between oral health reviews for all patients should be 3 months	A recall interval of less than 3 months is not normally needed for a routine dental recall A patient may need to be seen more frequently for specific reasons such as disease management, ongoing courses of treatment, emergency dental interventions, or episodes of specialist care, which are outside the scope of an oral health review
The longest interval between oral health reviews for patients younger than 18 years should be 12 months	There is evidence that the rate of progression of dental caries can be more rapid in children and adolescents than in older people, and it seems to be faster in primary teeth than in permanent teeth. Periodic developmental assessment of the dentition is also required in children Recall intervals of no longer than 12 months give the opportunity for delivering and reinforcing preventive advice and for raising awareness of the importance of good oral health. This is particularly important in young children, to lay the foundations for lifelong dental health
The longest interval between oral health reviews for patients aged 18 years and older should be 24 months	Recall intervals for patients who have repeatedly demonstrated that they can maintain oral health (low risk) and who are not considered to be at risk of or from oral disease may be extended over time up to an interval of 24 months. Intervals of longer than 24 months are undesirable because they could diminish the professional relationship between dentist and patient, and people's lifestyles may change. It is also possible that other health conditions may change, and factors such as medications that reduce salivary function come into play changing the person from low risk to high caries risk

19.1.5 Caries Management by Risk Assessment

By utilizing all of the information described above in this chapter and relevant sections of other chapters, the practitioner can now carry out "Caries Management by Risk Assessment" as an individualized process for every patient. The steps are straightforward and are described in detail in published works (Featherstone et al. 2007; Ramos-Gomez et al. 2007).

The steps are (1) medical and dental history, (2) caries clinical exam including detection of lesions to determine whether non-cavitated lesions can be reversed or arrested, (3) caries risk assessment, (4) treatment plan including chemical therapy appropriate to the assessed risk level and minimal intervention dentistry for needed restorative work, (5) follow-up and recall, and (6) ongoing monitoring and risk assessment at recall.

There are numerous possible chemical therapeutic regimens appropriate to the different caries risk levels, and these will depend on product availability in each country, government regulations, guidelines in each country, available evidence, and agreement by the patient.

A detailed table of suggested therapies and additional information, such as recall intervals, x-ray frequency, pH control, etc., are given in the CAMBRA recommendations and have been used and assessed by outcomes studies (Featherstone et al. 2007; Chaffee et al. 2015b; Jenson et al. 2007; Ramos-Gomez et al. 2007). In simple terms, for patients aged over 6 years, chemical therapeutic recommendations are:

1. Low-risk individuals: over-the-counter fluoride toothpaste (1,000 ppm F or higher) twice daily
2. Moderate-risk individuals: 2xdaily fluoride toothpaste (1,000 ppm F or higher) and 2xdaily fluoride mouthrinse (0.05 % NaF) or 2xdaily high-concentration (5,000 ppm F) toothpaste
3. High-risk individuals: 2xdaily 5,000 ppm F toothpaste, 0.12 % or 0.2 % chlorhexidine gluconate mouthrinse once daily for one week every month, or xylitol gum or lozenges daily

4. Extreme-risk individuals: 2xdaily 5,000 ppm F toothpaste, 0.12% or 0.2% chlorhexidine gluconate mouthrinse once daily for one week every month, xylitol gum or lozenges daily, or baking soda (sodium bicarbonate) mouthrinse (10 g in 250 ml water) as needed throughout the day for pH control

Numerous other possible combinations are possible, but the above therapies were designed to increase the caries-preventive effect as the risk increases. Treatments can be individualized over time depending on patient compliance and response to therapy.

19.1.6 Key Messages for Dental Practitioners

- CRA and the determination of individual risk factors allow the establishment of an individualized treatment plan for each patient to prevent the onset or progression of the disease. Preventive strategies and targeted therapeutic management can then be established with the objective of optimizing outcomes.
- Together with the use of fluoride and optimal oral hygiene, the control of sugar intake makes an important contribution to the multifaceted strategy for caries prevention.

References

Ahovuo-Saloranta A, Saloranta A, Forss H, et al. Sealants for preventing dental decay in the permanent teeth. Cochrane Database Syst Rev. 2013;3, CD001830.

Albino J, Tiwari T. Preventing childhood caries: a review of recent behavioral research. J Dent Res. 2016; 95(1):35–42.

American Association of Paediatric Dentistry. Guideline on infant oral health care. Pediatr Dent. 2008;30(7 Suppl):90S–3.

American Association of Paediatric Dentistry. Guideline on caries-risk assessment and management for infants, children, and adolescents. Pediatr Dent. 2013;35(5):E157–64.

American Dental Association. Non-fluoride caries preventive agents. Full report of a systematic review and evidence-based recommendations. A report of the Council on Scientific Affairs. 2011. http://ebd.ada.org/~/media/EBD/Files/clinical_recommendations_non_fluoride_caries_preve.ashx. Accessed 17 Jan 2016.

Australian Dental Association. Outcome of fluoride consensus workshop 2012 to review Fluoride Guidelines from 2005. 2012 https://www.adelaide.edu.au/arcpoh/dperu/fluoride/Outcome_of_fluoride_consensus_workshop_2012.pdf. Accessed 17 Jan 2016.

Bader JD, Vollmer WM, Shugars DA, et al. Results from the xylitol for adult caries trial (X-ACT). J Am Dent Assoc. 2013;144(1):21–30.

Beirne P, Clarkson JE, Worthington HV. Recall intervals for oral health in primary care patients. Cochrane Database Syst Rev. 2007;4, CD004346.

Berchier CE, Slot DE, Haps S, et al. The efficacy of dental floss in addition to a toothbrush on plaque and parameters of gingival inflammation: a systematic review. Int J Dent Hyg. 2008;6(4):265–79.

Bratthall D, Hansel Petersson G. Cariogram: a multifactorial risk assessment model for a multifactorial disease. Community Dent Oral Epidemiol. 2005;33(4):256–64.

Campus G, Cagetti MG, Sale S, et al. Six months of high-dose xylitol in high-risk caries subjects-a 2-year randomised, clinical trial. Clin Oral Investig. 2013;17(3):785–91.

Chaffee BW, Cheng J, Featherstone JD. Baseline caries risk assessment as a predictor of caries incidence. J Dent. 2015.

Chaffee BW, Cheng J, Featherstone JD. Non-operative anti-caries agents and dental caries increment among adults at high caries risk: a retrospective cohort study. BMC Oral Health. 2015b;15(1):111.

Chong LY, Clarkson JE, Dobbyn-Ross L, et al. Slow-release fluoride devices for the control of dental decay. Cochrane Database Syst Rev. 2014;11, CD005101.

Collègue des Enseignants en Odontologie Pédiatrique. Fiches pratiques d'odontologie pédiatrique. Paris: CdP – Initiatives Santé; 2014.

da Silva Bastos Vde A, Freitas-Fernandes LB, Fidalgo TK, et al. Mother-to-child transmission of Streptococcus mutans: a systematic review and meta-analysis. J Dent. 2015;43(2):181–91.

Doméjean S, Featherstone JDB, White J. Validation of the CDA CAMBRA caries risk assessment – a six-year retrospective study. J Calif Dent Assoc. 2011;39(10):709–15.

Douglass JM, Li Y, Tinanoff N. Association of mutans streptococci between caregivers and their children. Pediatr Dent. 2008;30(5):375–87.

Ekstrand KR, Poulsen JE, Hede B, et al. A randomized clinical trial of the anti-caries efficacy of 5,000 compared to 1,450 ppm fluoridated toothpaste on root caries lesions in elderly disabled nursing home residents. Caries Res. 2013;47(5):391–8.

Elderton RJ. Iatrogenesis in the treatment of dental caries. Proc Finn Dent Soc. 1992;88(1–2):25–32.

Elderton RJ. Treating restorative dentistry to health. Br Dent J. 1996;181(6):220, 221–225.

European Association of Paediatric Dentistry. Guidelines on the use of fluoride in children: an EAPD policy document. Eur Arch Paediatr Dent. 2009;10(3): 129–35.

Featherstone JD. The caries balance: contributing factors and early detection. J Calif Dent Assoc. 2003;31(2): 129–33.

Featherstone JD, Domejean S. Minimal intervention dentistry: part 1. From 'compulsive' restorative dentistry to rational therapeutic strategies. Br Dent J. 2012;213(9):441–5.

Featherstone JD, Domejean-Orliaguet S, Jenson L, et al. Caries risk assessment in practice for age 6 through adult. J Calif Dent Assoc. 2007;35(10):703–7, 710–713.

Featherstone JD, White JM, Hoover CI, et al. A randomized clinical trial of anticaries therapies targeted according to risk assessment (caries management by risk assessment). Caries Res. 2012;46(2):118–29.

Fédération Dentaire Internationale. Minimal intervention in the management of dental caries – FDI policy statement, in Assemblée générale de la Fédération Dentaire Internationale (FDI) Vienne; 2002. http://www.fdiworldental.org/media/11275/Minimal-intervention-in-the-management-of-dental-caries-2002.pdf. Accessed 17 Jan 2016.

Fédération Dentaire Internationale. The challenge of oral disease – a call for global action. The oral health atlas. 2nd ed. Geneva: FDI World Dental Federation; 2015. http://www.fdiworldental.org/media/77552/complete_oh_atlas.pdf. Accessed 17 Jan 2016.

Ferrazzano GF, Amato I, Ingenito A, et al. Anti-cariogenic effects of polyphenols from plant stimulant beverages (cocoa, coffee, tea). Fitoterapia. 2009;80(5):255–62.

Ferrazzano GF, Roberto L, Amato I, et al. Antimicrobial properties of green tea extract against cariogenic microflora: an in vivo study. J Med Food. 2011; 14(9):907–11.

Fontana M, Gonzalez-Cabezas C. Minimal intervention dentistry: part 2. Caries risk assessment in adults. Br Dent J. 2012;213(9):447–51.

Gore DR. The use of dental sealants in adults: a long-neglected preventive measure. Int J Dent Hyg. 2010;8(3):198–203.

Haute Autorité de Santé. Appréciation du risque carieux et indications du scellement prophylactique des sillons des premières et deuxièmes molaires permanentes chez les sujets de moins de 18 ans. 2005. http://ansm.sante.fr/var/ansm_site/storage/original/application/7db1d82db7f5636b56170f59e844dd3a.pdf. Accessed 17 Jan 2016.

Hiiri A, Ahovuo-Saloranta A, Nordblad A, et al. Pit and fissure sealants versus fluoride varnishes for preventing dental decay in children and adolescents. Cochrane Database Syst Rev. 2010;3, CD003067.

Holmgren C, Gaucher C, Decerle N, et al. Minimal intervention dentistry II: part 3. Management of non-cavitated (initial) occlusal caries lesions – non-invasive approaches through remineralisation and therapeutic sealants. Br Dent J. 2014;216(5):237–43.

Jamoulle M. Quaternary prevention, an answer of family doctors to overmedicalization. Int J Health Policy Manag. 2015;4(2):61–4.

Jenson L, Budenz AW, Featherstone JD, et al. Clinical protocols for caries management by risk assessment. J Calif Dent Assoc. 2007;35(10):714–23.

Johansson I, Holgerson PL, Kressin NR, et al. Snacking habits and caries in young children. Caries Res. 2010;44(5):421–30.

Kraivaphan P, Amornchat C, Triratana T, et al. Two-year caries clinical study of the efficacy of novel dentifrices containing 1.5% arginine, an insoluble calcium compound and 1,450 ppm fluoride. Caries Res. 2013; 47(6):582–90.

Lapidos A, Shaefer HL, Gwozdek A. Toward a better understanding of dental appointment-keeping behavior. Community Dent Oral Epidemiol. 2016;44(1): 85–91.

Li J, Xie X, Wang Y, et al. Long-term remineralizing effect of casein phosphopeptide-amorphous calcium phosphate (CPP-ACP) on early caries lesions in vivo: a systematic review. J Dent. 2014;42(7):769–77.

Li X, Zhong Y, Jiang X, et al. Randomized clinical trial of the efficacy of dentifrices containing 1.5% arginine, an insoluble calcium compound and 1450 ppm fluoride over two years. J Clin Dent. 2015;26(1):7–12.

Lin HK, Fang CE, Huang MS, et al. Effect of maternal use of chewing gums containing xylitol on transmission of mutans streptococci in children: a meta-analysis of randomized controlled trials. Int J Paediatr Dent. 2016;26(1):35–44.

Lingström P, Birkhed D, Ruben J, et al. Effect of frequent consumption of starchy food items on enamel and dentin demineralization and on plaque pH in situ. J Dent Res. 1994;73(3):652–60.

Lingström P, van Houte J, Kashket S. Food starches and dental caries. Crit Rev Oral Biol Med. 2000; 11(3):366–80.

Lingstrom P, Holm AK, Mejare I, et al. Dietary factors in the prevention of dental caries: a systematic review. Acta Odontol Scand. 2003;61(6):331–40.

Liu BY, Lo EC, Chu CH, et al. Randomized trial on fluorides and sealants for fissure caries prevention. J Dent Res. 2012;91(8):753–8.

Macritchie HM, Longbottom C, Robertson M, et al. Development of the Dundee Caries Risk Assessment Model (DCRAM) – risk model development using a novel application of CHAID analysis. Community Dent Oral Epidemiol. 2012;40(1):37–45.

Marinho VC, Higgins JP, Logan S, et al. Fluoride varnishes for preventing dental caries in children and adolescents. Cochrane Database Syst Rev. 2002a;3, CD002279.

Marinho VC, Higgins JP, Logan S, et al. Fluoride gels for preventing dental caries in children and adolescents. Cochrane Database Syst Rev. 2002b;2, CD002280.

Marinho VC, Higgins JP, Logan S, et al. Topical fluoride (toothpastes, mouthrinses, gels or varnishes) for preventing dental caries in children and adolescents. Cochrane Database Syst Rev. 2003;(4):CD002782.

Marinho VC, Higgins JP, Sheiham A, et al. Fluoride toothpastes for preventing dental caries in children and adolescents. Cochrane Database Syst Rev. 2003b;1, CD002278.

Marinho VC, Higgins JP, Logan S, et al. Fluoride mouthrinses for preventing dental caries in children and adolescents. Cochrane Database Syst Rev. 2003c;3, CD002284.

Marinho VC, Higgins JP, Sheiham A, et al. One topical fluoride (toothpastes, or mouthrinses, or gels, or varnishes) versus another for preventing dental caries in children and adolescents. Cochrane Database Syst Rev. 2004a;1, CD002780.

Marinho VC, Higgins JP, Sheiham A, et al. Combinations of topical fluoride (toothpastes, mouthrinses, gels, varnishes) versus single topical fluoride for preventing dental caries in children and adolescents. Cochrane Database Syst Rev. 2004b;1, CD002781.

Marinho VC, Worthington HV, Walsh T, et al. Fluoride varnishes for preventing dental caries in children and adolescents. Cochrane Database Syst Rev. 2013;7, CD002279.

Marinho VC, Worthington HV, Walsh T, et al. Fluoride gels for preventing dental caries in children and adolescents. Cochrane Database Syst Rev. 2015;6, CD002280.

Marthaler TM. Successes and drawbacks in the caries-preventive use of fluorides: lessons to be learnt from history. Oral Health Prev Dent. 2003;1(2):129–40.

Martignon S, Ekstrand KR, Gomez J, et al. Infiltrating/sealing proximal caries lesions: a 3-year randomized clinical trial. J Dent Res. 2012;91(3):288–92.

Mejare I, Axelsson S, Dahlen G, et al. Caries risk assessment. A systematic review. Acta Odontol Scand. 2014;72(2):81–91.

Ministry of Health New Zealand. New Zealand Guidelines Group – Guidelines for the use of fluorides. 2009. http://www.health.govt.nz/publication/guidelines-use-fluorides. Accessed 17 Jan 2016.

Morgan MV, Adams GG, Bailey DL, et al. The anticariogenic effect of sugar-free gum containing CPP-ACP nanocomplexes on approximal caries determined using digital bitewing radiography. Caries Res. 2008;42(3):171–84.

Morou-Bermudez E, Billings RJ, Burne RA, et al. Caries risk pyramid: a practical biological approach to caries management by risk assessment. P R Health Sci J. 2011;30(4):165–6.

Muller-Bolla M, Courson F. Toothbrushing methods to use in children: a systematic review. Oral Health Prev Dent. 2013;11(4):341–7.

National Institute for Clinical Excellence. Dental recall: recall interval between routine dental examinations. 2004. http://www.nice.org.uk/guidance/cg19. Accessed 17 Jan 2016.

Nongonierma AB, Fitzgerald RJ. Biofunctional properties of caseinophosphopeptides in the oral cavity. Caries Res. 2012;46(3):234–67.

Nordstrom A, Birkhed D. Preventive effect of high-fluoride dentifrice (5,000 ppm) in caries-active adolescents: a 2-year clinical trial. Caries Res. 2010;44(3):323–31.

Patel S, Bay RC, Glick M. A systematic review of dental recall intervals and incidence of dental caries. J Am Dent Assoc. 2010;141(5):527–39.

Peres MA, Sheiham A, Liu P. et al. Sugar consumption and changes in dental caries from childhood to adolescence. J Dent Res. 2016;95(4):388–94.

Petersen PE, Lennon MA. Effective use of fluorides for the prevention of dental caries in the 21st century: the WHO approach. Community Dent Oral Epidemiol. 2004;32(5):319–21.

Ramos-Gomez FJ, Crall J, Gansky SA, et al. Caries risk assessment appropriate for the age 1 visit (infants and toddlers). J Calif Dent Assoc. 2007;35(10):687–702.

Ramos-Gomez FJ, Crystal YO, Domejean S, et al. Minimal intervention dentistry: part 3. Paediatric dental care: prevention and management protocols using caries risk assessment for infants and young children. Br Dent J. 2012;213(10):501–8.

Raphael S, Blinkhorn A. Is there a place for Tooth Mousse in the prevention and treatment of early dental caries? A systematic review. BMC Oral Health. 2015; 15(1):113.

Re D, Augusti G, Battaglia D, et al. Is a new sonic toothbrush more effective in plaque removal than a manual toothbrush? Eur J Paediatr Dent. 2015;16(1):13–8.

Reddy A, Norris DF, Momeni SS, et al. The pH of beverages in the United States. J Am Dent Assoc. 2016;147(4):255–63.

Reynolds EC, Cai F, Cochrane NJ, et al. Fluoride and case in phosphopeptide-amorphous calcium phosphate. J Dent Res. 2008;87(4):344–8.

Riley P, Moore D, Ahmed F, et al. Xylitol-containing products for preventing dental caries in children and adults. Cochrane Database Syst Rev. 2015;3, CD010743.

Rodríguez G, Ruiz B, Faleiros S, et al. Probiotic compared with standard milk for high-caries children: a cluster randomized trial. J Dent Res. 2016.

Sampaio FC, Levy SM. Systemic fluoride. Monogr Oral Sci. 2011;22:133–45.

Scottish Intercollegiate Guidelines Network. SIGN 138 – dental interventions to prevent caries in children. 2014. http://www.sign.ac.uk/pdf/SIGN138.pdf. Accessed 17 Jan 2016.

Seki M, Yamashita Y, Shibata Y, et al. Effect of mixed mutans streptococci colonization on caries development. Oral Microbiol Immunol. 2006;21(1):47–52.

Sheiham A. Minimal intervention in dental care. Med Princ Pract. 2002;11 Suppl 1:2–6.

Sitthisettapong T, Phantumvanit P, Huebner C, et al. Effect of CPP-ACP paste on dental caries in primary teeth: a randomized trial. J Dent Res. 2012;91(9):847–52.

Slot DE, Dörfer CE, Van der Weijden GA. The efficacy of interdental brushes on plaque and parameters of periodontal inflammation: a systematic review. Int J Dent Hyg. 2008;6(4):253–64.

Spratt DA, Daglia M, Papetti A, et al. Evaluation of plant and fungal extracts for their potential antigingivitis and anticaries activity. J Biomed Biotechnol. 2012;2012:510198.

Srinivasan M, Shetty S, Ashworth D, et al. High-fluoride toothpaste: a multicenter randomized controlled trial in adults. Community Dent Oral Epidemiol. 2014;42(4):333–40.

Tellez M, Gomez J, Pretty I, et al. Evidence on existing caries risk assessment systems: are they predictive of future caries? Community Dent Oral Epidemiol. 2013;41(1):67–78.

Thomas A, Thakur S, Mhambrey S. Comparison of the antimicrobial efficacy of chlorhexidine, sodium fluoride, fluoride with essential oils, alum, green tea, and garlic with lime mouth rinses on cariogenic microbes. J Int Soc Prev Community Dent. 2015;5(4):302–8.

Tinanoff N, Kanellis MJ, Vargas CM. Current understanding of the epidemiology mechanisms, and prevention of dental caries in preschool children. Pediatr Dent. 2002;24(6):543–51.

Tubert-Jeannin S, Auclair C, Amsallem E, et al. Fluoride supplements (tablets, drops, lozenges or chewing gums) for preventing dental caries in children. Cochrane Database Syst Rev. 2011;12, CD007592.

Twetman S. Consistent evidence to support the use of xylitol- and sorbitol-containing chewing gum to prevent dental caries. Evid Based Dent. 2009;10(1):10–1.

Twetman S. Are we ready for caries prevention through bacteriotherapy? Braz Oral Res. 2012;26 Suppl 1:64–70.

Twetman S. Caries risk assessment in children: how accurate are we? Eur Arch Paediatr Dent. 2015a;2015.

Twetman S. The evidence base for professional and self-care prevention – caries, erosion and sensitivity. BMC Oral Health. 2015b;15 Suppl 1:S4.

Twetman S, Keller MK. Probiotics for caries prevention and control. Adv Dent Res. 2012;24(2):98–102.

Twetman S, Fontana M, Featherstone JDB. Risk assessment – can we achieve consensus? Community Dent Oral Epidemiol. 2013;41(1):e64–70.

Vieira AR, Modesto A, Marazita ML. Caries: review of human genetics research. Caries Res. 2014;48(5):491–506.

Walsh T, Worthington HV, Glenny AM, et al. Fluoride toothpastes of different concentrations for preventing dental caries in children and adolescents. Cochrane Database Syst Rev. 2010;(1):CD007868.

Walsh T, Oliveira-Neto JM, Moore D. Chlorhexidine treatment for the prevention of dental caries in children and adolescents. Cochrane Database Syst Rev. 2015;4:CD008457.

Yaacob M, Worthington HV, Deacon SA, et al. Powered versus manual toothbrushing for oral health. Cochrane Database Syst Rev. 2014;6:CD002281.

Zenkner JE, Alves LS, de Oliveira RS, et al. Influence of eruption stage and biofilm accumulation on occlusal caries in permanent molars: a generalized estimating equations logistic approach. Caries Res. 2013;47(3):177–82.

Zhan L, Cheng J, Chang P, et al. Effects of xylitol wipes on cariogenic bacteria and caries in young children. J Dent Res. 2012;91(7 Suppl):85S–90.

Zheng X, Cheng X, Wang L, et al. Combinatorial effects of arginine and fluoride on oral bacteria. J Dent Res. 2015;94(2):344–53.

MIX
Papier aus verantwortungsvollen Quellen
Paper from responsible sources
FSC® C105338

If you have any concerns about our products,
you can contact us on
ProductSafety@springernature.com

In case Publisher is established outside the EU,
the EU authorized representative is:
Springer Nature Customer Service Center GmbH
Europaplatz 3, 69115 Heidelberg, Germany

Printed by Libri Plureos GmbH
in Hamburg, Germany